The Human Placenta:
Proteins and Hormones

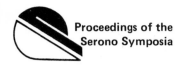 **Proceedings of the Serono Symposia**

---

*At the time of going to press these titles were in preparation.

The Human Placenta: Proteins and Hormones

Proceedings of the
Serono Symposia, Volume 35

Edited by

Arnold Klopper

Department of Obstetrics and Gynaecology,
University of Aberdeen,
Royal Infirmary,
Foresterhill, Aberdeen, Scotland

Andrea Genazzani

Cattedra di Patologia, Obstetrica e Ginecologia,
Università degli Studi,
15300 Siena, Italy

Pier Giorgio Crosignani

Section of Endocrinology,
Department of Obstetrics and Gynaecology,
University of Milan,
20122 Milan, Italy

1980

ACADEMIC PRESS
A Subsidiary of Harcourt Brace Jovanovich, Publishers

London New York Toronto Sydney San Francisco

ACADEMIC PRESS INC. (LONDON) LTD.
24–28 OVAL ROAD
LONDON NW1

U.S. Edition published by
ACADEMIC PRESS INC.
111 FIFTH AVENUE
NEW YORK, NEW YORK 10003

British Library Cataloguing in Publication Data
Human Placenta—Proteins and Hormones. (*Conference*),
   Siena 1979
   The human placenta.—(Proceedings of the Serono
   Foundation symposia; no. 35 ISSN 0308-5503).
   1. Placenta—Congresses
   I. Title   II. Klopper, Arnold
   III. Genazzani, A   IV. Crosignani, Pier
   Giorgio   V. Series
   612.6'47   QP281   80–40686

   ISBN 0-12-416150-2

Typeset by Reproduction Drawings Ltd., Sutton, Surrey
Printed in Great Britain by
T. J. Press (Padstow) Ltd., Padstow, Cornwall

PREFACE

This book is the outcome of a meeting held in Siena in July 1979 in the Serono Symposia series. The title, then as now, was an all embracing one—The Human Placenta: Proteins and Hormones. Not surprisingly, the contributions which were offered ranged widely. Through all, however, ran the thread of clinical concern with the assessment of placental function, which we hope will bind together the writings in this book as it did our deliberations in that midsummer's week.

The programme of the conference did not lend itself to the layout of a book and we have not attempted to follow it. We have instead brought together related material under categories of our own devising. Inevitably this has led to the appearance of a miscellaneous group in the contents list. We do not intend to imply that these contributions were irrelevant to the subjects under discussion; merely that they do not fit into our arbitrary classification.

The writings stem from three sources. Firstly, a number of investigators were invited to present reviews of aspects of their work. Secondly, most, but not all, the free communications given at the meeting were accepted for publication. Thirdly, the authors of some of the posters, which seemed to us to be of particular interest, were asked to prepare their contribution in written form.

The authors have been allowed a fairly free hand within the limits of what Academic Press could tolerate, but we have attempted to standardize on English as opposed to American usage. The range is wide; that is in the nature of open conferences. We hope that the writing reflects what European obstetricians were doing and thinking in 1979.

August 1980

ARNOLD KLOPPER
ANDREA GENAZZANI
PIER GIORGIO CROSIGNANI

CONTENTS

vii

Contents

Section Two: New Placental Proteins and Oestriol in the Assessment of Placental Function

Section Three: Tests of Placental Function

Section Four: Protein Synthesis in the Placenta

Section Five: Placental Morphology

Section Six: Prolactin

Section Seven: Maternal Proteins

Section Eight: Abortion

Section Nine: Miscellaneous

FOREWORD: REFLECTIONS OF A RESEARCH WORKER

Baccio Baccetti

Instituto di Zoologia, Università di Siena, Siena, Italy

In the winter of 1978–79, in Siena, an exhibition was organized of the works of Dario Neri, a Sienese painter active during the first half of this century. One is impressed not only by the rich landscape theme of the exhibition, but also by the singular human figure of this personage who alternated art with his job as an industrial entrepreneur, going on to become, for many years, director of the Sclavo Serotherapeutical Institute. Neri always complained about this period lost to painting, declaring unequivocally in a very poignant letter of 1942, "at least it will serve to explain why, at my age, I still haven't concluded much", and further on, "I promise that from now on I shall not waste any more time", and, "these business affairs do not do my art much good", and at the end, "now I don't want to do anything other than paint". The point is made that if an artist wants to achieve the best results he should only be an artist, and nothing else.

At first sight, it would seem obvious that the same argument should apply to all the most demanding human occupations. But strangely, the research scientist does not abide by this rule. Tradition would have the latter as an ascetic figure, withdrawn from the world, holed up in his laboratory, living on very little, just like the poet or philosopher, achieving the best results in conditions of maximum concentration and isolation. However, the real state of affairs means instead that to pursue a discovery of real worth at international level, in the highly sophisticated competition that now exists in all fields, requires spending a lot of one's time, and talent, groping among the confusion of various financing bodies with the aim of gleaning large amounts of money every year, since no serious piece of research costs less, trying to keep together, and in agreement, a large number of assistants, because no really demanding research can be done alone; travelling all over the world and mastering languages, because otherwise you miss the really essential points of various subjects. And furthermore, still dedicating as much time as possible to study, and thus maintaining those characteristics of culture, criticism, imagination, tenacity and precision which have always been the qualities of a scientist.

When, as a child, I began to show a worrisome inclination towards the study of insects, those who examined me in every detail, before deciding to launch this singular *"enfant prodige"*, made sure that I had a good memory, intelligence, willingness to work and above all enthusiasm. One of them, the most practical, even wanted to find out whether my family's financial circumstances were such as to support me for a long period in the penniless career of entomologist for which I was yearning. But when I was weighed up like a thoroughbred, no-one wondered whether I would have had the ability to steer my way through political parties, or to find loans, or to withstand strikes, or to arouse public opinion, or advertise my product—all since which regularly found me out. In fact, disaster broke out for the scientist and a contemplative spirit unexpectedly found himself an industrial manager as well. The same combination of jobs which horrified the painter became the rule for the chemist, physicist and biologist who wanted to follow the difficult path of demanding research.

I often wonder whether or not this is fair. The question is obviously paradoxical. It would be as if Edson Arantes do Scimento, alias Pelè, apart from inside forward, had had to be trainer, sports instructor, team manager, president of the association, commentator at his own matches, observer at rival football fields, talent scout and, why not, masseur and father confessor as well. It would also be nice for a researcher to be able to be totally taken care of, organized and contented like a famous footballer. However, when an attempt was made to consign scientists to research alone, letting them be managed, coddled and publicized by officials from different fields, its purpose always failed, creating a series of additional bureaucratic shackles, making them waste more time than before in the need to make their needs filter through untrained ears, and ending up by squandering money and offending the highly delicate sensitivity of those who were supposed to be helped. Like it or not, the scientist must therefore accept the fact that he has to change his own characteristic features. The reality of the situation is in fact this: that all over the world, when you go to visit the place where a great discovery has been made, you find a kind of Christopher Columbus figure at the limits of nervous exhaustion, who had the courage to surround himself with trusting assistants, convince administrative offices and political parties, withstand sabotage and irony, work like a horse and go on dreaming.

Section One

THE NEW PLACENTAL PROTEINS

NEW PLACENTAL PROTEINS—BIOLOGY AND CLINICAL APPLICATIONS

T. Chard and J. G. Grudzinskas

Departments of Obstetrics and Gynaecology, and Reproductive Physiology, St. Bartholomew's Hospital Medical College and The London Hospital Medical College, London, U.K.

INTRODUCTION

The placenta secretes a variety of protein hormones and enzymes into the maternal circulation (Table I), and measurement of these is widely used as a diagnostic marker of the well-being of the fetus in both early and late pregnancy (Chard, 1977). The recent identification of a number of new specific placental proteins (Klopper and Chard, 1979) has led to considerable further work on this subject.

THE NEW PLACENTAL PROTEINS

These are shown in Table II and have in common that none are chemically analogous to any defined protein in the non-pregnant adult, and that none have any well-identified biological activity. A number of possible functions have been suggested for SP_1, including a role in carbohydrate metabolism (Tatra *et al.,* 1976a), a role as a carrier of steroid hormones and iron (Bohn and Kranz, 1973; Lin *et al.,* 1974), and an immunosuppressive action (Cerni *et al.,* 1977). There is, however, little evidence that any of these are significant in a normal pregnancy. The lack of biological activity probably explains why the discovery of the new

Serono Symposium No. 35, "The Human Placenta", edited by A. Klopper,
A. Genazzani and P. G. Crosignani, 1980. Academic Press, London and New York.

Table I. Protein hormones and enzymes secreted by the human placenta.

Protein (and synonyms)	Abbreviation	No. of subunits	Molecular weight (daltons)	Half-life	Refs
Human chorionic gonadotrophin	hCG	2	45 000–50 000	12–36 h	A
Human placental lactogen	hPL	1	21 000	15–20 min	B
(human chorionic somatomammotrophin)	(hCS)				
Human chorionic thyrotrophin	hCG	2	45 000	—	C
Human chorionic corticotrophin	hCCT	1	5000	—	D
Human chorionic gonadotrophin releasing hormone	hC-GnRH	1	1000	—	E
Human chorionic thyrotrophin releasing hormone	hC-TRH	1	360	—	E
Heat-stable alkaline phosphatase	HSAP			—	F
Cystine aminopeptidase (oxytocinase)	CAP			—	G
Diamine oxidase (histaminase)	DO	2	190 000	15–30 min	H

References: A: Bahl *et al.*, 1974; Canfield *et al.*, 1971; Zondek, 1929. B: Handwerger and Sherwood, 1974; Ito and Higashi, 1961; Josimovich and MacLaren, 1962. C: Hennen *et al.*, 1969; Hershman and Starnes, 1971. D: Opsahl and Long, 1951; Rees, *et al.* 1975. E: Gibbons *et al.*, 1975. F: Fishman and Ghosh, 1967; Sadowsky and Zuckerman, 1965. G: Tuppy and Nesvadba, 1957. H: Lin and Kerley, 1976.

Table II. Non-functional specific[a] proteins secreted by the human placenta.

Proteins (and synonyms)	Abbreviations	No. of subunits	Molecular weight (daltons)	Half-life	Refs
Schwangerschafts-spezifisches β$_1$-glycoprotein (Protein P)	SP$_1$	1	90 000–110 000[b]		A
Pregnancy-specific β$_1$-glycoprotein	PSβ$_1$ G				
Trophoblast β$_1$-glycoprotein	TBG				
Trophoblast-specific β-glycoprotein	TSG				
Pregnancy-associated plasma protein C (β$_1$-SP$_1$)	PAPP-C				
Pregnancy-associated plasma protein A	PAPP-A		750 000	3–4 days	B
Pregnancy-associated plasma protein B	PAPP-B			<1 day	B
Placental protein 5	PP$_5$		42 000	15–30 min	C

[a]'Specific' in this context is relative rather than absolute. Small amounts may be present in the non-pregnant state. The placenta also contains and may synthesize large amounts of other proteins, such as ferritin, which are identical to products of the normal adult.

[b]Teisner *et al.* (1978) have shown that SP$_1$ may be heterogeneous with high and low molecular weight forms reformed as SP$_1\alpha$ and SP$_1\beta$ respectively. SP$_1\beta$ is the principal form measured in current radioimmunoassays.

References: A: Thornes, 1958; Bohn, 1971; Towler *et al.*, 1976; Tatarinov and Masyukevich, 1970; Lin *et al.*, 1974b, 1976; Klopper *et al.*, 1978; Searle *et al.*, 1978; Tatarinov, 1978. B: Lin *et al.*, 1974b, 1976. C: Bohn, 1976; Obiekwe *et al.*, 1979.

placental proteins has been relatively late, and has depended entirely on physico-chemical and immunochemical methods.

The principal characteristics of the new placental proteins are also listed in Table II. They do not possess any unique properties relative to other and better-known placental products (Table I), and all appear to be synthesized mainly by the syncytiotrophoblast (Bohn and Sedlacek, 1975; Lin and Halbert, 1976; Horne *et al.*, 1976b).

MEASUREMENT OF THE NEW PLACENTAL PROTEINS

Because of the absence of biological activity, the only methods available for determination of circulating levels of the new placental proteins are immunoassays. These include both immunoprecipitation methods (radial immunodiffusion and "rocket" immunoelectrophoresis) and radioimmunoassay (RIA). The studies on SP_1 reported by us depended exclusively on RIA (Grudzinskas *et al.*, 1977a; Obiekwe *et al.*, 1979) because they are considerably more sensitive than immuno-precipitation systems and thus allow studies in the earliest stages of pregnancy. However, for late pregnancy, non-isotopic immunoassays are probably the method of choice. In the case of PP_5, only RIA is sufficiently sensitive to permit detection at *any* stage of pregnancy, and before the introduction of RIA (Obiekwe *et al.*, 1979) it was thought to be an exclusively intracellular protein (Bohn, 1976).

PLACENTAL PROTEINS AS INDICATORS OF FETAL WELL-BEING

The criteria for the use of a placental protein as an indicator of the well-being of the fetus have been set out at length elsewhere (Chard, 1976, 1977) (Table III). As there is no *a priori* reason for selecting any one given protein as superior to any other, it is worthwhile to define the properties which suggest that further study of the protein is a valuable exercise. For SP_1 and PP_5 these are as follows (see also Table 3):

1. SP_1 may be unique to pregnancy and therefore offer greater specificity in the diagnosis of early pregnancy than chorionic gonadotrophin (hCG) (which is immunologically and physiochemically similar to luteinizing hormone (hLH)).

2. The maternal levels of SP_1 in late pregnancy are higher in molar terms than those of any other placental product, and measurement should therefore be rapid and simple, and precise.

3. PP_5 has been described as an intracellular protein (Bohn, 1976) and might therefore reflect aspects of placental dysfunction which would not be apparent with a protein which is normally exported into maternal blood.

Other possible criteria of efficiency, such as day-to-day variation and half-life, do not distinguish SP_1 or PP_5 from other placental proteins (*see* Tables I, II and III).

Table III. The criteria for a biochemical test of fetal well-being, and the place of SP_1 and PP_5 in relation to these criteria.

Criterion	SP_1 and PP_5
1. The substance measured should differ qualitatively or quantitatively from materials present in the non-pregnant adult	Both are 'specific' to the placenta, though small amounts of SP_1 have been reported in some non-pregnant adults (Searle *et al.* 1978; Würz, 1979).
2. The substance should be present in an accessible fluid (maternal blood or urine, amniotic fluid)	Applies to SP_1, and with the recent development of RIA is known to apply to PP_5 (Obiekwe *et al.*, 1979). .
3. Measurement should be practical and precise	Applies to SP_1, which because of its very high levels should be the simplest of all placental proteins to measure in late pregnancy. Measurement of PP_5 requires a *sensitive* RIA which does not meet these criteria.
4. Variability of levels between subjects and between different times in the same subject should be as low as possible.	Variability of SP_1 is similar to that of hPL and less than that of blood oestrogens (Masson *et al.*, 1977). No data is available for PP_5.
5. Half-life should be short so that changes in production are rapidly reflected by circulating levels.	Doubtful as a criterion (Gordon and Chard, 1979). Unfavourable to SP_1 (half-life 30 h), favourable to PP_5 (half-life 15–30 min).
6. The levels should distinguish between normality and abnormality.	Evidence suggests that clinical application of SP_1 is similar to hPL, but because of high levels may extend into very early pregnancy. Preliminary studies on PP_5 are unpromising.

SP₁ IN NORMAL PREGNANCY

SP₁ could not be detected in culture medium from human pre-implantation embryos derived from extracorporeal fertilization (I. L. C. Ferguson, J. G. Grudzinskas, M. B. Brush and B. Gordon, unpublished observations). As shown in Fig. 1, SP₁ can be detected in maternal blood 18–23 days after the LH surge

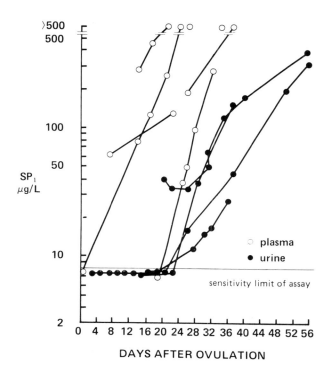

Fig. 1.   Concentration of SP₁ in urine and plasma from eight women in early pregnancy. (From Grudzinskas *et al.*, 1977a.)

(Grudzinskas *et al.*, 1977a,b). Thereafter there is an exponential rise, the levels doubling every 2–3 days; the slope decreases at 40 days (Grudzinskas *et al.*, 1979). By 10 weeks of gestation the concentration is 10–20 mg/l, and the levels rise progressively to a plateau at 36 weeks and after at a median level which has been variously estimated at 95–250 mg/l (Table IV). The day-to-day variation at this time is 6% as compared with 5% for hPL and 14–21% for oestrogens (Masson *et al.*, 1977). Fetal levels are 1000-fold less than maternal, and the levels in amniotic fluid are 100-fold less (Grudzinskas *et al.*, 1978). Small and variable amounts appear in urine.

Table IV. Circulating levels of **SP₁** in late pregnancy.[a]

Reference	No. of subjects	Mean (mg/l)	S.D.	Coefficient of variation	Method of assay[b]
Tatra et al., 1974	22	139	42.5	30.6	RID
Towler et al., 1976	16	199	53.9	27.1	RID
Gordon et al., 1977b	59	250	—	9[c]	RIA
Klopper et al., 1978	53	159	48.0	30.2	RID
Lin et al., 1974a	41	2200 IU/l	—	—	RID
Sorensen, 1978	20	199	—	—	EID
Heikenheim et al., 1979	51	95	—	—	RIA

[a]Note the wide range of levels due to use of different assay methods and standards.

[b]RID, radial immunodiffusion; RIA, radioimmunoassays; EID, electroimmunodiffusion ("rocket" immunoelectrophoresis).

[c]This figure was calculated after logarithmic transformation of results. As a skewed distribution appears to be universal for all placental proteins (Chard, 1976), including SP₁, analysis as arithmetic mean and standard deviations is probably not valid. Non-parametric analysis (median and percentiles) is the best approach.

SP$_1$ IN THE DETECTION OF EARLY PREGNANCY

Present assays for SP$_1$ are equivalent to, or marginally less sensitive than, those for the β-subunit of hCG in the detection of early pregnancy. In a recent study (Grudzinskas *et al.*, 1979), circulating hCG could be detected 10-16 days after the LH peak, and SP$_1$ at 18-23 days. Because the molar concentrations and rate of increase of SP$_1$ and hCG are almost identical in the first 4 weeks of gestation, it is likely that the principal factor influencing the choice between hCG and SP$_1$ will be the sensitivity of available techniques. Specificity is not likely to be a factor, since that of the hCG β-subunit assay is perfectly satisfactory, while recent studies (Searle *et al.*, 1978) have cast doubt on the total absence of SP$_1$ in the blood of the non-pregnant adult.

SP$_1$ IN ABNORMALITIES OF EARLY PREGNANCY

Highly sensitive methods for the measurement of hCG may detect "occult" pregnancies, i.e. those which abort around the time of the first missed menstrual period (Seppälä *et al.*, 1978a). A similar application has been proposed for SP$_1$ (Seppäla *et al.*, 1978c).

The estimation of SP$_1$ might prove effective as a diagnostic marker in threatened abortion, as has previously been proposed for both hCG (Dhont *et al.*, 1975) and hPL (Niven *et al.*, 1972). Decreased levels of SP$_1$ are associated with anembryonic pregnancy (Bennett *et al.*, 1978), and with threatened abortion in which the outcome of pregnancy is unsatisfactory (Jandial *et al.*, 1978; Schultz-Larsen and Hertz, 1978). However, it is likely that the true value of such tests does not appear until after 8-10 weeks of gestation (Schultz-Larsen and Hertz, 1978), and in our own preliminary studies experience with SP$_1$ prior to this time has been disappointing.

Circulating levels of both SP$_1$ and hCG decrease after prostaglandin-induced therapeutic abortion in the first trimester (Mandelin *et al.*, 1978); but the fall is not simultaneous, because in some subjects SP$_1$ was still detectable after 4 weeks, when hCG was not detectable.

SP$_1$ has been detected in vesicle fluid, tissue extracts, tissue sections and maternal blood and urine from cases of hydatidiform mole (Searle *et al.*, 1978; Seppälä *et al.*, 1978b; Tatarinov *et al.*, 1974, 1976; Horne *et al.*, 1977). The circulating levels fall rapidly after vaginal removal of tumour tissue. A case of chorio-carcinoma has been described in which circulating SP$_1$ was present while hCG was absent (Seppälä *et al.*, 1978b). If this discordance can be confirmed then estimation of SP$_1$ might become a valuable additional parameter in the diagnosis and treatment of trophoblastic tumours.

Ectopic production of SP$_1$ has been noted in some breast cancers (Horne *et al.*, 1976a), and other non-trophoblastic tumours (Tatarinov and Sokolov, 1977).

SP$_1$ IN ABNORMALITIES OF LATE PREGNANCY

Information on the value of SP$_1$ in the clinical management of late pregnancy is still relatively sparse, especially in relation to specific clinical conditions. However, there is general agreement that decreased levels of SP$_1$ are associated

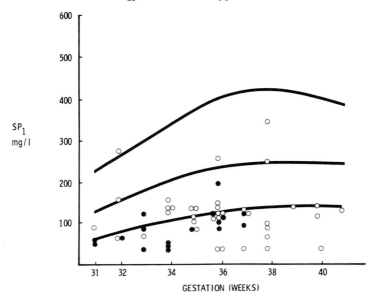

Fig. 2 Concentration of SP_1 in plasma from pregnancies with (•) and without (○) maternal hypertension in which there was growth retardation of the fetus. The solid lines show the median and 10th and 90th percentiles of the normal range for maternal plasma SP_1 . (From Gordon *et al.*, 1977a.)

with intrauterine growth retardation, both in the presence and absence of maternal hypertension (Chapman and Jones, 1978; Gordon *et al.*, 1977a; Grudzinskas *et al.*, 1977a; Lin *et al.*, 1974a; Sorensen, 1978; Towler *et al.*, 1977) (Fig. 2). In two of these studies low levels of SP_1 were found in 70% and 60% of cases in which the birthweight of the child was less than the 10th percentile of the normal population (Chapman and Jones, 1978; Gordon *et al.*, 1977a). The information on maternal SP_1 levels in relation to fetal distress during labour and neonatal asphyxia is confusing, probably because many cases of this type represent acute phenomena which are unrelated to long-standing nutritional deprivation of the fetus. Levels of SP_1 are raised in multiple pregnancy (Lin *et al.*, 1977; Tatra *et al.*, 1974; Towler *et al.*, 1976), and are normal in hypertension/pre-eclampsia (Chapman and Jones, 1978; Sorensen, 1978; Lin *et al.*, 1977) unless there are serious fetal complications (Tatra *et al.*, 1974). Increased levels of SP_1 in amniotic fluid have been described in conditions associated with excessive growth of the placenta (Tatra *et al.*, 1976a), including maternal Rhesus isoimmunization and diabetes. These observations suggest that the clinical interpretation of maternal SP_1 levels will probably be very similar to that of hPL (Chard, 1977), although a number of authors (*see above*) have proposed that SP_1 provides a rather clearer distinction between normality and abnormality.

PP₅ IN NORMAL PREGNANCY

The properties of PP_5 have been described in Table II. As maternal blood levels are very low it has only recently been possible to measure them using a specific

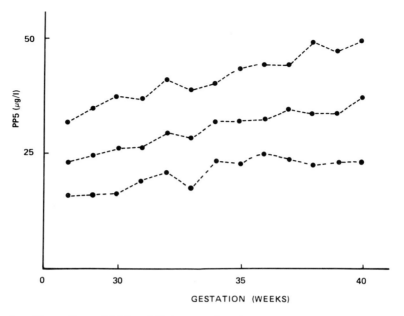

Fig. 3.   The median and 10th and 90th percentiles of maternal serum PP₅ after 28 weeks of gestation during normal pregnancy.

radioimmunoassay (Obiekwe *et al.,* 1979). Circulating PP_5 can be detected from about the 8th week of pregnancy and thereafter rises to reach a plateau at 36 weeks with a median level of 32 μg/l (Obiekwe *et al.,* 1979) (Fig. 3); this level is approximately 100-fold less than that of hPL at the same time.

PP_5 IN ABNORMAL PREGNANCY

As the levels of PP_5 are undetectable in early pregnancy using present methods, it cannot have any clinical use at this time. However, the presence of PP_5 has been reported in homogenates of trophoblastic tumours, in testicular teratomas, in mole vesicle fluid, and in the serum of some patients with hydatidiform mole (Grudzinskas *et al.,* 1979). There is no evidence to suggest that measurement of PP_5 would yield information which cannot be obtained by estimation of hCG or SP_1.

Preliminary studies on PP_5 in late pregnancy have shown no significant association between low levels (or high levels) and intrauterine growth retardation (B. Obiekwe, J. G. Grudzinskas, H. Bohn and T. Chard, unpublished observations). This may simply be due to the fact that circulating levels of PP_5 cannot be measured with the same precision as that of the very much higher levels of SP_1 and hPL; it has already been emphasized that detection efficiency and precision of assay are critically related (Chard, 1976) (Fig. 4).

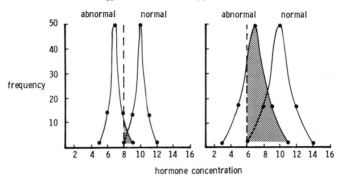

Fig. 4. The effect of assay variation on the distinction between normality and abnormality. On the left, population frequency distributions for levels of a placental hormone measured without any error: there is little overlap (shaded area) between normal and abnormal. On the right, the same frequency distributions with the addition of a further 10% variation due to error in measurement: there is now considerable overlap between the two populations. (From Chard, 1976.)

CONCLUSIONS: THE CLINCIAL USE OF MEASUREMENTS OF THE NEW PLACENTAL PROTEINS

In order to represent a significant clinical advance, the new proteins must have unique properties not possessed by materials which are already available. The special properties of SP_1 and PP_5 can now be considered in relation to specific clinical observations:

1. In contrast to the original claims, there is now some question as to whether SP_1 is unique to pregnancy (Searle *et al.*, 1978), and SP_1 determination seems no better than that of the β-subunit of hCG in the detection of early pregnancy or its non-neoplastic complications. However, it is possible that dissociation of synthesis of hCG and SP_1 by some trophoblast tumours might lead to a useful application for SP_1 measurements in this condition.

2. Measurement of maternal SP_1 levels in late pregnancy yields clinical information which in preliminary studies is rather better than that of hPL, but past experience suggests that more work is needed before this conclusion can be regarded as final. As the measurement of SP_1 could be simpler and more precise than that of hPL (although this has not yet been proven and the problem of heterogeneity (Teisner *et al.*, 1978) must be solved), it might be a valid alternative to hPL in the assessment of the well-being of the fetus in the third trimester.

3. Observations using a sensitive RIA for PP_5 suggest that there are no longer grounds for classifying this protein as an intracellular rather than a secretory product. Since precise measurement of the low circulating levels is difficult, and preliminary clinical studies have been unpromising, there seems no reason to suggest that PP_5 will be of unique clinical value.

In conclusion, measurement of SP_1 offers great promise as a clinical diagnostic tool in early and late pregnancy, while that of PP_5 does not.

REFERENCES

Bahl, O. P., Carlsen, R. B. and Bellisario, R. (1973). *Biochemical and Biophysical Research Communications* **48**, 416.

Bennett, M. J., Grudzinskas, J. G., Gordon, Y. B. and Turnbull, A. C. (1978). *British Journal of Obstetrics and Gynaecology* **85**, 348.

Bohn, H. (1971). *Archiv für Gynäkologie* **210**, 440.

Bohn, H. (1976). *In* "Protides of the Biological Fluids" (H. Peeters, ed.), p. 117, Pergamon, Oxford.

Bohn, H. and Kranz, T. (1973). *Archiv für Gynäkologie* **215**, 63.

Bohn, H. and Sedlacek, H. (1975). *Archiv für Gynäkologie* **220**, 105.

Canfield, R. E., Morgan, F. J., Kammerman, S., Bell, J. J. and Agosto, G. M. (1971). *Recent Progress in Hormone Research* **27**, 121.

Cerni, C., Tatra, G. and Bohn, H. (1977). *Archiv für Gynäkologie* **223**, 1.

Chapman, M. G. and Jones, W. R. (1978). *Australian and New Zealand Journal of Obstetrics and Gynaecology* **18**, 172.

Chard, T. (1976). *In* "Plasma Hormone Assays in Evaluation of Fetal Wellbeing" (A. Klopper, ed.), p. 1, Churchill-Livingstone, Edinburgh.

Chard, T. (1977). *In* "Recent Advances in Obstetrics and Gynaecology (12)" (J. Stallworthy and G. L. Bourne, eds), p. 146, Churchill-Livingstone, Edinburgh.

Dhont, M., Thiery, M., Vandekerckhove, D. and Van Cauwenberghe, A. (1975). *Tijdschrift voor Geneeskunde* **22**, 1097.

Fishman, W. H. and Ghosh, N. K. (1967). *Advances in Clinical Chemistry* **10**, 225.

Gibbons, J. M., Mitwick, M. and Chieffo, V. (1975). *American Journal of Obstetrics and Gynecology* **121**, 127.

Gordon, Y. B. and Chard, T. (1979). *In* "Placental Proteins" (A. Klopper and T. Chard, eds), p. 1, Springer-Verlag, Heidelberg.

Gordon, Y. B., Grudzinskas, J. G., Jeffrey, D., Chard, T. and Letchworth, A. T. (1977a). *Lancet i*, 331.

Gordon, Y. B., Grudzinskas, J. G., Lewis, J. D., Jeffrey, D. and Letchworth, A. T. (1977b). *British Journal of Obstetrics and Gynaecology* **84**, 642.

Grudzinskas, J. G., Lenton, E. A. and Obiekwe, B. C. (1979). *In* "Placental Proteins" (A. Klopper and T. Chard, eds), p. 119. Springer-Verlag, Heidelberg.

Grudzinskas, J. G., Gordon, Y. B., Jeffrey, D. J. and Chard, T. (1977a). *Lancet i,* 333.

Grudzinskas, J. G., Evans, D. G., Gordon, Y. B., Jeffrey, D. and Chard, T. (1978). *Obstetrics and Gynecology* **52**, 43.

Grudzinskas, J. G., Lenton, E. A., Gordon, Y. B., Kelso, I. M., Jeffrey, D., Sobowale, O. and Chard, T. (1977b). *British Journal of Obstetrics and Gynaecology* **84**, 740.

Handwerger, S. and Sherwood, L. M. (1974). *In* "Lactogenic Hormones, Fetal Nutrition and Lactation" (J. B. Josimovich, ed.), p. 33, John Wiley, New York.

Hennen, G., Pierce, J. G. and Freychet, P. (1969). *Journal of Clinical Endocrinology and Metabolism* **29**, 581.

Heikenheimo, M., Unnerus, H. A., Ranta, T., Jalanko, H. and Seppälä, M. (1978). *Obstetrics and Gynecology* **52**, 276.

Hershman, J. M. and Starnes, W. R. (1971). *Journal of Clinical Endocrinology and Metabolism* **32**, 52.

Horne, C. H. W. and Towler, C. M. (1978). *Obstetrics and Gynecology* **33**, 761.

Horne, C. H. W., Reid, I. N. and Milne, G. D. (1976a). *Lancet ii*, 279.
Horne, C. H. W., Towler, C. M. and Milne, G. D. (1977). *Journal of Clinical Pathology* 30, 19.
Horne, C. H. W., Towler, C. M., Pugh-Humphreys, R. G. P., Thomson, A. W. and Bohn, H. (1976b). *Experientia* 32, 1197.
Ito, Y. and Higashi, K. (1961). *Endocrinologia Japonica* 8, 279.
Jandial, V., Towler, C. M., Horne, C. H. W. and Abramovich, D. R. (1978). *British Journal of Obstetrics and Gynaecology* 85, 832.
Josimovich, J. B. and MacLaren, J. A. (1962). *Endocrinology* 71, 209.
Klopper, A. and Chard, T. (eds) (1979). "The Placental Proteins", Springer-Verlag, Heidelberg.
Klopper, A., Buchan, P. and Wilson, G. (1978). *British Journal of Obstetrics and Gynaecology* 85, 738.
Klopper, A., Masson, G. and Wilson, G. (1977). *British Journal of Obstetrics and Gynaecology* 84, 648.
Lin, C.-W. and Kerley, S. D. (1976). *In* "Protides of the Biological Fluids" (H. Peeters, ed.), p. 103, Pergamon, Oxford.
Lin, T. M. and Halbert, S. P. (1976). *Science, New York,* 193, 1249.
Lin, T. M., Halbert, S. P. and Spellacy, W. N. (1974a). *Journal of Clinical Investigation* 54, 576.
Lin, T. M., Halbert, S. P., Spellacy, W. N. and Berne, B. H. (1977). *American Journal of Obstetrics and Gynecology* 128, 808.
Lin, T. M., Halbert, S. P., Spellacy, W. N. and Gall, S. (1976). *American Journal of Obstetrics and Gynecology* 126, 382.
Lin, T. M., Halbert, S. P., Kiefer, D., Spellacy, W. N. and Gall, S. (1974b). *American Journal of Obstetrics and Gynecology* 118, 223.
Mandelin, M., Rutanen, E. M., Heikinheimo, M., Jalanko, H. and Seppälä, M. (1978). *Obstetrics and Gynecology* 52, 314.
Masson, G. M., Klopper, A. I. and Wilson, G. R. (1977). *Obstetrics and Gynecology* 50, 435.
Niven, P. A. R., Landon, J. and Chard, T. (1972). *British Medical Journal ii,* 799.
Obiekwe, B., Gordon, Y. B., Grudzinskas, J. G., Chard, T. and Bohn, H. (1979). *Clinica chimica acta* 95, 509.
Opsahl, J. C. and Long, C. N. H. (1951). *Yale Journal of Biology and Medicine* 24, 199.
Rees, L. H., Burke, C. W., Evans, S., Letchworth, A. T. and Chard, T. (1975). *Nature, London* 354, 620.
Sadowsky, E. and Zuckerman, H. (1965). *Obstetrics and Gynecology* 26, 211.
Schultz-Larsen, P. and Hertz, J. B. (1978). *European Journal of Obstetrics and Gynaecology and Reproductive Biology* 8, 5.
Searle, F., Leake, B. A., Bagshawe, K. D. and Dent, J. (1978). *Lancet i,* 579.
Seppälä, M., Lehtovirta, P. and Rutanen, E.-M. (1978a). *Acta endocrinologica, Copenhagen* 88, 164.
Seppälä, M., Rutanen, E. M., Heikinheimo, M., Jalanko, H. and Engvall, E. (1978b). *International Journal of Cancer* 21, 265.
Seppälä, M., Rutanen, E.-M., Jalanko, H., Lehtovirta, P., Stenman, U. G. and Engvall, E. (1978c). *Journal of Clinical Endocrinology and Metabolism* 47, 1216.
Sorensen, S. (1978). *Acta obstetrica et gynecologica scandinavica* 57, 193.
Tatarinov, Y. S. (1978). *Antibiotics Chemotherapy* 22, 125.
Tatarinov, Y. S. and Masyukevich, V. N. (1970). *Bulletin of Experimental Biology and Medicine of the U.S.S.R.* 69, 66.

Tatarinov, Y. S. and Sokolov, A. V. (1977). *International Journal of Cancer* **19**, 161.

Tatarinov, Y., Falaleeva, D. M. and Kalashnikov, V. V. (1976). *International Journal of Cancer* **17**, 626.

Tatarinov, V., Mesnyankina, N. V., Nikovlina, D. M., Novikova, L. A., Toloknov, B. O. and Falaleeva, D. M. (1974). *International Journal of Cancer* **14**, 548.

Tatra, G., Breitenecker, G. and Gruber, W. (1974). *Archiv für Gynäkologie* **217**, 383.

Tatra, G., Polak, S. and Placheta, P. (1976a). *Archiv für Gynäkologie* **221**, 161.

Tatra, G., Tempfer, H. and Placheta, P. (1976b). *European Journal of Obstetrics and Gynaecology and Reproductive Biology* **6**, 53.

Teisner, B., Westergaard, J. G., Folkersen, J., Husby, S. and Svenag, S.-E. (1978). *American Journal of Obstetrics and Gynecology* **131**, 262.

Thornes, R. D. (1958). M.D. thesis, Trinity College, Dublin (quoted by Horne and Towler, 1978).

Towler, C. M., Horne, C. H. W., Jandial, V., Campbell, D. M. and MacGillivray, I. (1976). *British Journal of Obstetrics and Gynaecology* **83**, 775.

Towler, C. M., Horne, C. H. W., Jandial, V., Campbell, D. M. and MacGillivray, I. (1977). *British Journal of Obstetrics and Gynaecology* **84**, 258.

Tuppy, H. and Nesvadba, M. (1957). *Monatshefte Chemie* **88**, 977.

Würz, H. (1979). *Archiv für Gynäkologie* **227**, 1.

Zondek, B. (1929). *Zentralblatt für Gynäkologie* **84**, 258.

THE NEW PLACENTAL PROTEINS: SOME CLINICAL APPLICATIONS OF THEIR MEASUREMENT

A. Klopper and G. Hughes

Department of Obstetrics and Gynaecology, University of Aberdeen, Aberdeen, Scotland

INTRODUCTION

Although a number of pregnancy-associated proteins have been isolated in recent years, enough data to assess the use of their measurement in obstetric practice has accumulated for only two of these; pregnancy-specific β_1-globulin (Tatarinov and Masyukevich, 1970) and pregnancy-associated plasma protein A (Lin *et al.*, 1974). In keeping with the suggestion made by Halbert (1979), we propose to use the designations of SP_1 (*Schwangerschafts* protein 1) (Bohn, 1972) and PAPP-A for these two proteins. Both these proteins have been localized to the syncytiotrophoblast by immunofluorescent staining and can be extracted from the placenta. There is thus strong, but not definitive, proof that they are placental in origin.

Both SP_1 and PAPP-A have long half-lives, over 24 h as compared to 13 min for placental lactogen (hPL) (Klopper *et al.*, 1978). The kind of clinical question to which SP_1 or PAPP-A measurements might provide answers is likely to be different from that which is applicable to hPL assays. SP_1 and PAPP-A concentrations are, however, very stable from time to time (Masson *et al.*, 1977). Their slow response to changes in placental input and their stability make it likely that SP_1 and PAPP-A assays will be more useful in a diagnostic, prognosticative sense than as an aid to immediate decision making in obstetric practice, based on

Serono Symposium No. 35, "The Human Placenta", edited by A. Klopper,
A. Genazzani and P. G. Crosignani, 1980. Academic Press, London and New York.

changing levels in serial assays. Our investigation has therefore been designed to examine how useful these assays might be in predicting the outcome of pregnancy if measurements are made some time before delivery.

PATIENTS AND METHODS

Blood samples were taken at random from 272 patients who presented at Aberdeen University Clinic for review at 34 weeks. Of these 176 remained normal throughout gestation and gave birth to normal babies with a birthweight above the 10th percentile for our population. Seventeen of the remaining 96 patients did not suffer from any of the forms of obstetric disorder included in this analysis and have been discarded. They include multiple pregnancy, essential hypertension, pre-eclamptic toxaemia and diabetes. The remaining 79 either presented at 34 weeks with signs of obstetric disease or subsequently developed them. These obstetric diseases were: pre-eclamptic toxaemia, antepartum haemorrhage, retarded fetal growth and premature labour. Some patients suffered from more than one disorder.

There were 39 patients with pre-eclampsia, only three of whom had albuminuria as well as hypertension. Of these 28 patients developed the pre-eclampsia after the 34 week specimen had been taken and 11 already had the disease at 34 weeks. The antepartum haemorrhage group consisted of 22 patients; 12 with bleeding before 34 weeks, often slight, and 10 with bleeding subsequent to the 34 week examination. There were 35 patients who gave birth to babies with a birthweight below the 10th percentile of birthweight for gestation (Thomson *et al.,* 1968). Twelve patients went into labour before 38 weeks of gestation and were classified as premature labour.

PAPP-A was measured by immunoelectrophoresis as described by Bischof *et al.* (1979). We used a monospecific antiserum raised against PAPP-A isolated from pregnancy blood and injected into rabbits. The standard was a pool of late pregnancy plasma calibrated against pure PAPP-A.

SP_1 was also measured by immunoelectrophoresis (Bruce and Klopper, 1978). The Behring commercial standards were used for reference and the antiserum was bought from Dako, Copenhagen.

RESULTS

The mean and standard deviations of the values in normal and abnormal pregnancy are listed in Tables I and II. Both PAPP-A and SP_1 have a skew distribution of normal values and logarithmic transforms were therefore used along with the Student t-test in determining the significances of the differences between groups.

PAPP-A values are significantly raised in pre-eclampsia, not only in patients suffering from the disorder but also in those who will only later develop the signs. PAPP-A levels are also raised in antepartum haemorrhage, although not significantly so in advance of the bleeding. It is difficult to know what to make of the raised levels of PAPP-A in association with premature labour. It is known that PAPP-A concentration rises with the onset of labour at term (Smith *et al.,* 1979),

Table I. Mean and standard deviation (in micrograms per millilitre) of PAPP-A in normal and abnormal pregnancy.

Normal	All PET	PET before 34 weeks	PET after 34 weeks	All APH	APH before 34 weeks	APH after 34 weeks	All IUGR	IUGR without PET or APH	Pre-mature labour
97.0 ±40.8 n = 176	154.9^a ±68.6 n = 39	170.2^a ±64.5 n = 11	149.2^b ±69.0 n = 28	130.0^c ±57.1 n = 22	132.7^c ±56.3 n = 12	126.7 ±59.7 n = 10	113.5 ±45.9 n = 35	104.7 ±42.1 n = 19	147.9^c ±77.6 n = 12

Abbreviations: PET, pre-eclamptic toxaemia; APH = antepartum haemorrhage; IUGR Intrauterine growth retardation.
^{a}2p > 0.0001; ^{b}2p > 0.001; ^{c}2p > 0.03; ^{d}2p > 0.05

Table II. Mean and standard deviation (in micrograms per millilitre) of SP$_1$ in normal and abnormal pregnancy.

Normal	All PET	PET before 34 weeks	PET after 34 weeks	All APH	APH before 34 weeks	APH after 34 weeks	All IUGR	IUGR without PET or APH	Pre-mature labour
115.0 ±32.8 n = 84	140.4 ±40.1 n = 12	103.4 — n = 2	149.3^a ±36.5 n = 10	94.1 ±23.1 n = 8	97.4 ±27.3 n = 6	85.0 — n = 2	122.0 ±38.8 n = 16	131.0 ±35.8 n = 8	137.1 ±28.0 n = 12

Abbreviations: See footnote to Table I.
^{a}2p > 0.03.

and there is some overlap between the premature labour group and other groups such as PET and APH which have a raised PAPP-A concentration. In addition, some of these cases of presumed premature labour could be due to mistaken dates, which would also account for their higher values at 34 weeks.

It was surprising and somewhat disappointing to find that neither PAPP-A nor SP_1 measurements gave any indication of retarded fetal growth. In this respect our findings are in contradistinction to those of Towler *et al.* (1977), who found that SP_1 values were significantly decreased in retarded fetal growth, particularly in association with pre-eclampsia. In view of the fact that we found raised values of SP_1 in pre-eclampsia and Towler *et al.* (1977) found them to be lowered, it would be as well if this condition were to be examined further.

Although the data in Tables I and II demonstrate that PAPP-A and SP_1 concentrations are raised in certain obstetric disorders, they do not indicate what proportion of such patients might be expected to show raised values. In the case of SP_1 it was found on examination of individual results that 30% of the pre-eclamptic patients showed values more than one standard deviation above the mean. In the case of PAPP-A the figure was 39%.

DISCUSSION

It is evident that neither PAPP-A nor SP_1 measurements at 34 weeks will give a completely reliable indication of what obstetric diseases might later become overt. Nevertheless, the proportion of patients with pre-eclampsia who show a raised PAPP-A value at 34 weeks is sufficiently high for this test to be useful in clinical practice. As the assays are so cheap and simple to do, there is a good case to be made for routine screening at 34 weeks with PAPP-A assays.

The raised concentration of PAPP-A in association with pre-eclampsia and antepartum haemorrhage is particularly interesting and deserves closer examination for any light it may throw on the physiological function of PAPP-A. Both these conditions are associated with disseminated intravascular coagulation (McKay, 1972) and raise strongly the possibility that PAPP-A may be a factor concerned in the clotting process.

It should not be too readily supposed that in PAPP-A and SP_1 we are certainly dealing with proteins elaborated by the syncytiotrophoblast and secreted directly into the maternal circulation; there to play some undetermined biological role. Some findings contradict this simplistic explanation. For one thing, SP_1 is almost certainly not one single protein, but two (Teisner *et al.*, 1978). It is just possible that in this case we are dealing with the placental receptor of a maternal protein and that the role of SP_1 is to mask placental antigens from maternal immunological surveillance, much as suggested by Faulk and Galbraith (1979) for transferrin. Both SP_1 and PAPP-A are in lower concentration in the retroplacental blood than in the maternal peripheral venous circulation: a finding which is very difficult to reconcile with the model of these proteins being directly secreted by chorionic villi into intervillous blood (Klopper *et al.*, 1979). Considerable amounts of trophoblast become separated from the main body of the placenta and are lysed in maternal tissues (Robertson *et al.*, 1976). It is possible that very little of either of these placental proteins is directly secreted by the villous trophoblast and that the high levels in the maternal circulation come from the lysis of maternal trophoblast, the protein accumulating in the maternal blood because of its slow removal. If this is true, it is unlikely that either SP_1 or PAPP-A have a hormone-like role to play in the maternal circulation. It would appear that their real role is a local one—at the point of contact between placental and maternal tissue. If so, the circulating material is biologically irrelevant.

ACKNOWLEDGEMENTS

Our thanks are due to Mrs P. Cunningham for technical assistance and to Miss G. Cowie for secretarial help. The expenses of the investigation were borne by a grant to one of us (A.K.) from the Medical Research Council.

REFERENCES

Bischof, P., Bruce, D., Cunningham, P. and Klopper, A. (1979). *Clinica chimica acta* **95**, 243.

Bohn, H. (1972). *Blut* **24**, 292.

Bruce, D. and Klopper, A. (1978). *Clinica chimica acta* **84**, 107.

Faulk, W. P. and Galbraith, G. M. (1979). *Proceedings of the Royal Society B* **204**, 83.

Halbert, S. P. (1979). *In* "Placental Proteins" (A. Klopper and T. Chard, eds), p. vii, Springer-Verlag, Berlin.

Klopper, A., Buchan, P. and Wilson, G. (1978). *British Journal of Obstetrics and Gynaecology* **85**, 738.

Klopper, A., Smith, R. and Davidson, I. (1979). *In* "Placental Proteins" (A. Klopper and T. Chard, eds), pp. 23–34, Springer-Verlag, Berlin.

Lin, T. M., Halbert, S. P., Kiefer, D. and Spellacy, W. N. (1974). *International Archives of Allergy and Applied Immunology* **47**, 35.

McKay, D. G. (1972). *Gynecological and Obstetrical Survey* **27**, 399.

Masson, G., Klopper, A. and Wilson, G. (1977). *Obstetrics and Gynecology* **50**, 435.

Robertson, W. B., Brosens, I. and Dixon, G. (1976). *European Journal of Obstetrics and Gynaecology and Reproductive Biology* **5**, 47.

Smith, R., Bischof, P., Hughes, G. and Klopper, A. (1979). *British Journal of Obstetrics and Gynaecology* **86**, 882.

Tatarinov, Y. S. and Masyukevich, V. N. (1970). *Bulletin for Experimental Biology and Medicine of the U.S.S.R.* **69**, 66.

Teisner, B., Westergaard, J. G., Folkersen, J., Husby, S. and Svenhag, S. C. (1978). *American Journal of Obstetrics and Gynecology* **131**, 262.

Thomson, A. M., Billewicz, W. and Hytten, F. (1968). *Journal of Obstetrics and Gynaecology of the British Commonwealth* **75**, 903.

Towler, C. M., Horne, C. H., Jandial, V., Campbell, D. M. and MacGillivray, I. (1977). *British Journal of Obstetrics and Gynaecology* **84**, 258.

PROTEIN ANTIGENS OF THE HUMAN PLACENTA

H. Bohn

Research Laboratories of Behringwerke AG, D-3550 Marburg,
German Federal Republic

PLACENTAL PROTEINS WITH KNOWN BIOLOGICAL ACTIVITY

The human placenta is a highly specialized organ which produces and contains a wide variety of active compounds, most of which are enzymes (Kyank, 1958). Thus far only a relatively small number of the biologically active proteins found in the placenta have been isolated to purity and characterized. Most of them apparently are identical or at least closely related to the corresponding functional proteins occurring in other human tissues or body fluids. For instance the placental fibrin stabilizing factor, a protransglutaminase isolated from human term placenta, turned out to be identical to the fibrin stabilizing factor from platelets, and closely related to the fibrin stabilizing factor occurring in human plasma (Bohn and Schwick, 1971); the placental tryptophanyl transfer ribonucleic acid synthetase, another well-characterized enzyme of the placenta, was found to be the same as the corresponding enzyme in the human skin (Penneys and Muench, 1974); and the isoenzymes A and B of placental N-acetyl-β-D -hexosaminidase could be immunochemically detected in other human tissues as well (Geiger *et al.*, 1975).

PLACENTAL PROTEINS WITH UNKNOWN FUNCTION

In addition to the proteins with known biological activity, a number of placental proteins with unknown function have been detected in pregnancy sera or in placental extracts by immunochemical methods.

Serono Symposium No. 35, "The Human Placenta", edited by A. Klopper,
A. Genazzani and P. G. Crosignani, 1980. Academic Press, London and New York.

Olivelli and Ruggieri (1958) described a placental α_2-globulin which could also be detected in sera from pregnant women. Krieg (1969) reported on an α_2-trophoblast cell antigen which he partly purified and which turned out to be a conjugated protein. Hofmann *et al.* (1970) detected five placental antigens which were also found to occur in sera from pregnant women. Tatarinov and Masyuke-vich (1970) reported on a "new β_1-globulin" which could be detected in sera from pregnant women only. Schultze-Mosgau and Fischer (1971) described the presence of three placental antigens in the sera of pregnant women. Lin *et al.* (1974), using antisera to pregnancy plasma, detected four pregnancy-specific proteins which they called PAPP-A, PAPP-B, PAPP-C and PAPP-D. In the same year, Gaugas *et al.* (1974) reported on the detection of four protein antigens, IPA-a, IPA-b, IPA-c and IPA-H, in the solubilized microsomal fraction of term placentae. Schwartz *et al.* (1974) isolated and partially characterized an insoluble lipoglycoprotein from the chorionic villi of term placentae. Petrunin *et al.* (1978) have recently described two chorionic microglobulins, one having the electro-phoretic mobility of an α_1-globulin the other of an α_2-globulin.

In our own laboratory more than 20 different soluble placental proteins and, in addition, 11 different solubilized, apparently membrane bound, antigens of the placenta have been detected by immunochemical methods in extracts from human term placentae (Bohn, 1971, 1972a, 1979a).

In 1971 we published a paper on the detection of four pregnancy proteins. These proteins could be detected in sera from pregnant women with the gel diffusion test of Ouchterlony (Bohn, 1971). The antisera used for their detection had been prepared by immunizing rabbits with protein fractions from human placentae and absorbed exhaustively with male serum to remove all antibodies directed against normal serum proteins.

One of these proteins turned out to be a new pregnancy-specific protein different from all other pregnancy-specific hormones and enzymes thus far known. This protein was shown to have the electrophoretic mobility of a β_1-globulin, a molecular weight of 90 000 daltons and a carbohydrate content of 29.3%; it therefore was named pregnancy-specific β_1-glycoprotein and abbreviated to SP_1 or PSβG.

SP_1 is synthesized in the syncytiotrophoblast (Horne *et al.*, 1976), whence it is secreted into the maternal blood stream in steadily increasing amounts with advancing pregnancy. The biological function of SP_1 and its physiological role during pregnancy are still unknown.

When we immunized rabbits with protein fractions from placental extracts, we not only obtained antibodies to pregnancy proteins such as SP_1, but also anti-bodies to antigens which occur neither in normal sera nor in sera from pregnant women. Most of these antigens turned out to be soluble protein constituents of the placental tissue which are not secreted into the maternal blood stream—at least not in concentrations which can be detected with the gel diffusion test.

Meanwhile, we have got antisera to more than 20 different soluble placental tissue proteins. A number of these proteins have already been isolated and charac-terized; they were designated as placental proteins, abbreviated to PP, and num-bered consecutively: PP_1, PP_2, PP_3, PP_4, PP_5, PP_6, PP_7, PP_8 and PP_{10}.

Table I summarizes the physicochemical properties of pregnancy protein SP_1 as well as of the placental tissue proteins PP_1–PP_8 and PP_{10}. These soluble placental

Table I.   Characteristics of the soluble placental proteins.

Placental protein	Name or function	Physicochemical properties			Amounts found in extracts of term placentae
		Electrophoretic mobility	Molecular weight (daltons)	Carbohydrate content (%)	(mg/placenta)
SP_1	Pregnancy-specific β_1-glycoprotein	β_1	90 000	29.3	30
PP_1		α_1	160 000	2.7	3
PP_2	Ferritin	α_2	500 000	—	18
PP_3		α_2	~ 100 000	?	?
PP_4		Albumin	~ 30 000	?	?
PP_5	Protease inhibitor	β_1	36 600	19.8	1.5
PP_6		α_1	1 000 000	6.6	100
PP_7		$\alpha_2 - \beta_1$	40 000	5.4	60
PP_8		α_1	45 000[a] 55 000[b]	4.1	7
PP_{10}		α_1	48 000[a] 65 000[b]	6.6	20

[a]Determined in the ultracentrifuge.
[b]Determined in sodium dodecyl sulphate–polyacrylamide gel.

antigens differ in their electrophoretic mobility, and their molecular weights range from 30 000 to 1 000 000 daltons. Mostly these proteins are glycoproteins: SP_1 contains almost 30% and PP_5 almost 20% of carbohydrate; the carbohydrate content of the other placental glycoproteins is less than 10%.

PP_2 has been identified as ferritin, which is an iron storage protein. PP_5 was found to inhibit plasmin and trypsin; its biological role, therefore, may be the inhibition of proteases. The function of the other placental proteins is still unknown.

The last column in Table I shows the amounts of the soluble placental proteins in the extracts of placental tissue; PP_6 and PP_7 appear to be the most abundant of these proteins in the human term placenta.

To find out whether these placental antigens are specific for the placenta or not, extracts from other human fetal and adult tissues have been investigated for these proteins. The results are shown in Table II. SP_1, PP_5 and PP_{10} were the only placental proteins which could not be detected in extracts from other organs. These antigens, therefore, are presumed to be specific for the placenta. The other proteins occur in other tissues as well; especially PP_7 and PP_8, which were present in relatively high concentrations in almost all tissue extracts thus far examined.

The solubilized protein antigens of the placenta have been obtained by extracting placentae with dissociating solvents, such as acidic buffers, chaotropic salt solutions and detergents, or by digestion with papain (see Table III). The antisera used for their detection have been prepared by immunizing rabbits with the

Table II. Occurrence of the placental protein antigens in extracts of other human tissues.

	SP$_1$	PP$_1$	PP$_2$	PP$_3$	PP$_4$	PP$_5$	PP$_6$	PP$_7$	PP$_8$	PP$_{10}$
Fetal tissues										
Heart	−	−	−	−	−	−	−	++	++	−
Kidney	−	+	−	−	−	−	−	++	++	−
Liver	−	+	−	−	−	−	−	++	(+)	−
Lung	−	+	+	−	−	−	(+)	++	++	−
Stomach	−	+	−	−	−	−	−	++	++	−
Brain	−	−	+	−	−	−	+	++	+	−
Adult tissues										
Heart	−	−	−	--	−	−	+	++	++	−
Lung	−	−	(+)	−	−	−	−	++	++	−
Skin	−	−	−	−	+	−	−	+	−	−
Stomach	−	−	+	(+)	+	−	+	++	++	−
Kidney	−	+	+	−	+	−	(+)	++	+	−
Uterus	−	−	(+)	−	−	−	−	++	++	−
Liver	−	+	+	−	−	−	+	++	++	−
Spleen	−	(+)	+	−	−	−	+	+	+++	−
Adrenal	−	−	−	−	(+)?	−	(+)	++	++	−
Colon	−	−	(+)?	−	−	−	−	++	+	−
Rectum	−	−	(+)?	−	−	−	−	++	−	−
Bladder	−	−	(+)?	−	−	−	−	++	++	−
Erythrocytes	−	−	−	−	−	−	(+)	(+)	−	−

Table III. Detection of solubilized placental tissue proteins.

Solubilization procedure	New solubilized antigens to which antibodies were formed
5% Glycine-HCl, pH 2.5	A,B,E
5% Glycine-HCl, pH 2.5, +2% mercaptoethanol	B,C
3 M KCl	D
2.8 M Kl	E,F
6 M Urea	E,F,G,I
0.5% SDS	F,K,H,I,L
5% Triton X–100	K,L
Papain	K

Abbreviations: KCl, potassium chloride; KI, potassium iodide; SDS, sodium dodecyl sulphate.

solubilized material obtained by these procedures. At least 11 different solubilized antigens, apparently derived from the placental membranes, could be detected (Bohn, 1979b); provisionally these antigens have been designated alphabetically by the letters A–L (Table III). But none of these solubilized placental proteins has been isolated and characterized thus far. The tissue specificity of these antigens also remains to be investigated.

PROTEIN ANTIGENS SPECIFIC TO THE PLACENTA

Of the numerous protein constituents of the placenta, only a few appear to be more or less specific to this reproductive tissue: some of them have the function of hormones like human chorionic gonadotrophin (hCG), human placental lactogen (hPL) and human chorionic thyrotrophin (hCT); others are enzymes like heat-stable alkaline phosphatase (HSAP), cystine aminopeptidase (CAP), 17β-hydroxy-steroid dehydrogenase (17β-BSD) and diamine oxidase (DAO). Among the placental proteins of unknown function, SP$_1$ (Bohn *et al.,* 1976), PP$_5$ (Bohn and Winckler, 1977a), PP$_{10}$ (Bohn and Kraus, 1979) and PAPP-A (Lin *et al.,* 1974), are the best characterized proteins which appear to be specific to the placenta. The physicochemical properties of all placenta-specific proteins thus far isolated and characterized are reported in Table IV.

The molecular weights of the placenta-specific proteins range from 21 000 to

Table IV. Characteristics of the placenta-specific proteins.

Placental proteins	Physicochemical properties		Amount in which they occur in	
	Molecular weight (daltons)	Carbohydrate content (%)	Term placentae (mg/placenta) (mean values)	Pregnancy sera (mg/100 ml) (maximal values)
hCG	47 000	31	< 1	< 1
hPL	21 600	0	150	< 1
hCT	~ 25 000	4.5	< 1	?
Heat-stable alkaline phosphatase	116 000	15	40	< 0.1
Cystine amino- peptidase	290 000	44	?	~ 1
17β-Hydro- steroid dehy- drogenase	68 000	0	4	?
SP$_1$	90 000	29.3	30	33
PP$_5$	36 600	19.8	1.5	< 0.1
PP$_{10}$	48 000	6.6	20	< 0.1
PAPP-A	~ 750 000	?	?	?

750 000 daltons. Most of these antigens are glycoproteins; CAP, hCG, SP_1 and PP_5 show the highest carbohydrate content. Table IV also shows the amounts of these proteins in human term placentae and in sera from pregnant women: hPL appears to be the most abundant placenta-specific protein in the placenta; it is followed by HSAP, SP_1 and PP_{10}.

During pregnancy most of the placenta-specific proteins are secreted into the maternal blood stream; the last column in Table IV shows the maximal values of the concentrations in which the placenta-specific proteins occur in sera from pregnant women. SP_1 reaches the highest level, namely 33 mg/100 ml; the concentrations of the other proteins are usually lower than 1 mg/100 ml or even lower than 0.1 mg/100 ml.

DIAGNOSTIC SIGNIFICANCE OF PLACENTAL PROTEINS

The placenta-specific proteins usually occur only in sera of pregnant women; measurement of these proteins in sera is used to detect pregnancy and to assess fetoplacental well-being. But placenta-specific proteins often appear in sera of patients with malignant diseases also. Their measurement, therefore, can also be useful in detecting tumours and in evaluating the therapy in tumour patients.

This leads us towards the diagnostic significance of the placental proteins in general and of the placenta-specific proteins in particular. But in this chapter I shall deal only with those new placental proteins which have been isolated and characterized in our laboratory and which have already been investigated for their clinical significance.

Pregnancy-specific β_1-Glycoprotein (SP_1, $PS\beta G$)

SP_1 is a placenta-specific protein which is synthesized in the human trophoblast and secreted into the maternal blood stream during pregnancy in steadily increasing amounts. *Post partum,* the protein disappears from the maternal circulation with a half-life of 30–40 h.

SP_1 was first isolated from aqueous extracts of human term placentae with common fractionation procedures (Bohn, 1972b); later it was prepared in highly purified form and in good yield by using an immunoadsorption technique in combination with hydroxyapatite chromatography (Bohn *et al.*, 1976).

The purified antigen was used for the preparation of specific antisera and for the development of sensitive assays to determine its concentration in sera and other body fluids and to evaluate the significance of measurement of this protein in pregnancy and tumour diagnostics.

SP_1 can be detected in the peripheral blood very soon (18–23 days) after conception; it appears little later than the β-subunit of hCG. Measurement of SP_1 therefore may become of value in the early diagnosis of pregnancy (Grudzinskas *et al.*, 1977).

Circulating concentrations of SP_1 rise steadily during gestation and tend to reach a plateau near term. The shape of the SP_1 curve during pregnancy closely resembles that of hPL; both seem to reflect the basic changes in placental function.

Levels of SP_1, like those of hPL, correlate well with the stage of gestation; measurement of SP_1 therefore may be of value as an index of fetal well-being in late pregnancy (Tatra *et al.*, 1974; Gordon *et al.*, 1977, Towler *et al.*, 1977) and appears to be useful in the early detection of fetal growth retardation, too. In this condition, measurement of SP_1 seems to have a better predictive value than hPL (Towler *et al.*, 1977; Chapman and Jones, 1978; Würz *et al.*, 1978).

SP_1 was found to occur not only in sera from pregnant women but also in sera from patients with diseases of the trophoblast: Tatarinov and Sokolov (1977) could detect SP_1 in almost 80% of cases with trophoblastic tumours. Seppälä *et al.* (1978), Searle *et al.* (1978) and Than *et al.* (1979) performed serial determinations of SP_1 simultaneously with measurement of hCG in such patients; they found that SP_1 is a useful parameter in monitoring trophoblastic diseases and can serve as an additional marker for the detection of residual tumour growth in patients with choriocarcinoma.

SP_1 can be produced by non-trophoblastic malignant tumours, too; it was demonstrated in the tissue of a variety of non-trophoblastic tumours, including breast cancer, adenocarcinoma of the gastrointestinal tract and bronchial carcinoma (Horne *et al.* 1979). The incidence was highest in breast carcinoma: Horne *et al.* (1976) identified SP_1, hPL and hCG in the tumour cells of 50 breast cancer patients. Of the proteins studied, SP_1 was present in 76% of cases, hPL in 82%, and hCG in 60%. Those women with cancers negative for SP_1 and hPL had significantly longer survival times compared with those whose cancers stained for these proteins; and SP_1 was the best indicator of prognosis.

SP_1 has also been detected in the sera of patients with a variety of malignant nontrophoblastic tumours, albeit in very low concentrations (3–20 μg/ml) (Tatarinov and Sokolov, 1977; Searle *et al.*, 1978; Würz, 1979). Follow-up studies of SP_1 in sera of patients with non-trophoblastic tumours were first performed by Würz (1979). She found that SP_1 levels that were elevated before surgery fell to the normal range within a few days after tumour removal and indicated that serial determinations of this protein could be of value in monitoring patients with non-trophoblastic tumours as well.

Placenta-specific Protein (PP₅)

PP_5, like SP_1, appears to be a protein specific to the placenta. In contrast to SP_1 it occurs mainly in the tissue; in the maternal circulation it is found only in trace amounts. The isolation and characterization of PP_5 have been described recently (Bohn and Winckler, 1977a). From one human term placenta an average amount of 1.5 mg PP_5 can be extracted. The protein is mainly localized in the syncytiotrophoblast. PP_5 was found to inhibit the proteolytic activity of plasmin and trypsin; therefore its biological function could well be to inhibit proteases.

The concentration of PP_5 in sera was studied by Obiekwe *et al.* (1979) and Seppälä *et al.* (1979) using sensitive radioimmunoassays. PP_5 is not present in normal sera; in pregnancy the protein becomes detectable in maternal serum 8 weeks after the last menstrual period. The levels increase with advancing gestation. The highest levels (mean 26–29 ng/ml) were seen in weeks 37–39 of pregnancy.

Seppälä *et al.* (1979) also investigated PP_5 levels in sera from patients with trophoblastic tumours and used immunohistochemical methods to study the occurrence and localization of PP₅ in the normal placenta as well as in hydatidiform mole, invasive mole, and choriocarcinoma. In testing the sera, only two out of 19 samples from patients with hydatidiform mole had demonstrable PP₅. All seven samples from patients with invasive mole were PP₅ negative and none of the 70 serum specimens from five patients with choriocarcinoma showed any detectable PP₅. In localizing PP₅ in the tissue, all 10 hydatidiform moles were stained with the peroxidase technique. In one out of 10 invasive moles a positive stain for PP₅ was seen; all six cases of true choriocarcinoma were constantly PP₅ negative when several tissue samples of the tumour were repeatedly examined.

These results demonstrate that PP₅ is expressed in the normal but not in the malignant syncytiotrophoblast; the absence of PP₅ in sera of patients with trophoblastic disease may have an implication for clinical practice as regards the differential diagnosis between normal pregnancy and invasive trophoblastic disease: in normal pregnancy PP₅, hCG and SP₁ are present, whereas in trophoblastic disease hCG and SP₁ levels are high but PP₅ is hardly detectable. In the light of the function of PP₅ as protease inhibitor the absence of PP₅ appears to be related to the invasive character of trophoblastic disease (Seppälä et al., 1979).

The Ubiquitous Tissue Proteins PP₇ and PP₈

PP₇ and PP₈ are ubiquitous tissue proteins; they were found to be present in relatively large amounts in almost all human tissues so far examined. From one human term placenta an average amount of 60 mg PP₇ and 7 mg PP₈ can be extracted. Isolation and characterization of these proteins have been reported recently (Bohn and Winckler, 1977b; Bohn, 1979b).

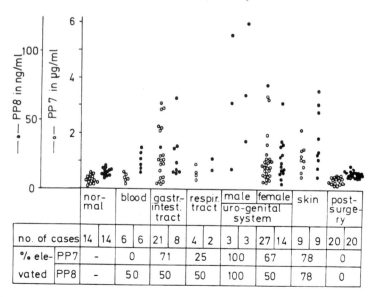

Fig. 1.   PP₇ and PP₈ in the serum of normal individuals and tumour patients.

A sensitive radioimmunoassay has been established to determine the concentration of PP_7 and PP_8 in sera of normal subjects as well as of patients suffering from a variety of different diseases in order to evaluate the diagnostic significance of measurement of the proteins (Lüben *et al.,* 1979). The normal circulating levels were found to be 100–500 ng/ml for PP_7 and 10–15 ng/ml for PP_8. In the sera of patients suffering from various kinds of tumours related to blood, stomach, intestine, respiratory tract, urogenital system and skin, the proteins PP_7 and PP_8 were shown to be mostly elevated above normal (Fig. 1). A number of post-cancer treatment sera taken from patients who had undergone tumour surgery have also been investigated; they almost invariably showed normal contents of PP_7 and PP_8. These findings indicate that these proteins may be of value as tumour markers and that their determination may be useful in cancer diagnosis and for monitoring tumour patients.

IMMUNIZATION AGAINST PLACENTAL ANTIGENS

Immunization against placental antigens is of special interest with regard to sterility and fertility regulation. It was shown that antibodies to placental antigens may arise spontaneously in women during pregnancy (Kaku, 1953; Hulka *et al.,* 1963). But at present there is no clear evidence of an association between gestosis or spontaneous abortion and antiplacental antibodies in women (Boss and Nelken, 1970; Edwards and Coombs, 1975).

In animals a number of experiments have been done to investigate the effects of immunization against placental antigens on fertility or pregnancy; these studies have been performed on a variety of animal species using both passive and active immunization with heterologous as well as homologous or isologous placental tissue as antigens. These investigations have shown that antibodies to placental antigens can induce abortion and reduce fertility in animals (Seegel and Loeb, 1940; Koren *et al.,* 1968; Behrman and Amano, 1972). Studies in this field have been extended during the last few years using purified placenta-specific proteins as antigens with the aim of finding new approaches to the regulation of fertility in humans (Harper, 1976).

In our laboratory we have investigated the antifertility effect of an immunization of female Cynomolgus monkeys with the human placenta-specific proteins SP_1, PP_5 and heat-stable alkaline phosphatase (Bohn, 1976; Bohn and Weinmann, 1974, 1976, and unpublished data). Some of the results obtained by the active immunization of female Cynomolgus monkeys are summarized in Table V. The placental proteins chemically modified with diazotized sulphanilic acid (DSA) served as antigens. Following immunization, the effect on reproduction in these animals was investigated. The ratio of matings to pregnancies resulting in normal birth was used as an indicator of the antifertility effect. The monkeys immunized with SP_1 and PP_5 showed a significant reduction in fertility, whereas immunization with heat-stable alkaline phosphatase (AP) appeared to be less effective.

The antifertility effect of immunization of monkeys with the placental hormones hPL and hCG was investigated by Stevens (1976). Of all the placenta-specific proteins so far tested, hCG appears at the moment the most promising antigen with regard to interference with fertility. The main problem arising with

Table V. Antifertility effect of active immunizations of Cynomolgus monkeys with placenta-specific proteins.

Antigens used for immunization	No. of animals	No. of matings	Abortions observed	Pregnancies resulting in normal birth	Matings per pregnancy
SP$_1$–DSA	6	22	5	5	4.4
PP$_5$–DSA	6	22	1	6	3.7
AP–DSA	6	13	–	5	2.6
Adjuvant alone (controls)	5	9	–	5	1.8

Abbreviations: DSA, diazotized sulphanilic acid; AP, heat-stable placental alkaline phosphatase.

the use of this placental hormone is its cross-reactivity with hormones of the pituitary gland. To overcome this difficulty, fragments of the peptide chain unique to the placental hormone have been prepared and used as antigens. Whether immunization against these peptides or other proteins specific to the placenta can lead to a new contraceptive method in humans awaits further investigation. Many problems are still to be surmounted before an immunological method of human fertility control can be considered as an alternative to those which are already available.

REFERENCES

Behrman, S. J. and Amano, Y. (1972). *Contraception* **5**, 357.

Bohn, H. (1971). *Archiv für Gynäkologie* **210**, 440.

Bohn, H. (1972a). *Archiv für Gynäkologie* **212**, 165.

Bohn, H. (1972b). *Blut* **24**, 292.

Bohn, H. (1976). *In* "Development of Vaccines for Fertility Regulation" (World Health Organization, ed.), pp. 111–126, Scriptor, Copenhagen.

Bohn, H. (1979a). *In* "Carcino-Embryonic Proteins" (F. G. Lehmann, ed.), Vol. 1, p. 289. Elsevier/North-Holland Biomedical Press, Amsterdam.

Bohn, H. (1979b). *In* "Protides of Biological Fluids" (H. H. Peeters, ed.) 27th Colloquium, pp. 879–882, Pergamon Press, Oxford.

Bohn, H. and Kraus, W. (1979). *Archiv für Gynäkologie* **227**, 125.

Bohn, H. and Schwick, H. G. (1971). *Arzneimittel-Forschung* **21**, 1432.

Bohn, H. and Weinmann, E. (1974). *Archiv für Gynäkologie* **216**, 347.

Bohn, H. and Weinmann, E. (1976). *Archive für Gynäkologie* **221**, 305.

Bohn, H. and Winckler, W. (1977a). *Archiv für Gynäkologie* **223**, 179.

Bohn, H. and Winckler, W. (1977b). *Archiv für Gynäkologie* **222**, 5.

Bohn, H., Schmidtberger, R. and Zilg, H. (1976). *Blut* **32**, 103.

Boss, J. H. and Nelken, D. (1970). *Fertility and Sterility* **21**, 508.

Chapman, M. G. and Jones, W. R. (1978). *Australian and New Zealand Journal of Obstetrics and Gynaecology* **18**, 172.

Edwards, R. G. and Coombs, R. R. A. (1975). *In* "Clinical Aspects of Immunology" (R. R. A. Coombs, P. G. H. Gell and P. J. Lachman, eds), pp. 561–598. Blackwell Scientific Publications, Oxford.

Gaugas, J. M., Wright, C. and Curzen, P. (1974). *British Journal of Experimental Pathology* **55**, 478.

Geiger, B. R., Navon, J., Ben-Yoseph and Arnon, R. (1975). *European Journal of Biochemistry* **56**, 311.

Gordon, Y. B., Grudzinskas, J. G., Jeffrey, D. and Chard, T. (1977). *Lancet i*, 331.

Grudzinskas, J. G., Gordon, Y. B., Jeffrey, D. and Chard, T. (1977). *Lancet i*, 333.

Harper, M. J. K. (1976). *In* "Development of Vaccines for Fertility Regulation" (World Health Organization, ed.), pp. 11–16, Scriptor, Copenhagen.

Hofmann, R., Brock, J. and Friemel, H. (1970). *Archiv für Gynäkologie* **208**, 266.

Horne, C. H. W., Towler, C. M., Pugh-Humphreys, R. G. P., Thomson, A. W. and Bohn, H. (1976). *Experientia* **32**, 1197.

Horne, C. H. W., Pugh-Humphreys, R. G. P. and Bremner, R. D. (1979). *In* "Carcino-Embryonic Proteins" (F. G. Lehmann, ed.), Vol. I, p. 301, Elsevier/North-Holland Biomedical Press, Amsterdam.

Hulka, J. F., Brinton, V., Schaaf, J. and Baney, C. (1963). *Nature, London* **198**, 501.

Kaku, M. (1953). *Journal of Obstetrics and Gynaecology of the British Empire* **60**, 148.

Koren, Z., Abrahams, G. and Behrman, S. J. (1968). *American Journal of Obstetrics and Gynecology* **102**, 340.

Krieg, H. (1969). *Medizinische Klinik* **64**, 1223.

Kyank, H. (1958). *Gynaecologia* **145**, 145.

Lin, T. M., Halbert, S. P., Kiefer, D., Spellacy, W. N. and Gall, S. (1974). *American Journal of Obstetrics and Gynecology* **118**, 223.

Lüben, G., Schütze, D. and Bohn, H. (1979). *In* "Protides of Biological Fluids" (H. H. Peeters, ed.) 27th Colloquium, pp. 253–255. Pergamon Press, Oxford.

Obiekwe, B. C., Pendlebury, D. J., Gordon, Y. B., Grudzinskas, J. G., Chard, T. and Bohn, H. (1979). *Clinica chimica acta* **95**, 509.

Olivelli, F. and Ruggieri, P. (1958). *Minerva ginecologica* **10**, 953.

Penneys, N. S. and Muench, K. H. (1974). *Biochemistry* **13**, 560.

Petrunin, D. D., Gryaznova, I. M., Petrunina, Yu. A. and Tatarinov, Yu. S. (1978). *Bulletin of Experimental Biology and Medicine of the U.S.S.R.* **35**, 600.

Schultze-Mosgau, H. and Fischer, K. (1971). *Archiv für Gynäkologie* **210**, 458.

Schwartz, E. S., Gang, N. F. and Gelfand, M. M. (1974). *American Journal of Obstetrics and Gynecology* **118**, 857.

Searle, F., Leake, B. A., Bagshawe, K. D. and Dent, J. (1978). *Lancet i*, 579.

Seegel, B. C. and Loeb, E. N. (1940). *Proceedings of the Society for Experimental Biology* **45**, 248.

Seppälä, M., Rutanen, E. M., Heikinheimo, M., Jalanko, H. and Engvall, E. (1978). *International Journal of Cancer* **21**, 265.

Seppälä, M., Wahlström, T. and Bohn, H. (1979). *International Journal of Cancer* **24**, 6.

Stevens, V. C., (1976). *In* "Development of Vaccines for Fertility Regulation" (World Health Organization, ed.), pp. 93–110, Scriptor, Copenhagen.

Tatarinov, Y. S. and Masyukevich, V. N. (1970). *Bulletin of Experimental Biology and Medicine of the U.S.S.R.* **69**, 66.

Tatarinov, Yu. S. and Sokolov, A. V. (1977). *International Journal of Cancer* **19**, 161.

Tatra, G., Breitenecker, G. and Gruber, W. (1974). *Archiv für Gynäkologie* **217**, 383.

Than, G. N., Bohn, H., Csaba, I. F., Karg, N. J. and Mann, V. (1979). *In* "Carcino-Embryonic Proteins". (F. G. Lehmann, ed.), Vol. II, p. 481, Elsevier/North-Holland Biomedical Press, Amsterdam.

Towler, C. M., Horne, C. H. W., Jandial, V., Campbell, D. M. and MacGillivray, I. (1977). *British Journal of Obstetrics and Gynaecology* **84**, 258.

Würz, H. (1979). *Archiv für Gynäkologie* **227**, 1.

Würz, H., Geiger, W., Künzig, H. J., Jabs-Lehmann, A. and Hoffmann, M. (1978). *Proceedings of the Xth International Congress of Clinical Chemistry, Mexico.*

TWO NEW HUMAN PLACENTA-SPECIFIC α-GLOBULINS: IDENTIFICATION, PURIFICATION, CHARACTERISTICS, CELLULAR LOCALIZATION AND CLINICAL INVESTIGATION

Y. S. Tatarinov, G. A. Kozljaeva, D. D. Petrunin and Y. A. Petrunina

Department of Biochemistry, Immunochemical Laboratory of the Second Moscow Medical Institute, Moscow, U.S.S.R.

INTRODUCTION

At the present time it is customary to distinguish at least three groups of placenta-specific antigens. The first group is represented by proteins with hormonal activity such as chorionic gonadotrophin, placental lactogen, chorionic thyrotrophin, uterotrophin and others (Saxena, 1971). The second group is represented by placental proteins with enzymatic activity. Among these proteins there is alkaline phosphatase, oxytocinase, steroid dehydrogenase and transglutaminase, which are the more carefully studied proteins (Bohn, 1975). The third group of placenta-specific antigens consists of quite a number of proteins, but the origin and functions of these are not yet determined. The secretion of some of these proteins occurs mainly into the maternal circulation, and presumably they perform some as yet unknown regulatory functions in pregnancy. The trophoblast-specific β_1-globulin (Tatarinov and Masuykevich, 1970), also called pregnancy-specific β_1-glycoprotein (Bohn, 1971), is the most carefully studied protein at the present time. The secretion of other proteins of this group takes place into amniotic fluid, where they apparently play a certain role in the process of fetation. These proteins are immunochemically identified, partially purified

Serono Symposium No. 35, "The Human Placenta", edited by A. Klopper, A. Genazzani and P. G. Crosignani, 1980. Academic Press, London and New York.

and are currently being subjected to comparative analysis (Bohn, 1972; 1975; Petrunin *et al.*, 1977; Sutcliffe *et al.*, 1978; Kalashnikov *et al.*, 1979).

In this report we shall review the latest results obtained in our laboratory on the study of the physicochemical properties, cellular localization and dynamics of two placenta-specific α-globulins in amniotic fluid.

MATERIALS AND METHODS

Immunochemical Identification

Immunodiffusional analysis in agar by Ouchterlony's method (Ouchterlony, 1948) was carried out with some modifications (Khramkove and Abelev, 1961). The immunoelectrophoresis technique of Grabar and Williams (1953) was also used in our work.

Placental Antigens

Placenta-specific α_1-microglobulin (PAMG-1) was isolated from amniotic fluid by combined salt precipitation with subsequent absorption chromatography. The final fraction of PAMG-1 contained about 90% of pure protein and was used as an antigen for the preparation of monospecific antisera. The placenta-specific α_2-microglobulin (PAMG-2) was partially purified from the chorionic tissue of early placentae by absorption chromatography followed by a final salt precipitation. This yielded a PAMG-2 preparation which contained about 45% of the pure protein and was used as an antigen for the preparation of antisera.

Antisera

Rabbits were immunized with partially purified preparations plus Freund's complete adjuvant injected over 4–5 weeks. In 1–3 months the rabbits were reimmunized with a single dose of PAMG-1 or PAMG-2 and on days 7–9 antisera were obtained. Antisera were absorbed with lyophilized, pooled, donors' plasma and extracts of various organs. Extracts for absorption were made from liver, kidneys, lungs, brain and muscular tissue. After absorption the antisera became monospecific, i.e. they reacted only with antigens which we identified.

Immunoelectrophoresis

Agarose electrophoresis was performed by the method of Grabar and Williams (1953). Tissue extracts and biological fluids were used in a native state, either immediately or after storage at 2 °C with addition of NaN_3. Monospecific antisera to PAMG-1 and PAMG-2, serum albumin (anti-hSA) and polyvalent antisera to donors' blood sera (anti-BSP) were used for immuno-identification. Anti-hSA and anti-BSP were used in order to control semipurified preparations of placental proteins and for the determination of electrophoretic mobility (Fig. 1). Pyronine and the dye T-1824 were also used as control reagents.

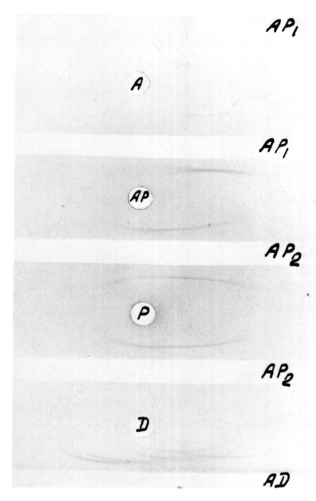

Fig. 1. Electrophoretic mobility of placenta-specific α-globulins. A, amniotic fluid (20 weeks), AP, mixture of amniotic fluid (20 weeks) and extract of immature placenta; P, extract of immature placenta, AP_1, anti-PAMG-1, AP_2, anti-PAMG-2, AD, anti-hSA.

Immunodiffusion

The double immunodiffusion in gel was done by the method of Ouchterlony (1948) with the modifications of Khramkova and Abelev (1961). Monospecific antisera to PAMG-1 and PAMG-2 and standards of the purified antigens were used. The sensitivity of the method was within 1–3 µg/ml of standard. The line of precipitation of the standard test system was changed (Fig. 2). Extracts of placentae and of various organs from healthy subjects, or homogenates of various tumours, were used as antigens.

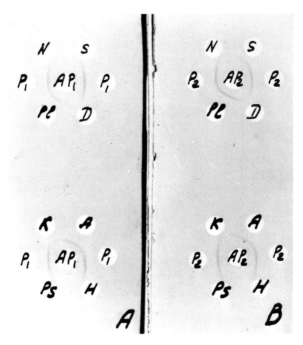

Fig. 2. Immunodiffusion reactions of antisera to PAMG-1 and PAMG-2 with biological fluids and extracts of organs.

(a) Immunodiffusion with standard PAMG-1. P_1, standard antigen PAMG-1; AP_1, anti-PAMG-1; A,Pl, positive reaction.

(b) Immunodiffusion with antisera to PAMG-2. P_2, standard antigen PAMG-2; AP_2, anti-PAMG-2; S,Pl,A, positive reaction.

Other abbreviations: S, sperm; D, pooled donors' serum; Pl, extract of immature placenta; N, newborn's serum; A, amniotic fluid; H, extracts of liver; Ps, pooled serum of pregnant women; K, extract of kidneys.

Homogenates

The tissue, together with Tris–glycine buffer (pH 8.3) and detergents (Triton X-100 and Tween-80), was homogenized with glass powder. The homogenate was frozen and thawed three times and then centrifuged at 8000 **g**. The supernatant was lyophilized. Extracts containing about 5 g% of the protein were used in immunodiffusion analysis.

Identification

Monospecific antisera to known proteins were used for comparison in immunodiffusion experiments. We used antisera to chorionic gonadotrophin, placental lactogen, ferritin, alkaline phosphatase, pregnancy-associated proteins SP_2 and SP_3 (Bohn, 1971), PAPP-A and PAPP-B (Lin *et al.*, 1974), trophoblast-specific β_1-globulin (Tatarinov and Masyukevich, 1970), EPA-2, $E\alpha_2 G$ and $A\alpha_1 G$ (Kalashnikov *et al.*, 1979).

Physicochemical Properties

The molecular weight was determined by thin layer chromatography (Petrunin *et al.*, 1978) on Sephadex G-100 and G-200. Electrophoretic mobility was detected by the method of Uriel (1963). The relations of PAMG-1 and PAMG-2 to trypsin, deoxyribonuclease, ribonuclease and neuraminidase were determined. The precipitation reactions were studied using ammonium sulphate, rivanol, perchloric acid and trichloroacetic acid.

Immunofluorescence

The samples of placental tissue (3–5 mm) were fixed in a cold mixture of 100% ethanol with acetic acid (99/1, v/v) by Hamashima's method (Hamashima *et al.*, 1964). Paraffin sections were made by Sante-Marie's method (Saint-Marie, 1962). The antibodies purified on glutaraldehyde by Avramaes and Ternynck's method (Avramaes and Ternynck, 1969) were obtained from the following rabbit antisera: (1) antiserum against PAMG-1 (anti-PAMG-1); (2) antiserum against PAMG-2 (anti-PAMG-2); (3) antiserum against human serum albumin (anti-hSA). The serum albumin was taken as a control protein to determine the non-specific absorption since the placenta does not produce albumin.

Table I. Comparative physical and chemical characteristics of placenta-specific α-microglobulins.

Properties	PAMG-1	PAMG-2
Molecular weight (daltons)	20 000 ± 2000	25 000 ± 2000
Relative electrophoretic mobility	0.85 ± 0.01	0.65 ± 0.01
Stain for glycoproteins	Not stained	Not stained
Changes of electrophoretic mobility by treatment with neuraminidaze	Not changed	Not changed
Stability to trypsin treatment	Destroyed	Destroyed
Stability to deoxyribonuclease treatment	Not destroyed	Not destroyed
Stability to ribonuclease treatment	Not destroyed	Not destroyed
Precipitation by ammonium sulphate, (% of saturation)	30–50%	25–60%
Precipitation by rivanol (%)	0.4%	0.4% (90%)
Precipitation by perchloric acid	0.6 M (85%)	0.3 M
Precipitation by trichloroacetic acid	2%	2%
Temperature stability	Full loss of antigenic activity at 85 °C	Retains antigenic activity at 100 °C

RESULTS

Comparative immunoelectrophoretic analysis of PAMG-1 and PAMG-2 is shown in Fig. 1. PAMG-1 is localized in the α_1-globulin zone, PAMG-2 in the α_2-globulin zone. As seen in Table I, the physicochemical properties of these proteins have many close similarities, although immunochemically they are different. They differ from known placental proteins and certain pregnancy-associated proteins which are found in pregnancy serum or amniotic fluid, i.e. chorionic gonadotrophin, placental lactogen, ferritin, alkaline phosphatase,

Table II. Isolation of placenta-specific α_1-microglobulin.

Stages of purification	Residual PAMG-1 (%)	Purity (%)
Amniotic fluid of 16–25 weeks	100	4
Precipitation by lanthanum perchlorate	90	25
Precipitation by semisaturated ammonium sulphate	70	35
Precipitation by lithium sulphate of 60% saturation	60	50
Absorption chromatography with calcium pyrophosphate	30	90

Table III. Isolation of placenta-specific α_2-microglobulin.

Stages of purification	Residual PAMG-2 (%)	Purity (%)
Extracts of early chorion	100	2
Absorption chromatography with silica gel	60	15
Absorption chromatography with hydroxyapatite	40	35
Precipitation with ammonium sulphate (55% saturation)	30	45

pregnancy-associated proteins SP_2 and SP_3, PAPP-A and PAPP-B, trophoblast-specific β_1-globulin, EPA-2, $E\alpha_2 G$ and $A\alpha_1 G$.

Tables II and III show steps in the isolation and purification of PAMG-1 and PAMG-2. PAMG-1 shows a relatively high degree of purification with simple procedures, but PAMG-2 requires more sophisticated measures for its isolation.

Table IV. Content of placenta-specific α-microglobulins in organs and biological fluids.

Investigated material	No. of tests	No. of positive tests	
		PAMG-1	PAMG-2
Placenta	25	25	25
Liver	20	0	0
Kidney	19	0	0
Spleen	16	0	0
Lung	14	0	0
Brain	11	0	0
Heart	12	0	0
Adrenal gland	14	0	0
Mucous membrane of gastro-intestinal tract	21	0	0
Bone	4	0	0
Cartilage	2	0	0
Muscle	2	0	0
Ovary	6	0	0
Testes	7	0	0
Endocrine glands	18	0	0
Myometrium	6	0	0
Endometrium	22	0	8
Blood serum	84	0	0
Biological fluids	13	0	0
Sperm	8	0	8
Menstrual blood	6	0	6
Total	330	25	47

Table V. Content of placenta-specific α-microglobulins in tumours.

Kind of tumour	No. tests	No. positive tests	
		PAMG-1	PAMG-2
Uterine chorionepithelioma	25	0	6
Other uterine tumours	26	0	3
Carcinoma of ovary	54	0	2
Carcinoma of liver	7	0	0
Carcinoma of kidney	28	0	0
Carcinoma of gastrointestinal tract	21	0	0
Carcinoma of lung	13	0	0
Carcinoma of mammary gland	16	0	0
Teratocarcinoma testis	8	0	0
Tumours of nervous tissue	24	0	0
Carcinoma of bone and soft tissues	8	0	0
Others	18	0	0
Total	248	0	11

Table VI.   Changes in placenta-specific α-microglobulin content
in amniotic fluid and in the placenta during gestation.

Investigated material	Content of PAMG-1 (μg/ml)	Content of PAMG-2 (μg/ml)
Amniotic fluid		
1st trimester	178.2 ± 18.4	18.7 ± 2.3
2nd trimester	166.4 ± 15.8	9.8 ± 1.7
3rd trimester	4.3 ± 0.3	–
Placenta extracts		
1st trimester	5.1 ± 0.5	407.6 ± 26.2
2nd trimester	4.2 ± 0.4	16.8 ± 2.1
3rd trimester	3.0 ± 0.4	5.6 ± 0.3

These preparations were nevertheless adequate for the immunization of rabbits
and yielded monospecific antisera to both PAMG-1 and PAMG-2.

As shown in Table IV, both proteins are present only in placental homogenates,
and immunodiffusion proved to be unable to reveal them in homogenates of other
organs. In addition, PAMG-2 was found in sperm, in extracts of endometrium (all
curettages made in the last 5 days before menstruation) and in menstrual blood.
PAMG-2 was also found in trophoblastic tumours, but neither of these proteins
were found in other malignant tumours (Table V). High concentrations, especially
of PAMG-1, were found in amniotic fluid during the first and second trimesters.
The concentration of both proteins in amniotic fluid during the third trimester
comes down to 1–3 μg/ml, while the maximum PAMG-1 concentration is 178.2
μg/ml (Table VI). The placental proteins which we described did not appear in
the serum of pregnant women, with the exception of some subjects with pre-
eclamptic toxaemia, when small quantities of PAMG-1 could be recorded by
immunodiffusion. Specific immunofluorescence due to PAMG-1 and PAMG-2
was found in the cytotrophoblastic and syncytiotrophoblastic cells of immature
chorion of 8–12 weeks (Fig. 3). The control sections, including those processed
with anti-hSA, did not show fluorescence. None of the non-trophoblastic tumour
samples showed specific fluorescence. Some of the chorionepithelioma sections had
specific fluorescence to PAMG-2 (Fig. 4).

DISCUSSION

Two placenta-specific α-microglobulins were immunochemically identified in
our laboratory (Petrunin *et al.*, 1976, 1977). These placental proteins are mainly
secreted into the amniotic fluid of pregnant women. One of these proteins—placenta-
specific α_1-microglobulin (PAMG-1), with a molecular weight of about 20 000
daltons—accumulates in amniotic fluid during the first and the second trimesters,
but is not found in the blood serum of normal pregnant women. In some cases of

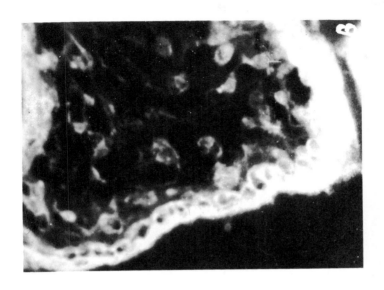

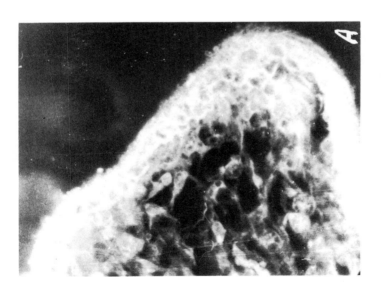

Fig. 3. Localization of PAMG-1 and PAMG-2 in immature placenta, × 80. Incubation with anti-PAMG-1 (A) or anti-PAMG-2 (B) and anti-rabbit γ-globulin labelled with fluorescein isothiocyanate (anti-RGGF).

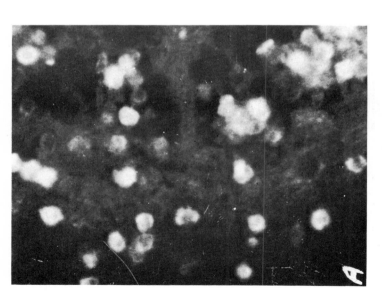

Fig. 4. Localization of PAMG-2 in chorionepithelioma of uterus, × 80. Incubation with anti-PAMG-2 and anti-RGGF; specific fluorescence in trophoblastic cells (A). Incubation with anti-hSA and anti-RGGF (B).

pregnancy toxaemia, PAMG-1 is increased in the blood serum and it becomes detectable by immunodiffusion. In tissues of adults, in fetal tissues and in tumour tissues, PAMG-1 was not found. It is apparent that this microglobulin has high specificity for chorion since it becomes possible to find specific immunofluorescence in cyto- and syncytiotrophoblast.

Another placental protein with a molecular weight of about 25 000 daltons and an electrophoretic mobility of α_2-globulin was named placenta-specific α_2-microglobulin or PAMG-2. This protein was not found in the majority of adult and fetal tissues, with the exception of endometrium, particularly during the premenstrual period. About 5 days before menstruation PAMG-2 is present in the endometrial extract and in samples of menstrual blood. We also found small amounts of this microglobulin in the sperm of men. PAMG-2 was found in the tumour tissue of uterine chorionepithelioma and in ovarian carcinoma. The relation of PAMG-2 to chorionepithelioma can be explained by its placental origin. As far as the presence of PAMG-2 in ovarian tumours is concerned, it can possibly be attributed to its ectopic synthesis.

Until now we have been unable to relate the placenta-specific antigens with hormonal or enzymatic activity, although the small molecular dimensions of both proteins are possibly an indication of their hormonal nature. Nothing is known about their biological or physiological importance in pregnancy. They are known to be actively accumulating during the first and second trimesters and then their concentration in amniotic fluid decreases towards term. The fact that these proteins are present in chorionic trophoblast may show either the site of their synthesis or the site of their active absorption and metabolism. Further study is necessary to reveal their role in the normal function of the placenta.

REFERENCES

Avramaes, S. and Ternynck, T. (1969). *Immunochemistry* 6, 53–57.
Bohn, H. (1971). *Archiv für Gynäkologie* 210, 440–457.
Bohn, H. (1972). *Blut* 24, 292–302.
Bohn, H. (1975). *Klinische Wochenschrift* 53 , 547–554.
Grabar, P. and Williams, C. A. (1953). *Biochimica et biophysica acta* 10, 193–194.
Hamashima, J., Harter, J. C. and Coohs, A. H. (1964). *Journal of Cell Biology* 20, 271–279.
Kalashnicov, V. V., Vasiliev, M. Yu., Voloschuk, S. G., Falaleeva, D. M. Rikunov, E. I. and Tatarinov, Yu. S. (1979). In press.
Khramkova, N. I. and Abelev, G. I. (1961). *Bulletin of Experimental Biology and Medicine of the U.S.S.R.* 52, 107–111.
Lin, T. M., Halbert, S. P., Kiefer, D. and Spellacy, W. N. (1974). *International Archives of Allergy and Applied Immunology* 47, 35–53.
Ouchterlony, O. (1948). *Acta pathologica et microbiologica scandinavica* 25, 186.
Petrunin, D. D., Gryaznova, I. M., Petrunina, Yu. A., Tatarinov, Yu. S. (1976). *Bulletin of Experimental Biology and Medicine of the U.S.S.R.* 7, 803–804.
Petrunin, D. D., Gryaznova, I. M., Petrunina, Yu. A., Tatarinov, Yu. S. (1977). *Akusherstvo i Gynekologija U.S.S.R.* 1, 64–65.
Petrunin, D. D., Gryaznova, I. M., Petrunina, Yu. A. and Tatarinov, Yu. (1978). *Bulletin of Experimental Biology and Medicine of the U.S.S.R.* 5, 600–602.

Sainte-Marie, G., (1962). *Journal of Histochemistry and Cytochemistry* **10**, 250-256.

Saxena, B., (1971). *Vitamins and hormones* **29**, 96-151.

Sutcliffe, R. G., Brock, D. J., Nicholson, L. V., Dunn, E. (1978). *Journal of Reproduction and Fertility* **54**, 85-90.

Tatarinov, Yu. S. and Masyukevich, V. N. (1970). *Bulletin of Experimental Biology and Medicine of the U.S.S.R.* **69**, 66-68.

Uriel, C. (1960). *In* "Analyse immuno-electrophoretique" (P. Grabar and P. Burtin, eds), Masson, Paris.

OBSERVATIONS ON THE ISOLATION OF MACROMOLECULES
OF PLACENTAL ORIGIN

P. Bischof*

*Department of Obstetrics and Gynaecology, University of Aberdeen,
Aberdeen, Scotland*

INTRODUCTION

The trophoblast produces and secretes into the maternal circulation a number of proteins other than the well-known hormones (like human chorionic gonadotrophin or human placental lactogen) or enzymes (like heat-stable alkaline phosphatase or oxytocinase).

At least four, of a growing list of newly described placental proteins, are considered as pregnancy specific. These, pregnancy-associated plasma proteins A and B (PAPP-A and PAPP-B) (Lin *et al.*, 1974), *Schwangerschafts* protein 1 (SP_1) (Tatarinov and Masyukevich, 1970; Bohn, 1972) and placental protein 5 (PP_5) (Bohn and Winckler, 1977) have been detected in the sera of pregnant women but are not measurable or are present only in minute amounts in the sera of non-pregnant women.

All four proteins are produced in increasing concentrations in the maternal blood as pregnancy progresses, but only small amounts make their way into the fetal circulation. PP_5, however, is essentially a placenta-specific protein (Bohn and Winckler, 1977), which means that it is essentially localized in placental tissue.

---

*Present address: Department of Obstetrics and Gynaecology, University of Geneva, Geneva, Switzerland.

Serono Symposium No. 35, "The Human Placenta", edited by A. Klopper,
A. Genazzani and P. G. Crosignani, 1980. Academic Press, London and New York.

Although the biological functions of these proteins are still unknown, the fact that they are secreted almost entirely into the maternal blood led us to examine the possibility of using them as parameters for assessing the functional state of the fetoplacental unit. For this purpose, we undertook the purification of PAPP-A, PAPP-B and SP$_1$ and devised methods to measure them (Bischof *et al.* 1979; Bruce and Klopper, 1978).

The purpose of this communication is to describe the purification and biochemical characteristics of PAPP-A, together with some preliminary results about the possible biological role of this protein.

THE PURIFICATION OF PAPP-A

The purification procedure adopted will only be described briefly; the reader is referred elsewhere for further details (Bischof, 1979*a,b*).

After precipitating some of the proteins in a pool of late pregnancy plasma with ammonium sulphate (final concentration 60% saturation), the redissolved precipitate was applied to a DEAE Sephadex A-50 column. This ion exchange step separates proteins according to their electric charge. Under our conditions, PAPP-A was tightly bound to the column and could be eluted with 0.4–0.5 M NaCl well after the bulk of contaminating proteins. After this step the resulting preparation contained only 5% of the initial concentration of protein, but 70% of the starting amount of PAPP-A (Table I).

Since PAPP-A has been described as a glycoprotein (Lin *et al.*, 1974), it was hoped that PAPP-A would bind to concanavalin-A (Con-A), a protein which has the interesting property of binding certain carbohydrates. A Con-A–Sepharose column was prepared and the PAPP-A containing preparation applied to it. PAPP-A did bind to the column and could be eluted with a gradient of methyl-α-D-mannopyranoside.

The eluate containing PAPP-A was then submitted to a gel filtration step on a Sepharose Cl 4B column. This separation procedure acts as a reversed molecular sieve, letting through large molecules and retarding smaller ones. PAPP-A is of a molecular size which is somewhat retarded on this column and thus separated

Table I. Purification of PAPP-A.

Pools	Total PAPP-A (mg)	Purity (%)
Pregnancy plasma	61	0.07
DEAE Sephadex	42.1	4.7
Con A–Sepharose	14.4	28.2
Sepharose Cl 4B	10.5	60.0
Anti-human serum–Sepharose	1.7	> 98.0

from faster running large proteins. There were, however, still impurities left in the PAPP-A eluate from this gel filtration column.

Because PAPP-A is specific to pregnancy it will not bind to antibodies raised against non-pregnant human serum. Such an antiserum was bound to a Sepharose matrix and the PAPP-A pool applied to this column.

PAPP-A was eluted as a single peak of unbound proteins free from other contaminating proteins which remained bound to the column.

The overall result of the purification is summarized in Table I. Although the yield of this purification method is low, it is of the same order of magnitude as for the purification of SP_1 (Bohn, 1972). The purification steps which increased the purity of the preparation by an important factor (Con A–Sepharose, anti-human serum–Sepharose) are those where the losses are the greatest. This might be due to non-specific binding of PAPP-A to these columns.

BIOCHEMICAL CHARACTERIZATION

Molecular Weight Determinations

The molecular weight of PAPP-A has been measured by different methods as shown in Table II. When the elution volume of PAPP-A on the Sepharose column is compared with elution volumes of proteins of known molecular weights (MW), PAPP-A is found to have a MW of 820 000 daltons. On polyacrylamide gradient gels PAPP-A migrates as a 740 000 dalton protein. The discrepancy between the two methods in assessing the MW of the whole molecule is probably due to the presence of carbohydrates which interfere with the migration on polyacrylamide. When the PAPP-A molecule is treated with 4 M urea, thus splitting it into subunits, a MW of 453 750 ± 83 800 daltons is obtained in four different measurements on 3% polyacrylamide gels in the presence of sodium dodecyl sulphate (SDS).

The reduction of PAPP-A with mercaptoethanol separates the protein into polypeptide chains. Under these conditions and on 5% polyacrylamide gels with SDS, PAPP-A has a MW of 218 330 ± 18 930 daltons.

Table II. Molecular weight determination.

Technique	Medium	Molecular weight (daltons) (mean ± S.D.)
Sepharose Cl 4B calibration	Phosphate pH 7.4	820 000
Polyacrylamide gradient gel electrophoresis	Tris-HCl pH 8.5	740 000
Polyacrylamide gel electrophoresis (3% and 5% gels)	Phosphate pH 7.2, SDS and urea	453 750 ± 83 800
	Phosphate pH 7.2, SDS and mercaptoethanol	218 330 ± 18 930

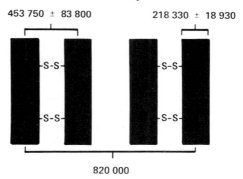

453 750 ± 83 800   218 330 ± 18 930

820 000

Fig. 1. Proposed molecular structure for PAPP-A with indication of molecular weight.

These results would imply that PAPP-A is a dimer of around 800 000 daltons, with each monomer of about 400 000 daltons being composed of two polypeptide chains of 200 000 daltons, as represented in Fig. 1. If this model is correct, then PAPP-A is very similar to a well-known serum protein: α_2-macroglobulin ($\alpha_2 M$)

Electrophoretic Mobility

As shown in Fig. 2, the electrophoretic mobility of PAPP-A and $\alpha_2 M$ have been measured by immunoelectrophoresis. Both proteins have similar if not identical mobilities.

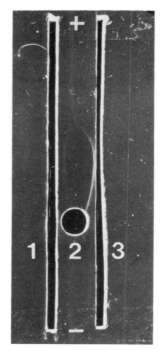

Fig. 2. Immunoelectrophoresis of PAPP-A and α_2-macroglobulin. 1, Antiserum to PAPP-A; 2, pregnancy plasma; 3, antiserum to α_2-macroglobulin.

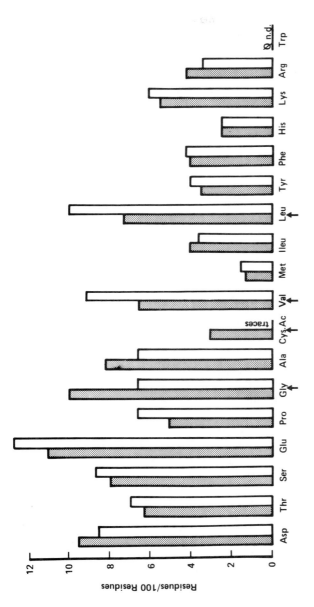

Fig. 3. Comparative amino acid composition between PAPP-A and α₂-macroglobulin. Open bars, α_2-macroglobulin; shaded bars, PAPP-A.

Amino Acid Composition

The amino acid composition of PAPP-A has been determined with an amino acid analyser after hydrolysis of the protein in HCl or performic acid (determination of cysteic acid). The proportionate amino acid composition of PAPP-A is shown compared with that of α_2M as published by Hamberg et al. (1973) (Fig. 3). Except for glycine, cysteic acid, valine and leucine, the composition of both proteins is very similar.

The striking similarity between PAPP-A and α_2M does not, however, include common antigenic determinants since, on immunodiffusion, PAPP-A does not react with an antiserum raised against α_2M. This result also indicates that our preparation of PAPP-A is not contaminated by α_2M.

INVESTIGATIONS ON THE BIOLOGICAL FUNCTION OF PAPP-A

It was hoped that by looking for common antigenic determinants between PAPP-A and proteins of known biological function a clue might be found to the physiological role of PAPP-A. The results of this investigation were negative since PAPP-A did not react with antisera raised to human thyroid stimulating hormone, luteinizing hormone, follicle stimulating hormone, prolactin, placental lactogen, alpha-fetoprotein, SP_1, SP_3, α_2M, antithrombin III, α_1-antitrypsin, plasminogen and prothrombin.

Because of the very slow disappearance rate of PAPP-A after delivery (Lin et al., 1976; Bischof and Klopper, 1979; Smith et al., 1979), it was thought that PAPP-A could be a steroid binding protein, thus extending the short half-life of these hormones. Binding studies were undertaken with tritium-labelled progesterone, oestrone, oestradiol, oestriol, testosterone and corticosterone. None of these likely pregnancy steroids were bound to PAPP-A.

The biochemical similarity between PAPP-A and α_2M, as pointed out earlier, led us to investigate possible similarities in their biological functions.

α_2M is known as a potent inhibitor of serine proteinases such as plasmin, urokinase, kallikrein, etc. It has also been described as a binder of most if not all endopeptidases (for a review, see Barrett and Starkey, 1973). The possibility that PAPP-A could exert similar functions on plasmin and urokinase was investigated using the casein assay as described by Crawford et al. (1976) and the fibrin plate method of Astrup and Müllerts (1952).

Bovine serum albumin (BSA) or PAPP-A (5 μg) was incubated with plasmin. Casein was then added as a substrate to be degraded by plasmin which did not bind to PAPP-A. The amount of digested casein, directly proportional to the unbound plasmin, was measured at 640 nm.

As compared to BSA, PAPP-A inhibits the caseinolytic activity of plasmin, as shown in Fig. 4.

Urokinase, a urinary plasminogen activator, splits the inactive precursor plasminogen and generates plasmin, which in turn digests fibrin. When 5 CTA units of urokinase are placed on a fibrin plate, an area of lysed fibrin can be measured after 24 h. If PAPP-A (5 μg) is added together with urokinase the lysed area is smaller by about 30%, as shown in Fig. 5.

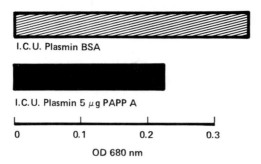

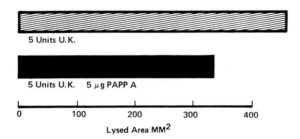

I.C.U. Plasmin BSA

I.C.U. Plasmin 5 μg PAPP A

0   0.1   0.2   0.3

OD 680 nm

Fig. 4. Inhibition of plasmin activity. 1 CU = 1 casein unit.

5 Units U.K.

5 Units U.K.   5 μg PAPP A

0   100   200   300   400

Lysed Area MM^2

Fig. 5. Inhibition of urokinase activity.

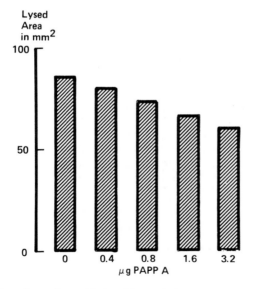

Lysed
Area
in mm^2

Fig. 6. Inhibition of complement-induced haemolysis.

These preliminary *in vitro* results tend to suggest that a possible function of PAPP-A would be to reduce the fibrinolytic activity of the blood. It is not known as yet if these observations have any physiological significance. However, it is well documented that the fibrinolytic activity of the blood decreases as pregnancy progresses and is rapidly restored after delivery of the placenta, but not the infant. This points to the presence of fibrinolytic inhibitors in the placenta, and such inhibitors have been shown to exist (Astedt, 1972).

Crude PAPP-A preparations have immunosuppressive properties; phytohaemag-glutinin-induced lymphoblastogenesis is inhibited by these preparations (Kiefer, 1979). These possible immunosuppressive properties were tested with pure PAPP-A in a complement inhibition assay.

Complement is the main effector pathway of the humoral immune response. Invading cells are identified by antibodies and lysed by the complement. An *in vitro* model was used. Antibodies to sheep red blood cells (SRBC) were bound to SRBC according to Kabat and Mayer (1961) and an aliquot of the cell suspension was then added to molten agarose and poured on a glass plate. When guinea-pig complement is added in a well cut in the agarose, an area of haemolysis develops around the well. If PAPP-A is added together with the guinea-pig complement, a dose-related reduction of the haemolytic area can be measured (Fig. 6).

This apparent inhibition of the haemolytic activity of the complement induced by PAPP-A supports the immunosuppressive properties demonstrated by Kiefer (1979). It is, however, unknown if these observations are of physiological significance.

ACKNOWLEDGEMENTS

The author is indebted to Dr J. E. Fothergill, Dr L. A. Fothergill and to Professor A. Klopper for helpful discussions and suggestions and to Miss G. Cowie for typing the manuscript and for secretarial assistance. This work has been supported by a grant from the Royal Society.

REFERENCES

Astedt, B. (1972). *Acta obstetricia et gynecologica scandinavica* Suppl. 18, 1.
Astrup, T. and Müllertz, S. (1952). *Archives of Biochemistry and Biophysics* **46**, 346.
Barrett, A. J. and Starkey, P. M. (1973). *Biochemical Journal* **133**, 709.
Bischof, P. (1979*a*). *In* "Placental Proteins" (A. Klopper and T. Chard, eds), pp. 105–118, Springer, Heidelberg.
Bischof, P. (1979*b*). *Archiv für Gynäkologie* **227**, 315.
Bischof, P. and Klopper, A. (1980). *Acta obstetricia et gynecologica scandinavica* in press.
Bischof, P., Bruce, D., Cunningham, P. and Klopper, A. (1979). *Clinica chimica acta* **95**, 243.
Bohn, H. (1972). *Blut* **24**, 292.
Bohn, H. and Winckler, W. (1977). *Archiv für Gynäkologie* **233**, 179.
Bruce, D. and Klopper, A. (1978). *Clinica chimica acta* **84**, 107.

Crawford, G. P. M., Ogston, D. and Douglas, A. S. (1976). *Clinical Science and Molecular Medicine* **51**, 215.

Hamberg, U., Stelwagen, P. and Ervast, M. S. (1973). *European Journal of Biochemistry* **10**, 439.

Kabat, E. A. and Mayer, M. M. (1961). *In* "Experimental Immunochemistry" (E. A. Kabat and M. M. Mayer, eds), pp. 133–145, C. C. Thomas, Springfield, Ill.

Kiefer, D. J. (1979). *Ph. D. thesis*, University of Miami.

Lin, T. M., Halbert, S. P., Spellacy, W. N. and Gall, S. (1976). *American Journal of Obstetrics and Gynecology* **124**, 382.

Lin, T. M., Halbert, S. P., Kiefer, D. J., Spellacy, W. N. and Gall, S. (1974). *American Journal of Obstetrics and Gynecology* **118**, 223.

Smith, R., Bischof, P., Hughes, G. and Klopper, A. (1979). *British Journal of Obstetrics and Gynaecology* **86**, 882.

Tatarinov, Y. S. and Masyukevich, V. N. (1970). *Bulletin of Experimental Biology and Medicine of the U.S.S.R.* **69**, 66.

STUDIES ON HUMAN PREGNANCY-ASSOCIATED PLASMA PROTEIN A

R. G. Sutcliffe, J. B. Hunter and S. Gibb and A. B. MacLean[1]

Institute of Genetics, University of Glasgow, and [1]Department of Midwifery Queen Mother's Hospital, Glasgow, Scotland

INTRODUCTION

Human pregnancy-associated plasma protein A (PAPP-A) was described in Lin *et al.* (1974) and by Lin and Halbert (1976) as a large molecular weight protein probably of placental origin. We have been impressed by the apparent similarities in size and electrophoretic mobility of PAPP-A and α_2-macroglobulin (α_2M). We describe a purification of PAPP-A and report on some comparative studies into the structure and antigenicity of the two proteins.

PURIFICATION OF PAPP-A

Maternal serum obtained at term was fractionated with neutral ammonium sulphate. The serum was adjusted to 1.2 M $(NH_4)_2SO_4$ and centrifuged (5000g for 10 min) to remove the precipitated protein. PAPP-A was then precipitated by increasing the concentration of $(NH_4)_2SO_4$ to 2.0 M. This precipitate was resuspended in phosphate-buffered saline (PBS) and was dialysed exhaustively. The recovery of PAPP-A from this step was greater than 95%. Individual aliquots of this material at 4 °C were passed over a Sepharose 4B column (150 ml) on which had previously been immobilized sheep antibody raised against PAPP-A

Serono Symposium No. 35, "The Human Placenta", edited by A. Klopper,
A. Genazzani and P. G. Crosignani, 1980. Academic Press, London and New York.

(Sutcliffe *et al.* 1979). PAPP-A was eluted from the column using 1.5 M KI in PBS and the eluate was dialysed against an excess of 0.05 M potassium phosphate at pH 7.5 for 3 days. After the elution the affinity column was regenerated with PBS prior to the next cycle. After 6–8 cycles the dialysed eluates were adsorbed on a 170 ml column (2.4 cm diameter) of DEAE Sepharose Cl6B and eluted with a linear salt gradient in phosphate buffer from 0.05 M NaCl at pH 7.5 to 0.4 M NaCl at pH 6.5. PAPP-A eluted as a peak at 0.25–0.26 M NaCl. The majority of other proteins eluted between 0.05 and 0.15 M NaCl. In two experiments the recovery of PAPP-A from the affinity chromatography step alone was 21% and 26%. The recovery of PAPP-A from a cycle of six affinity steps followed by ion exchange chromatography was 16%. Quantitation of PAPP-A was carried out by antibody–antigen crossed electrophoresis (AACE) as described previously (Sutcliffe *et al.* 1979) except that 0.1 M Tris was added to the electrophoresis tank buffer and that the direction of electrophoresis in the tank was reversed after 4 h.

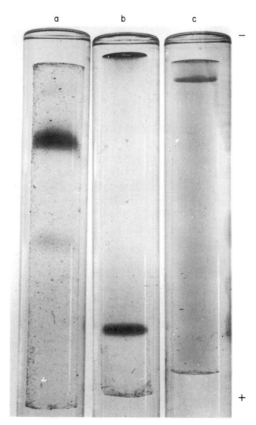

Fig. 1. Tris–glycine polyacrylamide tube gels of PAPP-A after affinity chromatography and ion exchange. (a) 3% non-denaturing gel; (b) 3% SDS gel; (c) 5% SDS gel. Origin and cathode at top.

ASSESSMENT OF PURITY OF PAPP-A

The ion exchange chromatography fractions which contained PAPP-A were pooled and concentrated prior to analysis. Immunoelectrophoresis of the protein revealed a single precipitin arc with sheep anti-PAPP-A and no precipitin arcs with an antiserum to non-pregnant human serum. A single protein band of slow electrophorectic mobility was found on electrophoresis in a 3% non-dissociating polyacrylamide gel (Fig. 1(a)). When similar gels were sliced longitudinally, it was found that the area of intense protein staining shown in Fig. 1(a) corresponded to the position of PAPP-A. This was assessed by embedding one longitudinal slice of gel in agarose and subjecting it to second-dimension electrophoresis into a gel of sheep anti-PAPP-A. On sodium dodecyl sulphate (SDS) polyacrylamide gels (Fig. 1(b) and (c)) the PAPP-A preparation again showed a

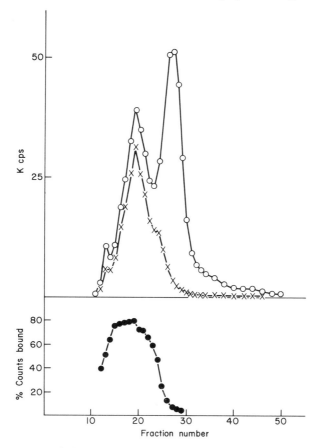

Fig. 2. Fractionation of ^{125}I-labelled PAPP-A on 45 cm × 0.9 cm column of Sepharose CL6B. Upper panel: total counts eluted from column (O–O) and counts precipitated by solid-phase anti-PAPP-A (x–x) over a 17 h incubation at room temperature with vigorous shaking. Lower panel: percentage of eluted counts bound to Sepharose (●–●).

single major band of slow mobility, with some very faint bands of faster mobility. These latter bands are probably contaminants, although we cannot rule out the possibility that some are degradation products of PAPP-A. The protein was then iodinated with low concentrations of chloramine T (0.7 mg/ml; neutralized by 2.67 mg/ml $Na_2S_2O_5$; in 40 μl) and further fractionated over Sepharose CL6B in 0.05 M potassium phosphate, pH 7.5, containing 2.0% horse serum (Welcome type V). Aliquots of the eluted fractions were mixed with aliquots of sheep anti-PAPP-A immobilized on Sepharose 4B. Figure 2 shows that up to 80% of the counts in the first major peak bound to anti-PAPP-A (under these conditions only 1–2% of counts bound to non-immune sheep serum immobilized on Sepharose). From these data it was concluded that a substantial purification of immunoreactive PAPP-A had been achieved.

PAPP-A IN MATERNAL SERUM AND PLASMA

The concentration of PAPP-A in maternal sera has been determined by AACE using a large pool of pregnancy serum at term as a reference standard. The concentration of PAPP-A in the standard has been determined by using the ion exchange preparations described above to estimate the quantity of PAPP-A (in milligrams) per millilitre of serum. The quantity of PAPP-A in the ion exchange preparations was measured by AACE and the quantity of PAPP-A protein was determined by the Folin reaction. Two separate ion exchange fractions of PAPP-A provided an estimated mean value of PAPP-A in the standard serum pool of 0.101 mg/ml

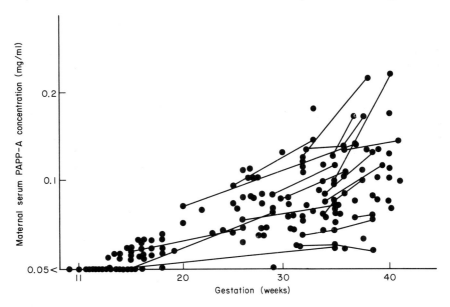

Fig. 3. Concentration of PAPP-A in sera from normal pregnancies delivered of normal singleton babies. The lines join up points from repeat assays on the same patient. PAPP-A measured in 2–20 μl by AACE.

(range of estimates in triplicate was 0.095–0.112 mg/ml). Figure 3 shows the concentration of PAPP-A in a series of women who were delivered of normal babies after normal pregnancies. The assays were carried out in quadriplicate one-dimensional AACE tests using 1.2% sheep anti-PAPP-A in the antibody gel. The lower limit of sensitivity of the assay was approximately 5 μg/ml. PAPP-A was detected in serum samples from 13 weeks of pregnancy onwards, although levels of less than 5 μg/ml were observed up to 18 weeks and even at 29 weeks without accompanying complications of pregnancy. At term, the concentration ranged from 15 μg/ml to 220 μg/ml. Between 38 and 40 weeks no significant difference was observed in PAPP-A levels with respect to the sex of the baby. In collaboration with Dr C. W. Horne we have measured the concentration of PAPP-A in the sera of 32 mothers with gestational diabetes and 14 mothers with insulin-treated diabetes. No substantial departures from the normal range (Fig. 3) were observed. Similarly, no substantial differences from control levels were observed in the serum PAPP-A levels from 26 patients with babies affected by intrauterine growth retardation;

The concentration of PAPP-A in serum and plasma was compared in paired blood samples from 12 patients at term. No significant difference in concentration was found between serum and plasma samples.

Variations in precipitin arc morphology have been repeatedly observed and commented on (Sutcliffe *et al.*, 1979).

EXTENT OF SIMILARITY BETWEEN PAPP-A AND α_2-MACROGLOBULIN

When maternal serum was fractionated over a 22 cm × 2.5 cm column of Sepharose CL6B, it was observed that PAPP-A eluted in the same volume as α_2-macroglobulin (α_2-macroglobulin (α_2M). α_2M has a molecular weight of approximately 725 000 daltons (Barret and Starkey, 1973; Jones *et al.*, 1972). Experiments in collaboration with Dr J. R. Coggins using SDS polyacrylamide electrophoresis indicated that the subunit molecular weight of PAPP-A is approximately 180 000–182 000 daltons. It indicates that PAPP-A is probably a tetramer of an approximate total molecular weight of 181 000 × 4 = 724 000 daltons. However, these figures are for empirical molecular weights and do not take into account the possible presence of carbohydrate groups which would retard the mobility of the protein in gel electrophoresis. This is probably relevant since we have found that PAPP-A binds to concanavalin-A Sepharose.

α_2M from normal, non-pregnant human serum was compared electrophoretically and immunologically with PAPP-A. The purification of α_2M was carried out by filtration through Ultragel AcA 34 followed by ion exchange chromatography (DEAE Sepharose CL6B) and then a final filtration through Sepharose CL6B. The resultant protein gave a single precipitin arc on immunoelectrophoresis with sheep anti-whole human serum. Purified PAPP-A and purified α_2M were run on 6% polyacrylamide SDS slab gels in the presence and absence of 2.0 M β-mercaptoethanol (Fig. 4, tracks 1–4). The figure shows that the apparent molecular weight of PAPP-A is somewhat greater than that of α_2M and that, for both proteins, β-mercaptoethanol tends to increase their apparent molecular weights. From this it was deduced that under the conditions of these experiments

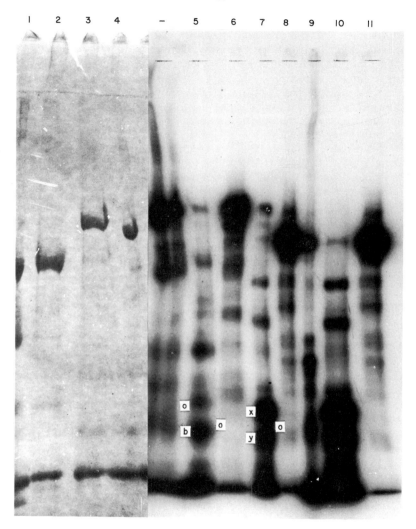

Fig. 4. 6% SDS polyacrylamide slab gels. Tracks 1–4 stained with Coomassie blue. Tracks 5–11, ^{125}I autoradiography. Samples loaded at top. Tracks 1–4: (1) α_2 M minus β-mercapto-ethanol (β-ME) in sample buffer; (2) α_2 M plus β-ME; (3) PAPP-A plus β-ME; (4) PAPP-A minus β-ME. Tracks 5–11: (5) ^{125}I-labelled PAPP-A plus V8; (6) ^{125}I-labelled PAPP-A minus V8; (7) and (10) ^{125}I-labelled α_2 M plus V8; (8) and (11) ^{125}I-labelled α_2 M minus V8. V8, V8 protease from *S. aureus*; incubation time, 20 min at 37 °C. Track 7 contains a small amount of spillover from track 6. This can be seen by comparing tracks 7 and 10 and observing the small high molecular weight contamination in track 7. *O* = albumin mobility (*see* text); for *a, b, x* and *y*, *see* text.

there was no evidence for interchain disulphide bonds. The apparent increase in molecular weight in the presence of β-mercaptoethanol is probably due to a reduction of intrachain disulphide bonds, leading to an extension of the polypeptide chain and a consequent fall in mobility.

PEPTIDE MAPPING

Peptide mapping was then used to investigate the possible structural relationship between PAPP-A and α_2M. The object of these experiments was to find out if there is any structural homology between the two proteins. Our initial studies were based on the method of Cleveland *et al.* (1977), which provides a rapid and simple technique for peptide mapping by limited proteolysis in SDS followed by analysis of the digestion products by SDS polyacrylamide slab gel electrophoresis. The proteins to be mapped were labelled with ^{125}I and 20 μg were digested in 50 μl of Tris-buffered SDS with 2 μg of *Staphylococcus aureus* V8 protease. This protease cleaves polypeptides at the COOH-terminal side of aspartic and glutamic acid residues (Houmard and Drapeau, 1972). Before proteolytic digestion of the proteins the iodinated proteins were subjected to electrophoresis on 4% polyacrylamide SDS gels and the respective peaks of radioactivity corresponding to PAPP-A and α_2M were separately eluted from the gel into Tris-buffered SDS. *S. aureus* V8 protease was then added and the mixture incubated for various times with controls at 27 °C. A stable pattern of cleavage products were observed at various sampling times between 7 min and 27 min at 37 °C. This pattern was relatively invariant for each protein, suggesting that the limiting digest had reached an end-point during this time. Figure 4 (tracks 5–11) shows a comparison between the digests of PAPP-A and α_2M in the presence and absence of *S. aureus* V8 protease. The proteins have been almost entirely converted to lower molecular weight species and there are substantial differences between the digest patterns for the two proteins. There is some similarity in the mobility of the doublet bands labelled *a* and *b* in PAPP-A (track 5) with bands *x* and *y* in tracks 7 and 10 for α_2M. However, comparison of the electrophoretic position of *a* and *b* relative to *x* and *y* has been made using serum albumin as an internal control. The position of serum albumin does not show up on the autoradiograph but is represented by the open circles beside the tracks in Fig. 4. From the position of the albumin markers it is clear that the *a* and *b* bands have a slightly greater apparent molecular weight than those of *x* and *y*.

The ability of *S. aureus* V8 peptide mapping to distinguish polypeptide homologies has been established for a limited number of proteins (Cleaveland *et al.*, 1977; Piperno and Luck, 1979). Cleaveland *et al.* (1977) have shown that quite different digestion patterns can be obtained from the proteins albumin, tubulin and alkaline phosphatase, which are presumed to be unrelated in structure. However, in itself a lack of correspondence in digest patterns does not completely rule out a polypeptide homology, since proteins may be homologous in some amino acid sequences which are not bounded by aspartic or glutamate acid residues which can be cleaved by V8. In this case it is necessary to make different partial digests using enzymes of different specificity. In the case of α_2M and PAPP-A, the undigested proteins differ in apparent molecular weight and this may obscure the presence of homologous peptide sequences in the two proteins by increasing the size of some polypeptides in the digest of PAPP-A. Thus the doublet bands *a* and *b* in PAPP-A (Fig. 4) could be homologous to the doublet bands *x* and *y* in α_2M. Experiments are under way to study the smaller molecular weight peptides generated by V8 and by tryptic digestion since the smaller peptides should not all be affected by local areas of non-homology, whether that be due to additional amino acids or alterations in other groupings such as carbohydrates.

IMMUNOLOGICAL STUDIES IN THE SEARCH FOR CROSS-REACTIVITY

The present sheep anti-PAPP-A serum has a titre of anti-PAPP-A of 1:50 000. It also has some anti-α_2M specificities at a titre of 1:5000. This raises the question as to whether PAPP-A and α_2M share specificities, or whether the anti-α_2M antibodies were raised against contaminating protein in the original immunization. The availability of PAPP-A in a high state of purity has permitted cross-immuno-electrophoretic studies on PAPP-A and α_2M using a mixture of rabbit anti-α_2M and sheep anti-PAPP-A. Figure 5 shows the results of such an experiment. The PAPP-A peaks have been arranged so as to be smaller than the α_2M peaks in order that the protein arcs can be easily distinguished. The left-hand end of the plate shows that PAPP-A contains no detectable α_2M. The right-hand series of inter-acting peaks reveals no reactions of partial or complete identity between α_2M and PAPP-A.

Because of the uncertainty about the sensitivity of precipitin tests of identity, competitive immunoassay tests were also carried out. Sheep anti-PAPP-A was immobilized on Sepharose and 50 μl of serially diluted antibody were reacted with 0.01 μg of ^{125}I-labelled PAPP-A in the presence and absence of α_2M (see Fig. 6). No displacement of PAPP-A counts was detected when α_2M was present in the reaction (Fig. 6(a)). The reciprocal experiment was carried out (Fig. 6(b)), in which solid-phase anti-α_2M was reacted with ^{125}I-labelled α_2M (0.01 μg) in the presence and absence of 3 μg PAPP-A. Here the presence of PAPP-A appeared to displace α_2M counts from a solid-phase anti-α_2M. The extent to which this latter experiment is significant depends upon the level of contamination of α_2M in the PAPP-A. The evidence from electrophoresis and immunoelectrophoresis is that no detectable contamination is present.

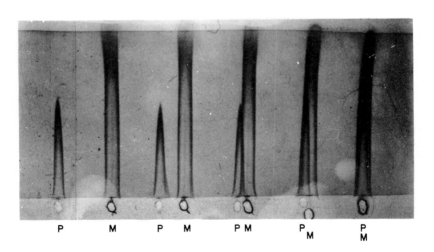

Fig. 5. AACE of α_2M and PAPP-A into a mixture of monospecific rabbit anti-α_2M and unadsorbed high titre sheep anti-PAPP-A. P, PAPP-A; M, α_2M.

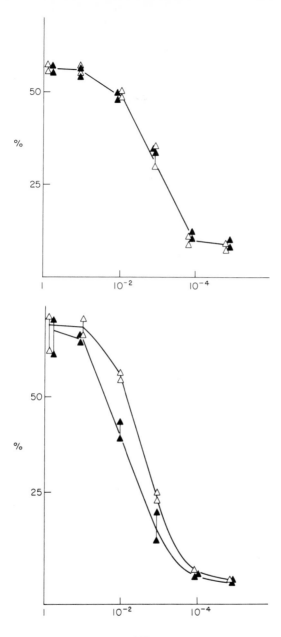

Fig. 6. Solid-phase immune precipitation of ^{125}I-labelled protein in the presence and absence of cold competitor (see text). (a) ^{125}I-labelled PAPP-A (0.01 μg) plus 50 μl of serial dilutions of solid-phase anti-PAPP-A in the absence ($\triangle$) and presence ($\blacktriangle$) of 7.5 μg α_2M. The results using 0.75 μg α_2M were similar to $\blacktriangle$. (b) ^{125}I-labelled α_2M (0.01 μg) plus 50 μl of serial dilutions of solid-phase anti-α_2M in the absence ($\triangle$) and presence ($\blacktriangle$) of 3 μg PAPP-A. Ordinate, percentage of counts bound to antibody; abcissa, dilutions of solid-phase antibody.

REFERENCES

Barrett, A. J. and Starkey, P. M. (1973). *Biochemical Journal* **133**, 709.

Cleveland, D. W., Fischer, S. G., Kirschner, M. W. and Laemmli, U.K. (1977). *Journal of Biological Chemistry* **252**, 1102.

Houmard, J. and Drapeau, G. R. (1972). *Proceedings of the National Academy of Sciences of the U.S.A.* **69**, 3506.

Jones, J. M., Creeth, J. M. and Kekwick, R. A. (1972). *Biochemical Journal* **127**, 187.

Lin, T. M. and Halbert, S. P. (1976). Science, *New York* **193**, 1249.

Lin, T. M., Halbert, S. P., Kicfer, D. J., Spellacy, W. N. and Gall, S. (1974). *American Journal of Obstetrics and Gynecology* **118**, 223.

Piperno, G. and Luck, D. J. L. (1979). *Journal of Biological Chemistry* **254**, 2187.

Sutcliffe, R. G., Kukulska, B. M., Nicholson, L. V. B. and Paterson, W. F. (1979). *In* "Placental Proteins" (A. Klopper and T. Chard, eds), pp. 55–70, Springer-Verlag, Heidelberg.

CLINICAL SIGNIFICANCE OF SP$_1$ IN PATHOLOGICAL PREGNANCIES

G. P. Mandruzzato, S. Zerilli and L. Radillo

Istituto per l'Infanzia, Trieste, Italy

INTRODUCTION

Among the many proteins that are produced by the trophoblast, some are used for the monitoring of pregnancy.

The discovery and isolation of SP$_1$ made us think that this new protein could be a useful tool from the clinical point of view. This assumption is a consequence of a series of considerations: SP$_1$ is produced only by the placenta (Bohn, 1971), and in normal conditions shows a constant progressive increase in concentration in maternal plasma (Cenciotti *et al.*, 1978). Furthermore, this protein has a smaller range of variability than other biochemical parameters (Klopper *et al.*, 1977). In addition, methods of assay for this protein have been introduced which are simple, precise, rapid and cheap. Obviously, due to the sensitivity of the radioimmuno-assay, this method can be used in the first trimester of pregnancy, while immuno-electrophoretic assay can be used during the second and third trimesters of pregnancy.

Considering the interesting prospects the assay of SP$_1$ level seems to offer, even without knowing its biological significance, we tried to examine its behaviour in pathological pregnancies so as to find whether its measurements are useful from a clinical point of view.

Patients and Methods

We studied 236 pregnant women between 24 and 42 weeks of gestation. Since samples were taken repeatedly from a number of patients, the total number of assays was 395. Of these, 191 patients did not show any clinical complication of

Serono Symposium No. 35, "The Human Placenta", edited by A. Klopper,
A. Genazzani and P. G. Crosignani, 1980. Academic Press, London and New York.

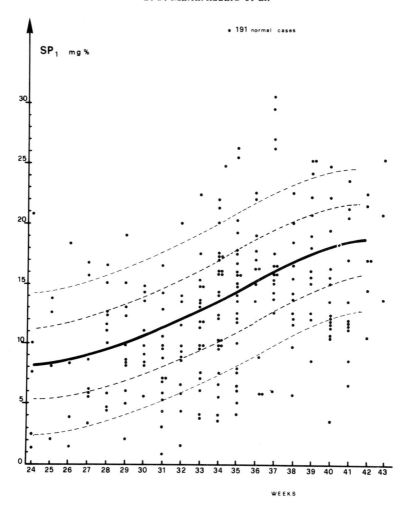

Fig. 1. Normal values for SP$_1$ during gestation. Solid line shows mean value and dotted lines show one and two standard deviations about the mean.

pregnancy, delivered at term or near term, and gave birth to babies whose weight was between the 10th and the 90th percentile as determined for our population (Mandruzzato *et al.,* 1973). These cases were therefore considered as normal.

The SP$_1$ concentration values of these patients were used to determine the normal range. These values are indicated in Fig. 1, which also shows the mean and one and two standard deviations about the mean.

A second group of 40 patients was considered as pathological because of clinical complications in pregnancy or because of abnormal neonatal weight. These comprized three cases of placenta praevia, 12 cases of pre-eclamptic toxaemia, seven cases of diabetes B (according to White's classification), three cases of Rh-iso-

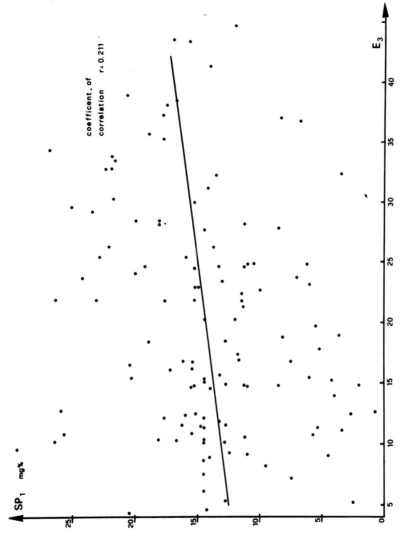

Fig. 2. The correlation between serum SP_1 value and urinary oestriol excretion.

immunization, and three cases with congenital malformations. Furthermore, we also studied 12 pregnancies in which an intrauterine growth retardation (IUGR) was noticed with no apparent cause.

Samples were taken from the cubital vein between 08.00 and 09.00, after the patients had fasted from midnight. The blood samples were centrifuged and the serum thus collected was stored at $-20\,^{\circ}$C. SP_1 concentration was measured by immunoelectrophoresis, according to Bruce and Klopper (1978).

In addition, we evaluated SP_1 concentrations in 26 pregnant women during an intravenous glucose tolerance test. One fasting blood sample was taken, followed by the rapid injection of glucose at the rate of 0.33 g/kg body weight. Thereafter, six samples were taken at 10 min intervals and a final one after 30 min.

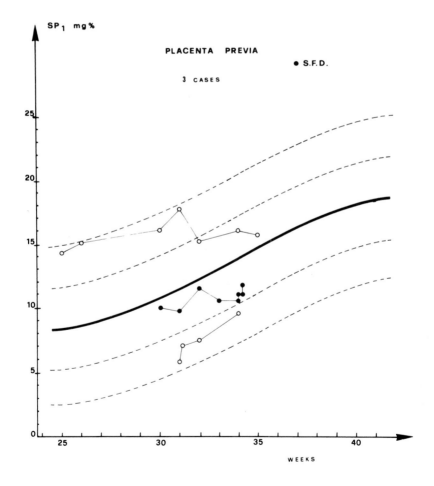

Fig. 3. Serial values of SP_1 in three patients with placenta praevia. Open circles represent patients who gave birth to babies of normal weight and solid circles show a case with intrauterine growth retardation.

RESULTS

In order to determine whether SP_1 concentration correlated with another well-known biochemical parameter, we measured urinary oestriol excretion. The regression line and the coefficient of correlation obtained by comparing these two parameters are shown in Fig. 2. The coefficient of correlation being 0.211, it is evident that the statistical significance is not strong (p value is between 0.05 and 0.01).

We also calculated the coefficient of correlation between SP_1 concentration and placental weight, and between SP_1 concentration and neonatal weight, taking the SP_1 measurement 1 week prior to delivery. There was no statistically significant correlation between SP_1 and either placental or neonatal weight.

Placenta Praevia

Figure 3 shows the trend of serial assays of SP_1 in the three cases of placenta praevia. Two of the patients gave birth to children of normal weight, i.e. between

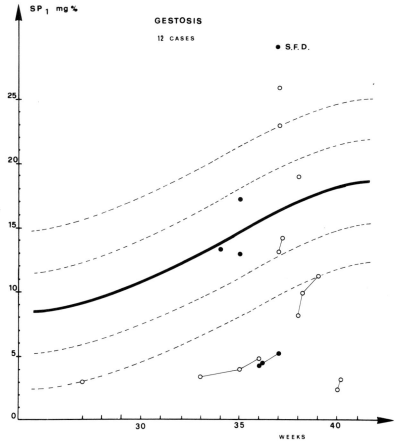

Fig. 4. SP_1 values in pre-eclampsia. Solid circles represent patients with intrauterine growth retardation.

the 10th and 90th percentiles as determined for our population. In the third case (solid circles) the weight of the baby was below the 10th percentile. It is evident that in all cases SP_1 values were within two standard deviations of the mean.

Pre-eclampsia

In Figure 4 the findings relative to the 12 cases of pre-eclampsia are shown.

Only in four cases were SP_1 values more than one standard deviation below the mean and in one case the SP_1 value fell on the minus two standard deviations line.

Four patients out of 12 delivered small for date neonates, but only in one of them did SP_1 values fall below the minus two standard deviations line.

Diabetes

Figure 5 shows the SP_1 values in the seven diabetic women. Only in one case were the values below the minus two standard deviations line. It must be said that

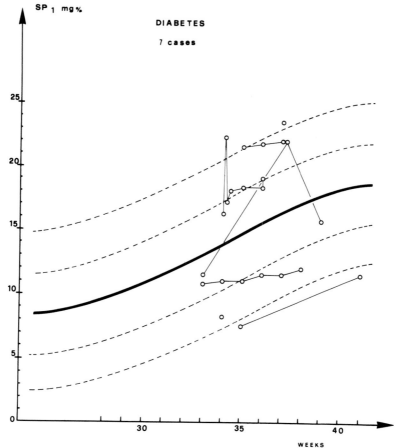

Fig. 5. SP_1 values in diabetic pregnancy. All subjects were White's class B.

diabetes was well controlled (the mean blood sugar was below 100 mg%) and the weights of the neonates were quite normal.

Isoimmunization

In Figure 6 the trends of SP_1 concentration in the three cases of Rh-isoimmunization are shown.

One case was over the plus two standard deviations line, one case was below the minus two standard deviations line, and one case was near the mean. In all three cases neonatal weight was normal, no intrauterine transfusion was necessary, and only neonatal treatment (exchange transfusion or phototherapy) was performed.

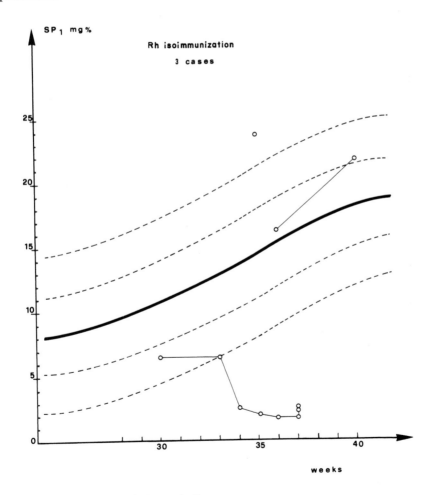

Fig. 6. SP₁ values in Rh-isoimmunization.

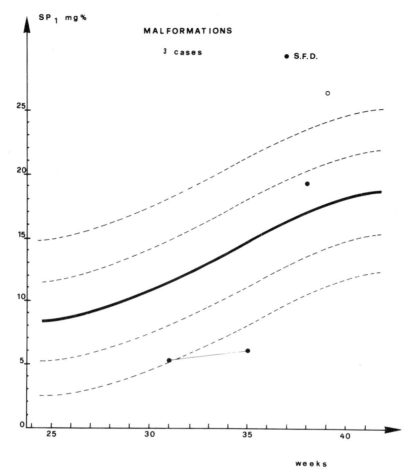

Fig. 7.   SP$_1$ values in congenital fetal malformation. Solid circles show cases who also had intrauterine growth retardation.

Malformations

Figure 7 shows SP$_1$ values obtained in the three cases of malformation.

One case was a lumbar rachyschysis with a normal birthweight. Its SP$_1$ value was over the plus two standard deviations line. In the other two cases the birth-weight was below the 10th percentile. The first was a case of multiple non-viable malformations, and the SP$_1$ value lay between the mean and plus one standard deviation line. The second was a case of microcephaly, and its SP$_1$ values were below the minus two standard deviations line.

IUGR

In the 12 cases of IUGR without any apparent cause, we noted a wide disper-sion of SP$_1$ values. In two cases SP$_1$ concentration was below the minus two standard deviations line. In another two cases values were over the plus two standard deviations line. In the remaining eight cases values were within normal limits.

Intravenous Glucose Tolerance Test and SP₁

In the 26 pregnant women who were submitted to an intravenous glucose tolerance test, the coefficient of utilization was calculated according to Conard *et al.* (1953). We divided the cases, according to that coefficient, into two groups.

In the first group (15 cases) the coefficient was equal to or higher than 2.04, which is the first standard deviation according to our data. In the second group (11 cases) the coefficient was lower than 2.04.

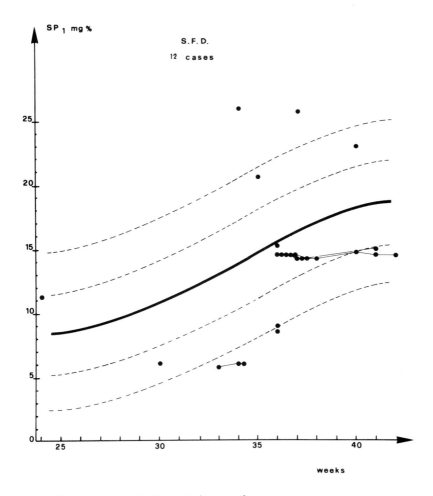

Fig. 8. SP₁ values in retarded intrauterine growth.

K ≥ 2.04	**K** < 2.04
(I DS)	
+ 38.82 %	+ 20.01%

Fig. 9. Percentage increase in SP_1 during glucose tolerance test according to the coefficient of utilization (K).

We therefore calculated the percentage increase in SP_1 concentration during the test. It is clear (Fig. 9) that there is a difference in increase between the two groups: the increase was higher in pregnant women with a higher coefficient.

DISCUSSION

Our results are as imprecise as the recorded findings of other workers.

We did not find any correlation between SP_1 concentration and neonatal weight or placental weight. This observation is in accordance with Lin et al. (1976) but not with the observations of Tatra et al. (1974) and Gordon et al. (1977). Klopper et al. (1977) considered the lack of such a correlation surprising, and think that the reason for this could be the fact that SP_1, like many other substances produced by the fetoplacental unit, is not strictly connected with fetal growth or other aspects of fetal well-being. This remark in itself contradicts the idea that SP_1 could be a sufficiently precise parameter for the evaluation of fetal well-being.

Nor is the correlation between SP_1 and urinary oestriol, although within statistical significance, particularly good. In fact we must remember that, for instance, the coefficient of correlation between urinary oestriol and neonatal weight was higher than the coefficient of correlation between SP_1 and neonatal weight, and therefore the former parameter might be more useful to monitor IUGR (Spanio et al., 1975).

There is no characteristic change of SP_1 in particular forms of pathological pregnancy, including IUGR.

The observations concerning the increase in SP_1 concentration following glucose load are of some interest. Our results are different from the observations made by Tatra at the Aberdeen meeting in 1978. He did not note any variation in SP_1 values after insulin-provoked hypoglycaemia. On the contrary, we found that SP_1 concentration increases no earlier than 30 min after the intravenous glucose load, and that this increase is higher in cases with a high coefficient of utilization. One might think that in these cases glucose placental perfusion is chronically insufficient. However, it is difficult to give an interpretation of this result.

CONCLUSION

In our experience the measurement of SP_1 concentration in maternal blood is of little aid as a diagnostic tool for monitoring the fetoplacental unit. This certainly seems to be true in cases of clinical maternal pathology and IUGR. Since we do not know the biological significance of this protein at present, it may be that better results will be obtained when this significance is discovered.

REFERENCES

Bohn, H. (1971). *Archiv für Gynäkologie* **210**, 440.

Bruce, D. and Klopper, A. (1978). *Clinica chimica acta* **84**, 107.

Cenciotti, L., Fortuna, A., Roncuzzi, R. and Abbondanza, G. C. (1978). *Minerva ginecologica* **30**, 251.

Conard, V., Franckson, J. R. M., Bastenie, P. A., Kestens, J. and Kovacs, L. (1953). *Archives internationales de pharmacodynamie et de thérapie* **93**, 277.

Gordon, Y. B., Grudzinskas, J. G., Lewis, J. D. and Jeffrey, D. (1977). *British Journal of Obstetrics and Gynaecology* **84**, 642.

Klopper, A., Masson, G. and Wilson, G. (1977). *British Journal of Obstetrics and Gynaecology* **84**, 648.

Lin, T.-M., Halbert, S. P. and Spellacy, W. H. (1976). *American Journal of Obstetrics and Gynecology* **125**, 17.

Mandruzzato, G. P., Macagno, F., Bellani, R., Carli, F., Carlomagno, G. and Sabbati, M. L. (1973). *Annali di ostetricia e ginecologia medicina perinatale* **9/10**, 595.

Spanio, P., Mandruzzato, G. P., Sabbati, M. C., Nisi, F., Macchia, M. and Persello, C. (1975). *In* "Therapy of Fetoplacental Insufficiency" (B. Salvadori, ed.), pp. 75–77. Springer-Verlag, Heidelberg.

Tatra, G., Breitenecker, G. and Gruber, W. (1974). *Archiv für Gynäkologie* **217**, 383.

PREGNANCY-SPECIFIC β_1-GLYCOPROTEIN (SP$_1$). MOLECULAR HETEROGENEITY AND MEASUREMENT

B. Teisner, J. G. Grudzinskas[1], P. Hindersson, J. Folkersen, J. G. Westergaard and T. Chard[1]

Institutes of Medical Microbiology, and Obstetrics and Gynaecology, Odense University, Odense, Denmark
and
[1]*Departments of Reproductive Physiology, and Obstetrics and Gynaecology, St. Bartholomew's Hospital Medical College, London, U.K.*

INTRODUCTION

The pregnancy-specific β_1-glycoprotein (SP$_1$ or PSβG) has been characterized as a β_1 electrophoretic mobile glycoprotein with a molecular weight of around 90 000 daltons. The clinical application of SP$_1$ measurements has been reviewed (Chard and Grudzinskas, 1979; Horne and Towler, 1979; Klopper *et al.*, 1979) and the preliminary results suggest that SP$_1$ measurements may be a useful marker of placental function and for monitoring of patients with trophoblastic tumours.

Measurement of SP$_1$ has so far been carried out mainly by immunoprecipitation and saturation assay techniques. Molecular heterogeneity of SP$_1$ has recently been shown, and the existence of a high molecular weight α_2-glycoprotein with SP$_1$ determinants demonstrated (Teisner *et al.*, 1978, 1979; Westergaard *et al.*, 1979a). The ratio between the originally described SP$_1$ (SP$_1\beta$) and the cross-reacting α_2-glycoprotein (SP$_1\alpha$) remains almost constant throughout the second and third trimesters of pregnancy but differs from individual to individual (Teisner

Serono Symposium No. 35, "The Human Placenta", edited by A. Klopper, A. Genazzani and P. G. Crosignani, 1980. Academic Press, London and New York.

et al., 1978; Westergaard *et al.*, 1979b). The aim of the present study was to evaluate the influence of $SP_1\alpha$ on $SP_1\beta$ measurement by immunoprecipitation techniques and radioimmunoassay.

MATERIALS AND METHODS

Sera

Pooled late pregnancy serum was used as starting material in the separation procedures. In the comparative study, serum samples were obtained from 47 pregnant women at 33–40 weeks of gestation. In order to compare the results obtained in rocket immunoelectrophoresis, quantitative crossed immunoelectrophoresis and radioimmunoassay, a pool of serum obtained from 40 women during the third trimester was used as a reference standard. The reference pool was defined as containing 100 arbitrary units (AU) per millilitre of SP_1 and was used for all assays where the SP_1 concentration was determined in native serum samples.

Anti-SP$_1$ Preparation

The immunoglobulin fraction of rabbit anti-human SP_1 antiserum (code 131, lot no. 018c) supplied by Dako Immunoglobulins, Copenhagen, Denmark was used in all assays.

Separation Procedures

Size Chromatography
Columns of 2.6 cm × 100 cm were packed with Ultrogel ACA 34 (L'Industrie Biologique Française, Clichy, France) in 0.05 M phosphate buffer, pH 7.4. Total bed volume (V_t) was 451 ml and void volume (V_0) estimated to be 158 ml.

Zone Electrophoresis
Preparative zone electrophoresis was done in 1% agarose (Indubiose A-37, L'Industrie Biologique Française, Clichy, France) using Tris-barbital buffer at pH 8.6 and ionic strength 0.02. This method is described in detail elsewhere (Teisner *et al.*, 1979).

Immunoelectrophoresis

Quantitative Rocket Immunoelectrophoresis (RIE)
RIE was performed in 1% agarose (Litex HSA, Litex, Glostrup, Denmark) in Tris-barbital buffer, ionic strength 0.02, pH 8.6. The agarose contained 1 μl anti-SP_1 antiserum/cm^2 and 2 μl of the samples (pregnancy serum or reference pool) were applied in duplicate or quadruplicate.

Crossed Immunoelectrophoresis (XIE)

Analytic XIE was performed in 1% Indubiose A-37 using the same buffer as mentioned above. The first-dimensional electrophoresis was run at 10 V/cm until a bromphenol blue-stained albumin marker had migrated 3 cm. The second-dimensional gel contained 1–2 μl anti-SP_1/cm^2 and 4% PEG to enhance the precipitation of $SP_1\alpha$ (Teisner *et al.*, 1979) and the second-dimensional electrophoresis was performed at 2.5 V/cm for 18 h. The $SP_1\alpha/SP_1\beta$ ratio was estimated as the ratio between the heights of the two precipitation arcs and compared to the ratio of the reference pool. Quantitative XIE was performed in 1% Litex agarose containing 1–2 μl anti-SP_1/cm^2 without addition of polyethylene glycol (PEG). The electrophoretic pattern was enlarged by projection (linear enlargement × 5) and SP_1 measured as the area enclosed under the precipitation arc. The samples were assayed in triplicate.

Mixing Experiments

Purified $SP_1\beta$ and $SP_1\alpha$ were analysed by RIE after being mixed using a constant volume of $SP_1\beta$, increasing amounts of $SP_1\alpha$ and a buffer volume to obtain the same volumes in all samples.

Radioimmunoassay (RIA)

The samples were assayed in duplicate and 16 selected samples in quadruplicate by RIA as described previously (Gordon *et al.*, 1977). The samples were assayed at a dilution of 1:30, or lower if the result was less than 30 μg/ml.

RESULTS

Immunoprecipitation Techniques

Using size chromatography and preparative zone electrophoresis as separation procedures, $SP_1\beta$ and $SP_1\alpha$ were isolated from late pregnancy serum. $SP_1\beta$ was assumed to be free of $SP_1\alpha$ contamination when the anodic part of the β-mobile precipitate extended down to the base line in XIE and no precipitate appeared in the α_2 region after addition of PEG to the second-dimensional gel. The $SP_1\alpha$ was assumed to be isolated from $SP_1\beta$ when a sharply pointed, strictly PEG-dependent immunoprecipitate appeared in rocket immunoelectrophoresis (Fig. 1). As seen from Fig. 1, addition of $SP_1\alpha$ to a constant amount of $SP_1\beta$ increased the heights of the precipitate more than 100% in conventional rocket immunoelectrophoresis, and purified $SP_1\alpha$ did not precipitate itself. When 4% PEG was added to the agarose, $SP_1\alpha$ formed immunoprecipitate and the mixed samples showed a double precipitation pattern (Fig. 1). The effect of addition of increasing amount of $SP_1\alpha$ to a constant amount of $SP_1\beta$ was found to be less pronounced in radial immunodiffusion than in RIE.

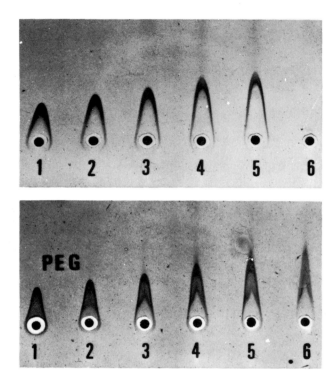

Fig. 1. Rocket immunoelectrophoretic analysis of $SP_1\beta$ (well no. 1), $SP_1\alpha$ (well no. 6) and $SP_1\beta/SP_1\alpha$ mixtures (wells no. 2–5). Wells no. 1–5 received the same amount of $SP_1\beta$. 4% PEG was added to the agarose in the plate marked PEG.

Monitoring of Size Chromatographic Fractionation of Late Pregnancy Serum by RIE and RIA

Fractions from size chromatographic separation of late pregnancy serum tested in RIE revealed three peaks of anti-SP_1 reactive material (Fig. 2). The immunoprecipitates in the high molecular weight peak appeared only when 4% PEG was added to the agarose. However, when the same fractions were subjected to RIA, only one peak was apparent (Fig. 3), and this peak corresponded to the molecular weight of $SP_1\beta$ (90 000 daltons). In addition, only trace amounts of anti-SP_1 reactive material were detected by RIA in fractions containing higher molecular weight material.

Measurement of SP_1 in Late Pregnancy Serum by RIE, RIA and XIE

The results of SP_1 measurement by RIE and RIA in serum samples from 47 women in the third trimester of pregnancy were compared and the correlation

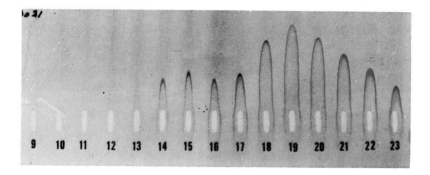

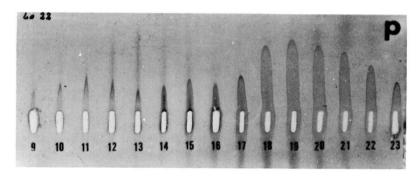

Fig. 2. Fractions from size chromatographic fractionation of pooled late pregnancy serum monitored by rocket immunoelectrophoresis. 4% PEG was added to the agarose in the plate marked P.

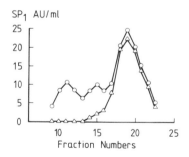

Fig. 3. Size chromatographic fractionation of late pregnancy serum (the same run as in Fig. 2) monitored by RIE (○) and RIA (△).

coefficient calculated to be 0.96. However, eight of the 47 samples with higher $SP_1\alpha/SP_1\beta$ ratio than the reference pool all gave higher values in RIE as compared to RIA, whereas the measurements for eight samples with lower $SP_1\alpha/SP_1\beta$ ratio than the reference fell on or below the line $x = y$. These 16 samples were further analysed in quantitative XIE. Comparison of the results obtained in RIE and XIE

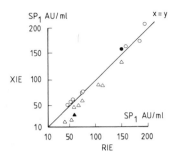

Fig. 4. A comparison of SP_1 measurement performed by XIE and RIE. △, Samples with estimated high $SP_1\alpha/SP_1\beta$ ratio; ○, samples with estimated low $SP_1\alpha/SP_1\beta$ ratio; ▲ and ●, concentrated fractions no. 14 and 21, respectively (*see* Fig. 2).

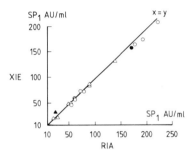

Fig. 5. SP_1 measurements performed by XIE and RIA on the same samples used for Fig. 4.

are shown in Fig. 4. The correlation coefficient was 0.98 and the eight samples with high $SP_1\alpha/SP_1\beta$ ratio had a higher apparent SP_1 content in RIE than in XIE, whereas no difference was observed in the samples with low $SP_1\alpha/SP_1\beta$ ratio. SP_1 levels in the 16 selected samples assayed in XIE and RIA are shown in Fig. 5. As can be seen from the figure, all 16 samples gave results on or very close to the 45° line, and the correlation coefficient was 0.99.

DISCUSSION

Following the initial demonstration of a molecular heterogeneity of SP_1 (Teisner *et al*, 1978), a high molecular weight α_2-glycoprotein ($SP_1\alpha$), immuno-logically cross-reacting with the originally described SP_1, i.e. $SP_1\beta$, has been isolated (Westergaard *et al.*, 1979a; Teisner *et al.*, 1979). The influence of isolated $SP_1\alpha$ on the estimation of $SP_1\beta$ is in agreement with results in an earlier report (Teisner *et al.*, 1979). Size chromatographic fractionation of late pregnancy serum permitted the identification by RIE of three peaks containing anti-SP_1 reactive material where the highest molecular weight material only precipitated in the presence of 4% PEG in the agarose. The intermediate peak has earlier been described as representing an area where both $SP_1\alpha$ and $SP_1\beta$ were present. It is, however, doubtful if the co-elution of $SP_1\alpha$ and $SP_1\beta$ can explain these results, and the possibility that it represents a third component should be considered. When the same fractions were analysed by RIA, only one peak corresponding to $SP_1\beta$ appeared, indicating that RIA predominantly measures $SP_1\beta$, and this finding seems to be confirmed by the result of SP_1 measurements in the 16 selected serum samples. This observation may find an explanation in the inherent nature of the various assays. Analysis by gel precipitation allows for the detection of high as well as low affinity interaction, while radioimmunoassays generally are dependent on high affinity interaction between antibody and antigen, and thus are less sensitive to inhibition by cross-reacting proteins. Estimation of SP_1 by RIE seems to give a result which reflects the total amount of SP_1 determinants, and the only immunoprecipitation technique which permits differential quantification is XIE; by contrast the measurement of SP_1 by RIA was not demonstrably affected by the presence of $SP_1\alpha$, suggesting that RIA measures predominantly $SP_1\beta$.

ACKNOWLEDGEMENTS

We gratefully acknowledge the support of F. L. Smidth and Co. A/S's Jubilæumsfond and Ferd. Hindsgauls Fond, and the technical assistance of Mrs J. Brandt and Mrs A. McCrae.

REFERENCES

Chard, T. and Grudzinskas, J. G. (1980). *Acta obstetrica et gynecologia scandinavica.*
Gordon Y. B., Grudzinskas, J. G., Jeffrey, D., Chard, T. and Letchworth, A. T. (1977). *Lancet i*, 331.
Horne, C. H. W. and Towler, C. M. (1979). *Obstetrics and Gynecology* **33**, 761.
Klopper, A. (1979). *In* "Placental Proteins" (A. Klopper, R. Smith and I. Davidson, eds), pp. 23–42, Springer Verlag, Berlin.
Teisner, B., Westergaard, J. G., Folkersen, J., Husby, S. and Svehag, S. E. (1978). *American Journal of Obstetrics and Gynecology* **131**, 262.
Teisner, B., Folkersen, J., Hindersson, P., Jensenius, J. C. and Westergaard, J. G. (1979). *Scandinavian Journal of Immunology* **9**, 409.
Westergaard, J. G., Folkersen, J., Hindersson, P., Svehag, S. E. and Teisner, B. (1979a). *In* "Carcino-Embryonic Proteins" (F. G. Lehman, ed.), Vol. II, p. 463, Elsevier/North Holland Biomedical Publishing Co., Amsterdam.
Westergaard, J. G., Teisner, B., Folkersen, J., Hindersson, P., Schultz-Larsen, P. and Svehag, S. E. (1979b). *Scandinavian Journal of Clinical and Laboratory Investigation* **39**, 351.

SYNTHESIS AND SECRETION OF PLACENTAL PROTEINS

J. G. Grudzinskas, J. N. Lee, B. Teisner[1] and T. Chard

Departments of Obstetrics and Gynaecology and Reproductive Physiology, St. Bartholomew's Hospital Medical College and the London Hospital Medical College, London, U.K. and
[1] *Institute of Medical Microbiology, Odense University, Odense, Denmark*

INTRODUCTION

The concentrations of pregnancy-"specific" placental proteins have been examined in a wide variety of physiological and pathophysiological situations. Yet there is virtually no information on the relationship between levels in maternal blood and tissue levels in the placenta itself, despite the fact that such information might provide a useful background to both biological and clinical studies on these materials. The evidence that these materials are produced by the trophoblast is based on the isolation of these molecules from the placenta, together with localization studies demonstrating their presence. Further evidence is provided by the existence of a gradient of concentration in the direction retroplacental space→ uterine vein→ peripheral circulation. This has been clearly demonstrated for placental lactogen (Klopper and Hughes, 1978), and it was surprising that studies on pregnancy-specific β_1-glycoprotein revealed no gradient, or even a gradient in the reverse direction (Klopper and Hughes, 1978).

In this study, we report concentrations of five placental proteins in maternal blood and placental homogenates collected in the first and third trimesters, and the concentrations of four placental proteins and a normal serum component in blood obtained from the retroplacental space and in the peripheral circulation at term delivery.

Serono Symposium No. 35, "The Human Placenta", edited by A. Klopper, A. Genazzani and P. G. Crosignani, 1980. Academic Press, London and New York.

MATERIALS AND METHODS

Venous blood was obtained from five patients immediately before surgical termination of pregnancy in the first trimester and from five patients at term delivery. Placental tissue obtained from these patients was washed in phosphate-buffered saline, homogenized and centrifuged. The supernatants were stored at $-20°C$ until assay. Peripheral venous blood was also obtained from 20 women immediately before delivery (vaginal, 9; Caesarean section, 11). Retroplacental blood was obtained by aspiration from the space immediately behind the placenta at Caesarean section, or from the maternal surface of the placenta after vaginal delivery. Serum was separated within 1 h of collection and stored at $-20°C$ until assay.

The measurement of human chorionic gonadotrophin (hCG), placental lactogen (hPL), placental protein 5 (PP_5), pregnancy-specific β_1-glycoprotein (SP_1) and ferritin (PP_2) were performed by radioimmunoassay (Gordon *et al.*, 1977; Grudzinskas *et al.*, 1977; Crowther *et al.*, 1979; Obiekwe *et al.*, 1979; Kramer *et al.*, 1979). α_2-macroglobulin was measured by "rocket" immunoelectrophoresis (Laurell, 1972) and $SP_1 \alpha$ was measured by crossed immunoelectrophoresis (Teisner *et al.*, 1978).

RESULTS

The circulating concentrations of hPL, SP_1, and PP_5 were higher during late pregnancy than in early pregnancy; that of hCG was lower, and ferritin levels showed no difference (Table I). Placental tissue levels of hPL and SP_1 were higher in late pregnancy, hCG levels were lower and ferritin and PP_5 showed no change (Table II).

The ratio of retroplacental to peripheral concentrations of the four placental proteins and α_2-macroglobulin is shown in Fig. 1. Levels of hPL and PP_5 in the retroplacental space were always higher than those in the peripheral blood, the median level being 3.39 for hPL and 4.83 for PP_5. Levels of SP_1 and hCG in the retroplacental space were lower than those in the peripheral blood, the median ratios being 0.84 for SP_1 and 0.83 for hCG. Furthermore, analytical crossed immunoelectrophoresis (XIE) showed that the ratio for $SP_1 \alpha$ was similar to that for $SP_1 \beta$ (Fig. 2)

DISCUSSION

The proteins examined in this study included four which are known to be specific products of the trophoblast (hCG, hPL, SP_1 and PP_5) and one, ferritin (PP_2), which is not specific although relatively high levels occur in the placenta. This fundamental difference is reflected by the fact that there were no obvious changes in either the blood or tissue levels of PP_2 during pregnancy, or in the ratio between them (Tables I, II, and III).

Of the trophoblast-specific proteins, the pattern of hCG is unique inasmuch as the levels in early pregnancy are considerably higher than those in late pregnancy (Tables I and II). Despite this, hCG shares with other trophoblast proteins the fact

Table 1. Levels (mean and range) of placental proteins in maternal serum in early and term pregnancy.

	No. of cases	Protein concentration (ng/ml)				
		hCG	hPL	SP$_1$	PP$_2$	PP$_5$
Early Pregnancy	5	3900 (2400–5000)	56.2 (14–122)	15 200 (6300–23 500)	25.3 (10.7–41.5)	< 2 < 2
Term Pregnancy	5	270.6 (96–628)	5300 (3000–7600)	318 000 (190 000–420 000)	21.4 (7.3–47.7)	27.7 (5.4–45)

Table II. Concentrations (mean and range) of placental proteins in placental tissue in early and term pregnancy

	No. of cases	Protein concentrations (μg/g wet weight)				
		hCG	hPL	SP$_1$	PP$_2$	PP$_5$
Early Pregnancy	5	88.4 (24.5–120)	54.3 (15.4–96)	25.3 (1.2–51.5)	63.3 (9.0–220)	2.2 (1.1–2.9)
Term Pregnancy	5	2.3 (1.3–4.5)	545.4 (404–732)	52.9 (29.9–91)	50.6 (15–75.5)	1.8 (1.4–2.1)

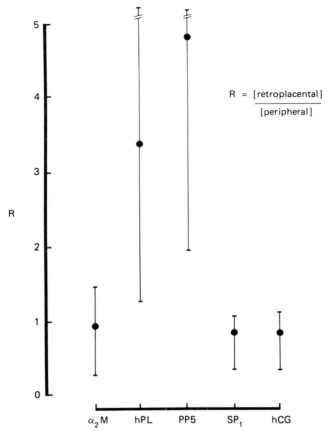

Fig. 1. The ratio of concentrations of α_2-macroglobulin (α_2M), hPL, PP5, SP$_1$, and hCG in retroplacental blood in relation to those in the peripheral circulation in 20 subjects.

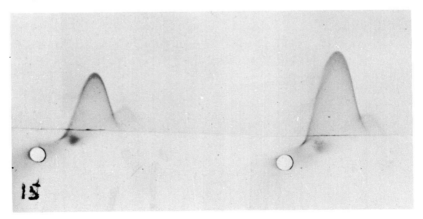

Fig. 2. Analytical crossed immunoelectrophoresis showing the relationship of SP$_1\beta$ (first arc) and SP$_1\alpha$ (second arc) in the retroplacental (a) and peripheral (b) blood in one particular subject.

that the ratio of maternal levels to placental tissue levels is greater in late than early pregnancy (Table III), presumably due to the increase in absolute mass of placental tissue.

The absolute tissue concentrations of hPL and SP_1 showed an apparent increase with gestation, those of hCG a decrease, and PP_5 showed no change (Table II). The findings with the first three are compatible with other information on these materials, while that on PP_5 is slightly surprising since the expected pattern should be similar to that of hPL and SP_1 (Obiekwe *et al.*, 1979). However, if the observations are correct, and it should be noted that the recorded PP_5 levels in placental tissue are very close to the sensitivity limits of the assay, they would indicate that PP_5 cannot be readily classified with other protein secretory products of trophoblast. It is of interest in this respect that Bohn (1976) originally described PP_5 as a non-secretory protein (although this is now disputed) (Obiekwe *et al.*, 1979), and that evidence has been presented that PP_5 may be related to coagulation processes in the intervillous space (Grudzinskas *et al.*, 1979a; Obiekwe *et al.*, 1979).

Table III. The ratio of mean serum concentrations to mean placental tissue concentration of placental proteins in early and term pregnancy.

	hCG	hPL	SP_1	PP_2	PP_5
Early Pregnancy	0.044	0.001	0.6	0.0004	<0.001
Term Pregnancy	0.117	0.0097	6.01	0.0004	0.0154

There is no simple explanation for the differences in blood–tissue ratios between hPL, hCG and SP_1. Superficially, it would be attractive if these were related to the half-lives of the hormones, yet this is clearly not the case since hCG and SP_1 have very similar clearance rates but very different blood–tissue ratios. Nor does the change in ratio during pregnancy relate to half-life since the change is least for hCG and greatest for SP_1. Furthermore, given that there must be an inverse relation between half-life and secretion, the rate of release of hPL (half-life 0.25–0.3 h) should be at least 100 times greater than that of SP (half-life 20–40 h). If there were a fixed ratio of secretion to tissue stores, then the blood–tissue ratio of SP_1 should be around 100 times that of hPL, yet in late pregnancy the actual ratio is greater than this (Table III).

If placental proteins are produced exclusively by the syncytiotrophoblast, there must be a gradient of concentration from the retroplacental space to peripheral blood. The slope of the gradient will vary with the clearance rate of the protein in the mother, being greatest for materials of short half-life (e.g. hPL and PP_5, half-life 15–20 min), and least for materials of long half-life (e.g. SP_1 and hCG, half-life 20–40 h). In the latter cases the actual rate of secretion is so low that the gradient may not be detectable given the imprecision of current assays. Materials secreted at sites other than the uterus and its contents should, of course, show no gradient.

The present studies show a clear gradient for the proteins with a short half-life, hPL and PP_5, and confirm previous findings on hPL (Klopper and Hughes, 1978). However, in agreement with earlier findings on SP_1 (Smith *et al.*, 1979), they show a *reverse* gradient for two proteins of long half-life, SP_1 and hCG, and a similar pattern with a non-placental protein, a_2-macroglobulin. Furthermore, the $SP_1 a$ levels showed a similar reverse gradient, which was surprising since the half-life of $SP_1 a$ is shorter than that of authentic SP_1 (Grudzinskas *et al.*, 1979a). There are three possible explanations of these findings. First, synthesis may occur in a site distal to the retroplacental space, though under these circumstances there would be no reason for a gradient in either direction. Second, the clearance of some placental proteins may be greater in the retroplacental space than in the peripheral circulation, and it is notable that both the placenta and myometrium are rich in enzymes. Third, there may be a technical artefact in collection, such as contamination with amniotic fluid. The last-mentioned is the most likely explanation, since the phenomenon was observed with two undoubtedly placental specific proteins, and one protein of totally different origin. These findings clearly indicate the need to interpret biochemical findings in the so-called 'retroplacental blood' with great care.

In conclusion, these studies show, albeit indirectly, that there are wide variations in the mechanism of secretion of different trophoblast proteins, and that there are striking changes at different stages of gestation. How these findings relate to the clinical interpretation of maternal blood levels is not known, but they contain at least the hint that there may be substantial differences between products, and that clinical results obtained with one material may not be easily extrapolated to another.

REFERENCES

Bohn, H. (1976). *Protides of Biological Fluids* **24**, 117.

Crowther, M. E., Grudzinskas, J. G., Poulton, T. and Gordon, Y. B. (1979). *Obstetrics and Gynecology* **53**, 59.

Gordon, Y. B., Grudzinskas, J. G., Jeffrey, D., Chard, T. and Letchworth, A. T. (1977). *Lancet i*, 331.

Grudzinskas, J. G., Gordon, Y. B., Jeffrey, D. and Chard, T. (1977). *Lancet i*, 333.

Grudzinskas, J. G., Charnock, M., Obiekwe, B. C., Gordon, Y. B. and Chard, T. (1979a). *British Journal of Obstetrics and Gynaecology* **86**, 642.

Grudzinskas, J. G., Teisner, B., Al-Ani, A. T. M., Chard, T. and Westergaard, J. (1979b). *American Journal of Obstetrics and Gynecology* in press.

Klopper, A. and Hughes, G. (1978). *Archiv für Gynäkologie* **225**, 171.

Kramer, McLean, R., Jones, H. M., Challand, G. S., Chard, T., Grudzinskas, J. G. and Charnock, M. (1979). *British Journal of Obstetrics and Gynaecology* in press.

Laurell, G. B. (1972). *Scandinavian Journal of Clinical and Laboratory Investigations* **29**, Suppl. 124, 21.

Obiekwe, B. C., Pendlebury, D., Gordon, Y. B., Grudzinskas, J. G. and Chard, T. (1979). *Clinica chimica acta* **95**, 509.

Smith, R., Klopper, A., Hughes, G. and Wilson, G. (1979). *British Journal of Obstetrics and Gynaecology* **86**, 119.

Teisner, B., Westergaard, J. G., Folkersen, J., Husby, S. and Svehag, S. E. (1978). *American Journal of Obstetrics and Gynecology* **131**, 262.

PROBLEMS IN THE QUANTIFICATION OF PREGNANCY-SPECIFIC β_1-GLYCOPROTEIN (SP$_1$) BY MEANS OF IMMUNOPRECIPITATION TECHNIQUES

P. Schultz-Larsen, J. Lyngbye, J. G. Westergaard and B. Teisner

Department of Clinical Chemistry, Herlev Hospital,
University of Copenhagen, Copenhagen, Denmark,
Department of Clinical Chemistry,
Frederiksborg Amts Sygehus In Hillerød, Hillerød, Denmark,
Department of Gynaecology and Obstetrics,
Odense Sygehus, Odense, Denmark, and
Institute of Medical Microbiology,
Odense University, Odense, Denmark

INTRODUCTION

The classical pregnancy-specific β_1-glycoprotein (SP$_1$) (Bohn, 1971) is described as having a molecular weight of about 90 000 daltons and β_1-mobility on electrophoresis. In sera from pregnant women at least one variant with anti-SP$_1$-reactive determinants (molecular weight of about 400 000 daltons and α_2-mobility) (Teisner *et al.*, 1978; Towler *et al.*, 1978) has been described. The ratio between the two SP$_1$ variants shows marked interindividual variation in native sera.

The heterogenic composition of antigenic determinants creates a number of problems when measuring SP$_1$ as the methods published so far are based on immunoprecipitation techniques: radial immunodiffusion (RID) (Bohn, 1971), rocket immunoelectrophoresis (RIE) (Schultz-Larsen, 1978), nephelometry (AIP)

Serono Symposium No. 35, "The Human Placenta", edited by A. Klopper,
A. Genazzani and P. G. Crosignani, 1980. Academic Press, London and New York.

(Wood *et al.*, 1978), radioimmunoassay (RIA) (Grudzinskas *et al.*, 1977; Towler *et al.*, 1977) and enzyme immunoassay (Grenner, 1978).

This study describes the influence that the various proportions of $SP_1 \alpha$ and $SP_1 \beta$ exert on the estimation of total SP_1 when measured by means of RID, RIE, API and RIA.

METHODS

Radial Immunodiffusion (RID)

A 5 μl sample or a standard is placed in the well punched in a 1% agarose gel containing 1% polyethylene glycol 6000 (PEG) and 2.25 μl anti-SP_1 per square centimetre. Diffusion period: 48 h.

Rocket Immunoelectrophoresis (RIE)

A 5 μl sample or a standard is placed in the wells punched in a 1% agarose gel containing 1% PEG and 2.25 μl anti-SP_1 per square centimetre. The electrophoresis is run at 3 V/cm for 14 h (Schultz-Larsen, 1978).

Nephelometry (AIP)

After pretreatment with PEG solution (200 g/l) and centrifugation the supernatant is diluted 1:10 and is ready for use in the nephelometer (Technicon, Auto Analyser II). Antibody is diluted 1:50 with a PEG solution (70 g/l NaCl) and filtered through an 0.22 μm filter (Millipore type GS) immediately before use.

Antibody and Standards in RID, RIE and AIP

In all three methods the same antiserum was used (Dakopatts, lot 018 B). The standards were male serum enriched with placental extract (Behringwerke, lot 2403).

Radioimmunoassay (RIA)

The labelling of purified SP_1 (from Dr H. Bohn) was carried out by means of ^{125}I and lactoperoxidase (Marchalonis, 1969).

A mixture containing (a) sample or standard, (b) radiolabelled SP_1 and (c) anti-SP_1 (Behringwerke) was incubated for 24 h. Separation of bound and free radiolabelled SP_1 was accomplished by means of immune complexes (normal rabbit serum/sheep anti-rabbit immunoglobulin) (Schultz-Larsen *et al.*, 1979).

Statistical Methods

The proportion of the two results from each individual sample is used in order to compare the two methods involved. The median and the confidence limits of the median of these proportions are calculated to test whether the two methods give identical results. The Mann–Whitney rank sum technique was used to test whether the proportions obtained from α-dominated sera are significantly different from those obtained from β-dominated sera.

RESULTS

Radioimmunoassay

Figure 1 shows dose–response curves for β-dominated sera (A and B) and for the Behring standard serum (S), as well as for three α-dominated sera C, D and E. The slopes of C, D and E are less steep than the slopes from A, B and S.

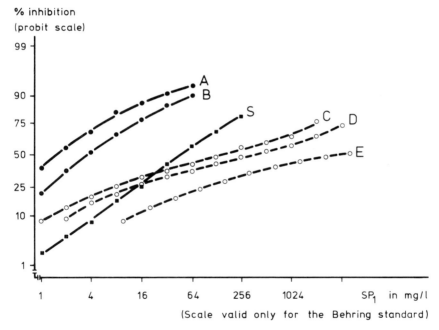

Fig. 1. Dose–response curves of β-dominated sera (A and B), the Behring standard (S) and α-dominated sera (C, D and E).

RID, RIE and AIP

Mixed Samples

In order to compare sera with varied contents of α- and β-component, a β-dominated sample was mixed in various proportions with an α-dominated sample. Figure 2 shows that the precipitation types of these samples correspond closely to the findings amongst individual native sera.

Figure 3 shows results of these mixtures when measured by means of RID,

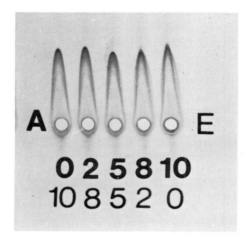

Fig. 2. Rocket immunoelectrophoresis on different mixtures of a β-dominated sample (A) and an α-dominated sample (E). Mixing proportions are indicated.

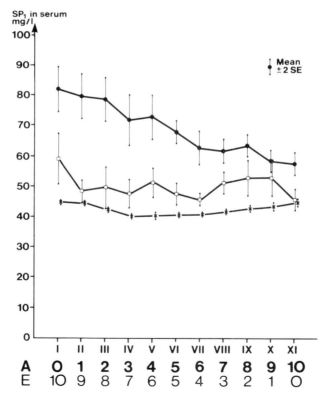

Fig. 3. Measurement of samples mixed from a β-dominated sample A and an α-dominated sample (E). Mixing proportions are indicated. ●—●, Radial immunodiffusion; □—□, nephelometry; x—x, rocket immunoelectrophoresis.

RIE and AIP. Deviation from a line drawn between the two original samples indicates a deviation from the result expected.

RIE shows a negative interaction of 10% maximum at a certain proportion of mixture. The same does not apply regarding RID or AIP.

Comparison of RID, RIE and AIP

In order to compare the RID, RIE and AIP results, 41 β-dominated sera and 14 α-dominated sera were analysed using all three methods. The results are shown in Table I. In β-dominated sera AIP and RIE showed identical values, but diverging results were found between RID and the two other methods (median proportions of 1.17 and 0.85). In α-dominated sera no accordance was demonstrated between any of the methods.

Likewise, Table I shows no accordance of the proportion of α- and β-dominated sera for any combination of methods.

Table I. Comparison[a] of serum SP₁ concentrations as measured by radial immunodiffusion (RID), rocket immuno-electrophoresis (RIE) and nephelometry (AIP).

Method combination	β-dominated sera	α-dominated sera
RID/RIE	1.17 (1.12–1.19)	1.40 (1.25–1.52)
AIP/RIE	1.00 (0.94–1.03)	0.85 (0.74–0.90)
AIP/RID	0.85 (0.81–0.89)	0.59 (0.57–0.60)

[a]Comparison expressed as the proportion of the two SP₁ concentrations from the methods involved. 95% confidence limits in parentheses.

DISCUSSION

Radioimmunoassay

Parallel dose–response curves between the calibration material and the unknown samples are required when using the RIA system for quantitation. Towler *et al.* (1978) demonstrated that serum SP₁ concentrations in α-dominated sera were falsely low when using one RIA system. We have demonstrated dose-response curves which—in α-dominated sera—were less steep than those of β-dominated sera. This might indicate that antigenic determinants react with a lower binding energy on α-components than on β-components.

RID, RIE and AIP

Mixed Samples

From a β-dominated and an α-dominated sample the conditions found in native sera could be produced. It is demonstrated that values up to 10% lower than expected are found in a RIE system in certain proportions of α- and β-components. For RID and AIP, such a deviation could not be found, one of the reasons being greater analytical variation.

Comparisons between RID, RIE and AIP

In this study inconsistency between the determinations of α- and β-dominated sera were demonstrated for all methods. This study shows that α- and β-dominated sera are determined differently in relation to each other as well as in relation to the result expected. The one exception is the determination of β-dominated sera using AIP and RIE.

Because of these methodological conditions a serum SP_1 concentration can only be compared to a reference value when both of them are determined using the same method.

REFERENCES

Bohn, H. (1971). *Archiv. für Gynäkologie* **210**, 440–457.

Grenner, G. (1978). *Fresenius' Zeitschrift für analytische Chemie* **290**, 99.

Grudzinskas, J. G., Gordon, Y. A., Jeffrey, D. and Chard, T. (1977). *Lancet* **i**, 333–335.

Marchalonis, J. J. (1969). *Biochemical Journal* **113**, 299–305.

Schultz-Larsen, P. (1978). *Scandinavian Journal of Immunology* Suppl. **8**, 591–597.

Schultz-Larsen, P., Sizaret, Ph., Martel, N. and Hindersson, P. (1979). *Clinica chimica acta* **95**, 347.

Towler, C. M., Horne, C. H. W., Jandial, V. and Chesworth, J. M. (1977). *British Journal of Obstetrics and Gynaecology* **84**, 580–584.

Teisner, B., Westergaard, J. G., Folkersen, J., Husby, S. and Svehag, S. E. (1978). *American Journal of Obstetrics and Gynecology* **131**, 262–266.

Towler, C. M., Glover, R. G. and Horne, C. H. W. (1978). *Clinica chimica acta* **87**, 289–296.

Wood, P. J., Cockett, D. and Mason, G. (1978). *Clinica chimica acta* **90**, 87–91.

DETERMINATION OF SP_1 AND hPL FOR PREDICTING PERINATAL ASPHYXIA

O. Bellmann, J. Tebbe, N. Lang and M. P. Baur

Department of Obstetrics and Gynaecology and Institute of Medical Statistics, Medical School, University of Bonn, German Federal Republic

INTRODUCTION

Early diagnosis of intrauterine growth retardation has been improved by the determination of human placental lactogen (hPL) and pregnancy-specific β_1-glyco-protein (SP_1) in the maternal serum (for a review, *see* Spellacy, 1976; Bohn, 1978). Both placental proteins are relatively closely linked to the nutritional function of the placenta. Previous investigations (Bellmann *et al.*, 1977) showed that in about 50% of all cases with intrauterine growth retardation the serum concentrations of hPL and SP_1 were below the normal range during the last 2 weeks prior to delivery, i.e. a 10-fold higher incidence of abnormally low values as compared to normal pregnancies. Furthermore, we observed that the frequency of cases with abnormally low serum concentrations increased with intrauterine growth retardation (Table I).

In contrast to the well-established relationship between hPL and intrauterine growth retardation, the relationship between hPL and perinatal asphyxia is less defined. According to the literature (Keller *et al.*, 1971; Letchworth and Chard, 1972; Spellacy *et al.*, 1972; England *et al.*, 1974; Kelly *et al.*, 1975; Edwards *et al.*, 1976; Spellacy, 1976; Letchworth *et al.*, 1978) this relationship varies considerably and is dependent on the nature of the complications of pregnancy causing fetal distress. On the other hand, any biochemical parameter which enables the reliable

Serono Symposium No. 35, "The Human Placenta", edited by A. Klopper, A. Genazzani and P. G. Crosignani, 1980. Academic Press, London and New York.

Table I. Incidence of pateints with abnormally low serum concentrations of SP_1 and hPL during the last 2 weeks before delivery in the group of intrauterine growth retardation.

	hPL			SP_1		
	n	(Total)	% of total	n	(Total)	% of total
All cases	45	(93)	48	42	(90)	47
SGA[a]	26	(71)	37	27	(68)	40
VSGA[b]	19	(22)	86	15	(22)	68

[a]SGA: small for gestational age, birthweight of the newborn below the 10th percentile of the Lubchenco diagram, but less than 3 weeks retarded with regard to the 10th percentile.
[b]VSGA: very small for gestational age, birthweight of the newborn below the 10th percentile of the Lubchenco diagram, and more than 3 weeks retarded with regard to the 10th percentile.

prediction of fetal risk during labour should be of great clinical interest. Presently, there is little information about the relation between changes in SP_1 values and perinatal asphyxia (Tatra *et al.*, 1974; Lin *et al.*, 1976).

In the present study the following investigations were carried out:

1. Determination of SP_1 serum levels in cases of perinatal asphyxia without any other complication of pregnancy.
2. Determination of SP_1 values with the aim of predicting perinatal asphyxia in high risk pregnancies.
3. Comparison of SP_1 with hPL serum concentrations with regard to their possible value in predicting perinatal asphyxia.

METHODS

The diagnosis of perinatal asphyxia was based on abnormalities of the cardiotocogram and/or on the colour of the amniotic fluid and/or on the Apgar score and/or on the behaviour of the newborn during the first postnatal week. Abnormalities were defined as follows:

1. Decrease of fetal heart rate variability in the cardiotocogram to less than 5 beats/min during the first stage of labour for at least 30 min and/or late decelerations.
2. Green staining of the amniotic fluid.
3. Apgar scores at 1 min of less than 7, or at 5 min of less than 8.
4. Acidosis and/or abnormalities of neurological or muscular function.

The relations between SP_1 and hPL in perinatal asphyxia were studied in 148 patients with an uneventful course of pregnancy. Cases with cord complications were excluded. The results were compared with a control group of 65 women who delivered healthy babies without any evidence of asphyxia and who had no complications of pregnancy. The value of SP_1 and hPL for predicting perinatal asphyxia in high risk pregnancies was studied in the following four groups:

Table II. Clinical data of the pregnant women divided into six groups.

Group	Number of patients	Number of blood samples for analyses of		Gestational week at delivery	Weight of the newborn (g. mean)		Perinatal asphyxia (% of total)
		hPL	SP_1				
Control group	65	324	306	40	3.343		0
Perinatal asphyxia	148	528	526	40	3.324		100
Intrauterine growth retardation	96	435	386	38	1.959		52
Twins	48	156	158	37	I 2.387 II 2.347		72
Premature labour	112	605	578	37	2.734		37
Rh-isoimmunization	65	297	279	36	2.696		40

1.   Intrauterine growth retardation (n = 96). The newborns in this group had a birthweight below the 10th percentile of the Lubchenco diagram.

2.   Twin pregnancies (n = 48).

3.   Threatened premature labour (n = 112). Premature contractions occurred at about 31 weeks gestation on the average. These patients were treated with the β-sympathicomimetic drug fenoterol for an average of about $3\frac{1}{2}$ weeks according to principles described by Bellmann *et al.* (1978).

4.   Rh-isoimmunization (n = 65). In this group 32 were mildly, 20 moderately, and eight severely affected (for definition see Bellmann *et al.*, 1975).

Table II gives detailed information about the number of patients, the size of the sample pool, the gestational week at delivery, the birthweight and the proportion of perinatal asphyxia for each of the six groups examined.

The determination of SP_1 in the serum was performed by means of radial immunodiffusion and that of hPL by means of radioimmunoassay (Bellmann *et al.*, 1977). The reagents for the assays were supplied by Behring Werke/Marburg and by Hoechst AG/Frankfurt, respectively.

For statistical analysis only one value for every pregnant woman was chosen at random. In this way the measurements were independent with respect to gestational week. A regression curve and its 90% tolerance limits were calculated using these values.

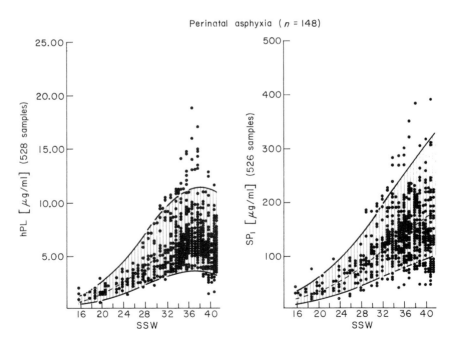

Fig. 1. Scattergram of all SP_1 and hPL values in the group with perinatal asphyxia. The hatched area delineates the 90% fiducial limits of the control group.

RESULTS

Maternal SP₁ and hPL values were analysed in more than 500 serum samples of the 148 patients who delivered newborns showing perinatal asphyxia. All pregnancies were otherwise uncomplicated. Figure 1 shows all SP₁ and hPL values distributed according to gestational age. The 90% fiducial limits of the normal controls are shown as a shaded area. For both parameters a trend to lower serum concentrations is obvious.

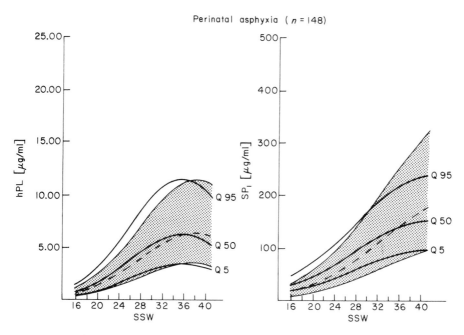

Fig. 2. The regression curves and the 90% tolerance limits for SP₁ and hPL in the group of perinatal asphyxia as compared to those of the control group.

Table III. Incidence of patients with abnormally low serum concentrations of SP₁ and hPL during the last 2 weeks before delivery in the group of perinatal asphyxia as compared to the control group.

	Perinatal asphyxia			Control group		
	n	(Total)	% of total	*n*	(Total)	% of total
hPL	11	(118)	9	2	(47)	4
SP₁	22	(115)	19	3	(44)	7
hPL and SP₁	3	(115)	3	1	(44)	2
hPL and/or SP₁	30	(115)	26	4	(44)	9

The regression curves of SP_1 and hPL show a slight difference between the two groups. The curve for hPL is slightly above and almost parallel to the corresponding curve of the control group until 32 weeks gestation (Fig. 2). Then the curve flattens out until 36 weeks gestation; thereafter it declines. The trend of the SP_1 regression curve is similar, but shows no decline.

Taking into account only the values obtained from the last 2 weeks prior to delivery, the patterns of SP_1 and hPL values are described as follows (Table III): In 19% of the cases one or more SP_1 values fell below the 90% tolerance region; for hPL the incidence was 9%. In comparison, the corresponding figures for the control group were 7% and 4%, respectively. Thus, in the group with perinatal asphyxia there was a two- to threefold increase of abnormally low serum levels of both SP_1 and hPL as compared to the control group.

After having established the relation between serum concentrations of these two placental proteins, and the occurrence of perinatal asphyxia in women with an uncomplicated course of pregnancy, the question was raised whether the determination of SP_1 and hPL in maternal serum could help to predict perinatal asphyxia in high risk pregnancies. Therefore, we tried to find out whether the incidence of perinatal asphyxia was greater in patients showing abnormal serum concentrations of SP_1 and hPL during the last 2 weeks prior to delivery than in those showing normal serum levels.

In the group of intrauterine growth retardation an incidence of asphyxia of 52% (Table IV) was found. In cases with abnormally low SP_1 values the incidence was 67%; in that with abnormally low hPL values it was 62%. Consequently, the determination of SP_1 or hPL in maternal serum did not give any additional information about the risk of perinatal asphyxia in cases of intrauterine growth retardation.

In the group of the twin pregnancies we found an incidence of perinatal asphyxia (one or both twins) of 72%. More than 50% of the values of both SP_1 and hPL fell above the 90% tolerance region. The cases with abnormally high values of SP_1 or hPL did not differ essentially from those with normal values

Table IV. Relationship between SP_1 and hPL in maternal serum and the incidence of perinatal asphyxia in the group with intrauterine growth retardation.

	Total of patients,	Patients with perinatal asphyxia	
	n	n	% of total
hPL analyses performed	93	48	52
High hPL	45	28	62
Low hPL	48	20	42
SP_1 analyses performed	90	47	52
High SP_1	42	28	67
Low SP_1	48	19	40

Table V. Relationship between SP_1 and hPL in maternal serum and the incidence of perinatal asphyxia in the group with twin pregnancies.

	Total of patients,	Patients with perinatal asphyxia of one or of both of the children	
	n	*n*	% of total
hPL analyses performed	43	31	72
High hPL	27	18	67
Low hPL	16	13	81
SP_1 analyses performed	43	31	72
High SP_1	20	15	75
Low SP_1	23	16	70

Table VI. Relationship between SP_1 and hPL in maternal serum and the incidence of perinatal asphyxia in the group with threatened premature labour.

	Total of patients,	Patients with perinatal asphyxia	
	n	*n*	% of total
hPL analysis performed	87	32	37
High hPL	14	6	43
Low hPL	73	26	36
SP_1 analysis performed	88	32	36
High SP_1	12	8	67
Low SP_1	76	24	32

as regards fetal asphyxia (Table V). Consequently, SP_1 and hPL do not help to predict perinatal asphyxia in twin pregnancies.

In the group of threatened premature labour the incidence of asphyxia was 37% (Table VI). This group was characterized by a tendency to abnormally high values of both parameters. Abnormally high values of SP_1 were associated with asphyxia in 67%, whereas abnormally high hPL values were associated with asphyxia in 43% of the cases. Although the incidence of fetal asphyxia occurred almost twice as often in patients with abnormally high SP_1 values than in those with normal SP_1 values, final conclusions cannot be drawn from this observation, as the size of the sample is too small.

In pregnancies complicated by mild or moderate Rh-isoimmunization, the serum levels of SP_1 and hPL did not differ from those in the control group. In all cases of severe Rh-isoimmunization a striking increase of the serum concentrations of both SP_1 and hPL could be observed before a hydropic degeneration

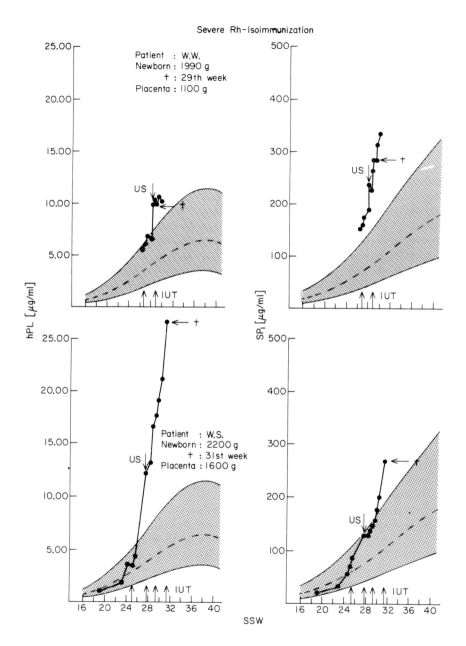

Fig. 3. The serum concentrations of SP_1 and hPL in two cases of severe Rh-isoimmunization. IUT, intrauterine transfusion; US, ultrasonographic examination establishing the diagnosis of hydrops fetus et placentae.

of the conceptus had been detected by ultrasonographic examination. Two of the severe cases are demonstrated in Fig. 3. Intrauterine transfusions had no influence on SP_1 and hPL serum levels. In all these cases, intrauterine death occurred. Consequently, both parameters give valuable information about the fetal risk in cases of severe Rh-isoimmunization.

CONCLUSIONS

1. The relations between SP_1 concentrations in maternal serum and perinatal asphyxia are much less pronounced than those between SP_1 and intrauterine growth retardation.

2. The relation between SP_1 and perinatal asphyxia does not differ to any great extent from that between hPL and perinatal asphyxia.

3. Both parameters are useful in prenatal screening for intrauterine growth retardation. In undisturbed pregnancies the prenatal screening for perinatal asphyxia by means of SP_1 and hPL appears to be of little value. The determination of SP_1 and hPL gives no information about the risk of asphyxia in cases of intrauterine growth retardation and in twin pregnancies. The clinical relevance of SP_1 determination in cases of threatened premature labour has still to be evaluated. In pregnancies complicated by Rh-isoimmunization, both parameters are of great value and should be part of the prenatal monitoring.

REFERENCES

Bellmann, O., Lang, N. and Baur, M. P. (1977). *In* "Gynäkologie und Geburtshilfe, Forschungs-Erkenntnisse" (H. Husslein, ed.), Vol, I, p. 107, Verlag H. Egermann, Wien.

Bellmann, O., Lang, N. and Baur, M. P. (1978). *In* "Fenoterol (Partusisten®) bei der Behandlung in der Geburtshilfe und Perinatologie" (H. Jung and E. Friedrich, eds), p. 44, Georg Thieme Verlag, Stuttgart.

Bellmann, O., Leyendecker, G., Nocke, W., Patt, V., Hansmann, M. and Lang, N. (1975). *Archiv für Gynäkologie* 219, 445.

Bohn, H. (1978). *Scandinavian Journal of Immunology* 7, Suppl. 6, 119.

Edwards, R. P., Diver, M. J., Davis, J. C. and Hipkin, C. J. (1976). *British Journal of Obstetrics and Gynaecology* 83, 229.

England, P., Lorrimer, D., Fergusson, J. C., Moffat, A. M. and Kelly, A. M. (1974). *Lancet* i, 5.

Keller, P. J., Baertschi, U., Bader, P., Gerber, C., Schmid, J., Soltermann, R. and Kopper, E. (1971). *Lancet* ii, 729.

Kelly, A. M., England, P., Lorimer, J. D., Ferguson, J. C. and Govan, A. D. T. (1975). *British Journal of Obstetrics and Gynaecology* 82, 272.

Letchworth, A. T. and Chard, T. (1972). *Lancet* i, 704.

Letchworth, A. T., Slattery, M. and Dennis, K. J. (1978). *Lancet* i, 955.

Lin, T. M., Halbert, S. P. and Spellacy, W. N. (1976). *American Journal of Obstetrics and Gynecology* 125, 17.

Spellacy, W. N. (1976). *In* "Management of High Risk Pregnancy" (W. N. Spellacy, ed.) p. 107, University Park Press, Baltimore.

Spellacy, W. N., Buhi, W. C., Birk, S. A. and Holsinger, K. K. (1972). *American Journal of Obstetrics and Gynecology* **114**, 803.

Tatra, G., Breitenecker, G. and Gruber, W. (1974). *Archiv für Gynäkologie* **217**, 383.

PREGNANCY-ASSOCIATED PLASMA PROTEIN A.
A MEASURE OF PLACENTAL AGEING

R. Smith, W. Cooper and M. A. R. Thomson

Department of Obstetrics and Gynaecology, University of Dundee, Ninewells Hospital and Medical School, Dundee, Scotland

INTRODUCTION

Plasma-associated plasma protein A (PAPP-A) is a large molecular weight protein initially isolated by Lin *et al.* (1974) and subsequently localized in the trophoblast by Lin and Halbert (1976). With Lin's antiserum, Klopper and co-workers were able to purify and measure PAPP-A (Bischof, 1979; Bischof *et al.*, 1979). Preliminary studies in normal pregnancy (Smith *et al.*, 1979) suggest a rising trend of this protein through the last trimester and into labour. Using the Aberdeen standard and antiserum, we addressed ourselves to a detailed appraisal of the rise of PAPP-A with the onset of labour. The change in the levels of PAPP-A are compared in normal onset and induced labour.

PATIENTS AND METHODS

Healthy volunteers were found from the routine antenatal clinic in Dundee. Six primigravidae with uncomplicated pregnancies, who went into labour spontaneously, had blood samples taken in the course of routine antenatal visits from 30 to 38 weeks and daily thereafter. Further samples were taken in advanced labour, i.e. between 5 cm and full dilatation of the cervix. Other samples were collected from 14 normal patients at their last antenatal visit and during advanced spontaneous labour. These were matched for the same time interval of sampling

Serono Symposium No. 35, "The Human Placenta", edited by A. Klopper, A. Genazzani and P. G. Crosignani, 1980. Academic Press, London and New York.

± 87.2 (s.d.) units per millilitre in advanced labour, and for the spontaneous labouring group 108 ± 69.0 rising to 113 ± 72.4 units of PAPP-A per millilitre. PAPP-A was measured by Laurell immunoelectrophoresis as described by Bischof *et al.* (1979) using the same standard. One arbitrary unit of PAPP-A is 1.5063 µg of PAPP-A. Serial data for the normal onset of labour patients have been expressed as a percentage of their 36 week value and, to allow for the variable duration of pregnancy, 36 weeks to delivery has been taken as a unit of time for each patient, in order to build a composite pattern of PAPP-A change until labour. To eliminate absolute values of PAPP-A in the induced versus normal groups, PAPP-A values in advanced labour were expressed as a percentage of the last antenatal value. Results were tested for statistical significance using a one-tailed *t*-test.

RESULTS

Figure 1 shows the patterns of change of PAPP-A in the six normal patients who had daily blood samples taken from the 38th week until the onset of labour. The composite pattern of change computed from these values is shown in Fig. 2.

There was little difference in the mean PAPP-A values from the 14 patients induced as compared with the 14 patients who went into labour spontaneously; that is, the last antenatal value of PAPP-A before the onset of labour in the induced group was 123 ±74.5 (s.d.) units PAPP-A per millilitre and rose to 126

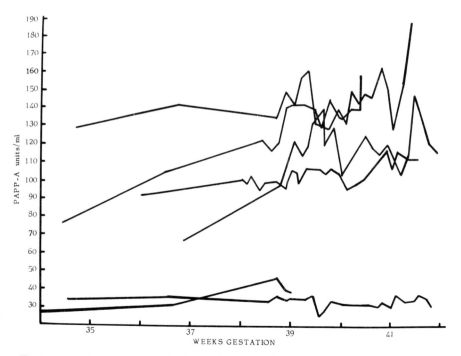

Fig. 1. PAPP-A concentrations in six primigravidae. The changes from late pregnancy to advanced labour are shown.

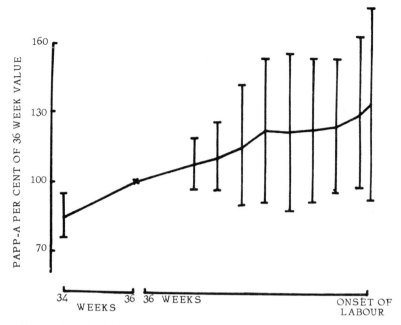

Fig. 2. Mean and standard deviation of PAPP-A in late pregnancy.

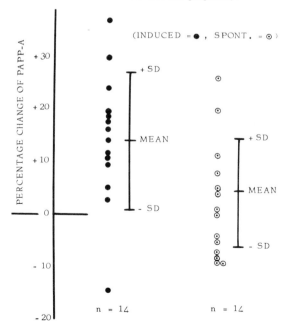

Fig. 3. The percentage change of PAPP-A in 28 patients from late pregnancy to advanced labour, induced and spontaneous onset.

to 14 patients with uncomplicated pregnancy, who were induced for social reasons or postmaturity. Plasma samples were stored at $-20\,^{\circ}$C until assayed. The mean interval between samples for each group was 3 ± 2.3 (s.d.) days. The mean duration of pregnancy was 282 ± 7.7 (s.d.) days for the spontaneous onset of labour group and 288 ± 7.0 (s.d.) days for the induced labour group ($p = 0.05$). The mean values of PAPP-A obscure the changes observed in the individuals from each group. This change is expressed in Fig. 3, as a percentage change from the last antenatal value to the advanced labour value. All but one of the induced group showed an increase of PAPP-A whereas half of the spontaneous labourers showed a decrease of PAPP-A. The mean percentage change was 14 ± 12.5 (s.d.)% for the induced patients and 4 ± 10.3 (s.d.)% for the spontaneous labouring patients ($p < 0.01$) (*see* Fig. 3).

DISCUSSION

Considering the six patients who had blood taken daily from the 38th week until the onset of labour, it is evident that there is a good deal of variation from one patient to another. When these values were manipulated in such a way as to eliminate absolute values and corrected for varying duration of each pregnancy, there would appear to be a rising trend of PAPP-A into labour in normal pregnancy on average. However, the in-labour value could be predicted by the pattern of change in the two previous samples in all but one example, although the trend was so small in three cases as to be insignificant in terms of the sensitivity of the assay. Of the remaining three, two showed a clear increase into labour and one a clear decrease.

The comparison of the rate of increase of PAPP-A between the 14 patients of the induced labour group and the patients in the spontaneous onset of labour group showed a higher percentage increase in the induced patients from the last antenatal sample to the in-labour sample. The trend was, with only one exception, an increase. The only clinical difference between these two groups of patients was the duration of pregnancy and the absence of spontaneous labour.

It has been suggested (Smith *et al.*, 1979) that PAPP-A might enter the circulation as trophoblastic microemboli, which subsequently die in the lungs over the next 2–3 days. Attwood and Park (1961) described such a phenomenon, indicating that it may be increased with uterine activity. Turnbull and Anderson (1971) describe the pattern of uterine activity in patients who labour spontaneously at term as commencing at about 36 weeks. This activity appears later in patients going past dates. We believe that our findings could be explained as follows. PAPP-A levels in late pregnancy increase with increasing placental size. As the placenta ages and its growth slows down, PAPP-A continues to rise as the mechanical trauma of uterine activity debrides the placenta of potential microemboli. In patients going into labour at term the PAPP-A trend is indicative of this process having occurred for several weeks before labour. In the induced, mainly post-dates pregnancies, the time scale is probably foreshortened and the placenta older. If these concepts are borne out, PAPP-A trends may indicate rates of embolism from the placenta, perhaps influenced by a variety of obstetric disease, which could provide a new approach for evaluating placental status.

ACKNOWLEDGEMENTS

We are indebted to Professor Klopper and Paul Bischof in Aberdeen for their help and the provision of antisera and standards, and to the Tayside Health Board for financial assistance for this work.

REFERENCES

Attwood, H. D. and Park, W. W. (1961). *Journal of Obstetrics and Gynaecology of the British Commonwealth* **68**, 61.

Bischof, P. (1979). Submitted for publication.

Bischof, P., Bruce, D., Cunningham, P. and Klopper, A. (1979). *Clinica chimica Acta* **95**, 243.

Lin, T. M., Halbert, S. P., Kiefer, D., Spellacy, W. N. and Gall, S. (1974). *American Journal of Obstetrics and Gynecology* **118**, 223.

Lin, T. M. and Halbert, S. P. (1976). *Science, New York* **193**, 1249.

Smith, R., Bischof, P., Hughes, G. and Klopper, A. (1979). *British Journal of Obstetrics and Gynaecology* **86**, 882.

Turnbull, A. and Anderson, A. (1971). *In* "Scientific Basis of Obstetrics and Gynaecology" (R. R. MacDonald, ed.), p. 64, J. & A. Churchill, Edinburgh.

A COMPARISON BETWEEN HUMAN PLACENTAL LACTOGEN (hPL) AND PREGNANCY-SPECIFIC β_1-GLOBULIN (SP$_1$)

J. Guibal, R. Donati, T. Oudghiri[1], J.-L. Viala[1] and J.-M. Bastide

Laboratory of Immunology, Faculté de Pharmacie, 34060 Montpellier, and [1] Obstetrics Clinic, 34000 Montpellier, France

INTRODUCTION

During pregnancy the placenta produces a variety of hormones and proteins whose levels increase gradually in maternal blood. Among these proteins of various importance, and whose role in many instances is unknown, human placental lactogen (hPL and pregnancy-specific β_1-globulin (SP$_1$) have attracted the interest of researchers and clinicians. Workers such as Cedard (1977), Gordon *et al.* (1977), Lin *et al.* (1977), Towler *et al.* (1976, 1977), Viala *et al.* (1979) have tried to establish a correlation between serum concentration and the fetoplacental unit. The results are based on statistical analysis and must be interpreted with great care in the light of new developments in the area. hPL has the advantage of having a known chemical structure and being detectable in serum as early as the 5th week of pregnancy by radioimmunoassay. Its serum level increases until the 37th week of pregnancy, after which it decreases progressively until delivery, as demonstrated by Lindberg and Nilsson (1973). The half-life of hPL is 10–30 min, which is relatively short. The hPL assay thus reflects immediate hormone production. Production of this hormone has a direct relationship to the placental weight according to Josimovich (1970) and Spellacy (1972). SP$_1$ is a glycoprotein detectable very early in maternal blood by radioimmunoassay (Bohn, 1978). However, the recent discovery by Teisner *et al.* (1978) of another pregnancy-associated serum protein which exhibits pregnancy-specific β_1-glycoprotein determinants may influence the results. SP$_1$ serum level increases parallel to hPL concentration,

Serono Symposium No. 35, "The Human Placenta", edited by A. Klopper,
A. Genazzani and P. G. Crosignani, 1980. Academic Press, London and New York.

but at a level 20 times higher. However, a strict correlation between hPL and SP_1 production has not been found by all researchers (Esteve and Foby, 1978; Gordon *et al.*, 1977; Towler *et al.*, 1976). The usual assay methods are radial immuno-diffusion and radioimmunoassay. Radioimmunoassays are more sensitive and allow early accurate detection of proteins, but must be performed in specialized laboratories where a gamma-counter is available. Radial immunodiffusion, although simple, lacks accuracy; the results are not useful before 20 weeks and are unreliable before 30 weeks. In addition it takes 48 h to reach the end-point. This is why we have developed a rapid, easy and reliable method using electroimmunodiffusion assay, that can be performed in any laboratory (Guibal *et al.*, 1976; Donati *et al.*, 1978). From results collected at various stages of pregnancy, we have established curves showing hPL and SP_1 concentrations as a function of time. Then we looked back at the outcome of the pregnancy to establish the value of the above method in the prognosis of high risk pregnancy.

MATERIALS AND METHODS

Sera

One thousand consecutive serum samples were obtained at the Montpellier Obstetrical Clinic from out-patients from the 6th week of pregnancy to term.

Reagents and Equipment

Barbitone buffer (pH 8.6) was used for gel preparation and for electrophoresis. Indubiose A 37 was supplied by I.B.F. Rabbit antisera to hPL and SP_1 were supplied by Behring Laboratories. Tannic acid (2%) was used to increase precipi-tation of the protein. Coomassie brilliant blue R solution was used for staining the precipitated protein. Electrophoresis was carried out in a U 77 Shandon with a Vokam CC power pack to stabilize the current. Plate sizes were 8 cm x 8 cm.

Technique

Rocket immunoelectrophoresis was performed in 1% indubiose A 37. Antisera concentration in agarose gels ranged from 0.8 to 1.2% (v/v) for SP_1 determination and from 0.3 to 0.6% for hPL determination (depending on batches).

The wells were cut 15 mm from the plate edges. For hPL determination the wells were made with a 5 mm cutter and 30 μl serum or standard put in each. For SP_1 determination the wells were made with a 1.5 mm cutter and 2 μl of serum or standard put in each.

A potential of 2.5 V/cm was applied. Electrophoresis was performed in barbi-tone buffer for 6 h for hPL and 5 h for SP_1.

After migration, the plates were removed and the precipitated proteins were intensified for 15 min in a 2% tannic acid bath or coloured with Coomassie brilliant blue R solution if the plates were to be preserved.

Measurements

Measurements of rockets were performed with a calibrating radial immuno-diffusion viewer from Transidyne General Corporation.

RESULTS AND DISCUSSION

As a preliminary study, our electroimmunodiffusion assay was compared with the radial immunodiffusion assay using Partigen plates supplied by Behring Laboratories. The correlation coefficient was $r = 0.945$ for SP_1 determination and $r = 0.945$ for hPL determination. There is thus an excellent correlation between the two methods.

The hPL and SP_1 curves increase gradually during pregnancy, but individual differences, most likely related to placental weight, are especially wide in the third trimester (see Figs 1 and 2). The statistical analysis, based on samples for each week, did not allow us to establish a curve corresponding to the superior

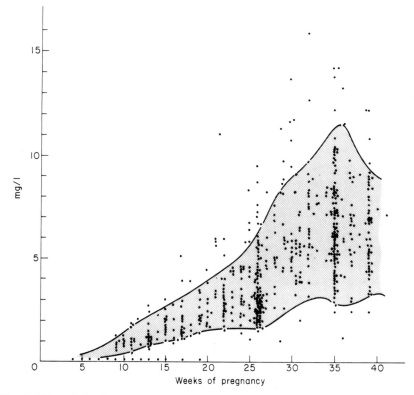

Fig. 1. hPL variation in maternal blood.

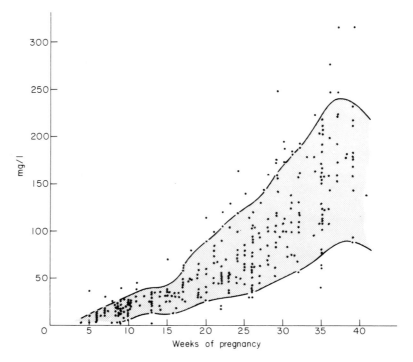

Fig. 2. SP$_1$ variation in maternal blood.

and inferior biological limits, within ± two standard deviations. This is probably due to a certain heterogeneity and also because some sample populations were, according to Sandor *et al.* (1970), too small (< 30). The results were expressed as a collection of points from which we defined a shaded zone, limited by two curves delimiting the upper and lower observed values. We consider that all values that are situated outside or near the edge of the shaded zone are doubtful. Our curves showing the hPL variations increase gradually until 34–36 weeks of gestation, stabilize, and then fall during the last 4 weeks. The curves that show the variation of SP$_1$ are similar to those showing the variations of hPL, but they fall in the 37th week.

Furthermore, we found an excellent correlation between the concentrations of hPL and those of SP$_1$ ($r = 0.916$).

In our study, 30 cases of high risk pregnancy, each providing more than five measurements, were analysed. Our conclusion is that SP$_1$ concentration is more representative of placental function than hPL concentration.

1. Among these 30 pregnancies there were two twin pregnancies for which the increase of SP$_1$ concentration was larger than for hPL.
2. Three low birthweight newborns were observed (a 2.600 kg female and two males of 2.450 kg and 2.090 kg) for which low concentrations were more significant. We also observed two cases in whom hPL concentrations were low

enough to expect low birthweight newborns, but with normal SP$_1$ concentrations. At delivery normal birthweight babies were born; this confirms the usefulness of SP$_1$ concentration as an aid in prognosis.

3.   There were two cases of non-viable births, one with a heart defect, the other one was a cyclops. Concentrations of SP$_1$ and hPL were in the low range, but again the drop in SP$_1$ concentration was more important.

4.   In the 21 other cases, pregnancy was normal up to delivery, with the birth of normal infants. SP$_1$ and hPL concentrations were within usual limits.

The measurement of circulating levels of hPL and SP$_1$ seems to be very useful for monitoring normal and abnormal pregnancies. It would be best to avoid single measurements. It seems reasonable to us to take multiple samples for a single pregnancy beginning in the 4th month for hPL and the 8th week for SP$_1$, being careful to consider as normal those values which fall in the centre of the shaded zone. We should consider doubtful those points falling outside or near the edge of the shaded zone, as well as a situation in which the concentrations of hPL and SP$_1$ do not increase in a parallel fashion.

REFERENCES

Bohn, H. (1978). *Scandinavian Journal of Immunology* 7, 119.

Cedard, L. (1977). *Gynecologie et obstétrique* 7, 105.

Donati, R., Guibal, J. and Scheiber, D. (1978). *Feuillets de biologie* 19, 101.

Esteve, M. and Foby, M. C. (1978). *Journal de gynécologie, obstétrique et biologie de la reproduction* 7, 419.

Gordon, Y., Grudzinskas, J., Lewis, J., Jeffrey, D. and Letchworth, A. (1977). *British Journal of Obstetrics and Gynaecology* 84, 642.

Guibal, J., Donati, R. and Bastide, J.-M. (1976). *Microbia* 2, 3.

Josimovich, J. B. (1970). *Obstetrics and Gynecology* 36, 249.

Lin, T. M., Halbert, S. M., Spellacy, W. N. and Berne, B. H. (1977). *American Journal of Obstetrics and Gynecology* 128, 808.

Lindberg, B. S. and Nilsson, B. A. (1973). *Journal of Obstetrics and Gynaecology of the British Commonwealth* 80, 619.

Sandor, G., Sandor, N. and Orley, C. (1970). *Annales de biologie clinique* 28, 309.

Spellacy, W. N. (1972). *In* "Lactogenic Hormones" (Wolstenholme and Knight, eds). Ciba Foundation Symposium p. 263, Elsevier/North Holland, Amsterdam.

Teisner, B., Westergaard, J., Folkersen, J., Husby, S. and Svehag, S. E. (1978). *American Journal of Obstetrics and Gynecology* 131, 262.

Towler, C. M., Horne, C. H. W., Jandial, V. and Campbell, D. M. (1976). *British Journal of Obstetrics and Gynaecology* 83, 775.

Towler, C. M., Horne, C. H. W., Jandial, V. and Campbell, D. M. (1977). *British Journal of Obstetrics and Gynaecology* 84, 258.

Viala, J. L., Bastide, J.-M., Guibal, J., Oudghiri, T. and Donati, R. (1979). *Journal de gynécologie, obstétrique et biologie de la reproduction* in press.

CIRCULATING LEVELS OF A HIGH MOLECULAR WEIGHT PREGNANCY-SPECIFIC PROTEIN (SP$_4$) IN NORMAL AND PATHOLOGICAL PREGNANCIES

J. G. Westergaard, J. Folkersen[1], P. Hindersson[1] and B. Teisner[1]

Department of Obstetrics and Gynaecology, Odense University Hospital, and [1] Institute of Medical Microbiology, Odense University, Odense, Denmark

INTRODUCTION

The preparation of monospecific antisera to a high molecular weight pregnancy-specific protein, SP$_4$, and the purification of this protein by affinity chromatography has been described elsewhere (Folkersen *et al.*, 1979a). Antisera to pregnancy-associated plasma protein A (PAPP-A) (Lin *et al.*, 1974a,b), kindly supplied by Drs Halbert and Lin, Miami, U.S.A., were shown to react with SP$_4$, and the two proteins are probably identical (Folkersen *et al.*, 1979a). A highly sensitive line radioimmunoelectrophoresis has been developed using purified radiolabelled SP$_4$ and monospecific rabbit SP$_4$ antiserum (Folkersen *et al.*, 1979b).

This report describes preliminary data on SP$_4$ measurements in consecutive serum samples from women with prospectively normal pregnancies compared to measurements of SP$_4$ in twin pregnancies and pregnancies with intrauterine growth retardation.

MATERIALS AND METHODS

The SP$_4$ concentration was measured in 705 serum samples drawn serially throughout pregnancy from 86 women admitted to the Department of Obstetrics

Serono Symposium No. 35, "The Human Placenta", edited by A. Klopper, A. Genazzani and P. G. Crosignani, 1980. Academic Press, London and New York.

and the Antenatal Clinic of Odense University Hospital. All women entering the study were white, born of Danish parents and free of chronic diseases before the pregnancy. Initially 61 women were selected using strict criteria of obstetric normality. In the event 51 of these had a normal pregnancy and went on to deliver a normal baby at term. Of the remaining 10 subjects, two presented with intra-uterine fetal death at 33 and 40 weeks. Neither showed any sign of maternal disease or congenital defect, but severe fetal growth retardation was observed in both instances. Six other women also delivered growth-retarded babies, i.e. a birthweight below the 5th percentile of the local normal range (Ulrich, 1979). Two of these also had severe pre-eclampsia with a diastolic blood pressure above 110 mm Hg, albuminuria greater than 300 mg/l and hypertonic retinal changes. The remaining two women both gave birth to twins after a normal pregnancy.

In addition, 147 serial serum samples from 25 women with clearly defined obstetric pathology were included in this study. Seventeen women gave birth to twins; five of these being delivered prematurely between the 32nd and the 36th week after otherwise uncomplicated pregnancies (99 samples). The remaining eight women delivered infants with growth retardation, and two of these preg-nancies were complicated with severe pre-eclampsia.

Sera

Blood samples were drawn weekly up to the 15th week from women entering the study in the first trimester of pregnancy, and thereafter at intervals of 2–6 weeks until delivery. For women entering the project in the second trimester, blood samples were taken at 20, 30, 32, 36, 38, 39 and 40 weeks of pregnancy. When the diagnosis of twins or intrauterine growth retardation was suspected, blood samples were drawn weekly. None of the blood samples examined were drawn from women in labour. Serum samples were divided into eight aliquots, four stored at $-20\,°C$ and four at $-60\,°C$; all serum samples in the study were stored at $-20\,°C$ until measurement.

Rocket Line Radioimmunoelectrophoresis

SP_4 was determined by rocket line radioimmunoelectrophoresis using mono-specific rabbit antiserum to SP_4 and ^{125}I-labelled SP_4, as described in detail elsewhere (Folkersen *et al.*, 1979b). The electrophoresis was performed in 10.5 cm × 20 cm glass plates with a 1.5 mm layer of 1% agarose (Indubiose A-37, L'Industrie Biologique Française, Clichy, France). The radiolabelled SP_4 was incorporated in a line gel (0.5 cm × 20.5 cm) cast on the lower part of the plate, and the antibody containing gel above the line gel. The electrophoresis was performed at 2.5 V/cm for 18 h using Tris-barbital buffer, pH 8.6; ionic strength 0.02. Six wells were filled by a dilution series of a pool of late pregnancy serum. Two wells were quality controls using serum samples from women in the 40th and 10th weeks of pregnancy diluted 1:32 and 1:2. A standard (diluted 1:32) prepared from pooled late pregnancy serum collected from 200 women in the third trimester of pregnancy was used. The standard was defined as containing 100 arbitrary units (AU) of SP_4 per millilitre. (1 AU equals 590 ng.) Consecutive samples from one woman were always examined on the same plate. The intrassay variation and the interassay variation was 3 and 7% respectively.

RESULTS

Normal Pregnancies

Using rocket line radioimmunoelectrophoresis, SP_4 was detectable in serum from the 6th week of pregnancy. Figure 1 shows the serum concentration of SP_4 in consecutive serum samples from 11 pregnant women with prospectively normal pregnancies. Until the 12th week of pregnancy, serum SP_4 increased about 100% per week, whereas the same relative increase occurred over a 2–3 week period between the 12th and 16th weeks. Pregnant women with SP_4 concentrations in the upper part of the range in the first trimester also showed the highest concentrations throughout the second and third trimesters of pregnancy (Fig. 1).

Figure 2 shows SP_4 concentrations from 40 prospectively normal pregnant women in the second and third trimester of pregnancy. In 49 of 51 normal pregnancies the serum SP_4 concentration continued to increase until delivery and a more marked increase in concentration was observed in the last 14 days before delivery (Figs 1 and 2).

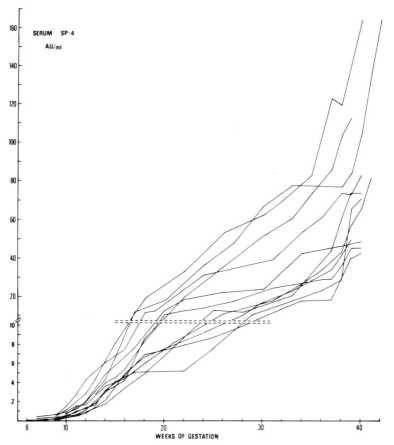

Fig. 1. Serial assays of SP_4 in serum from 11 prospectively normal pregnant women (183 samples, 11–21 samples per woman). Dashed line indicates change in the ordinate scale.

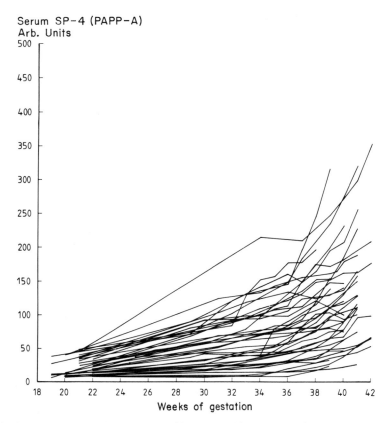

Fig. 2. SP$_4$ concentration in serum from 40 women with prospectively normal pregnancies; 301 samples drawn from the 20th week of pregnancy to delivery were examined.

Twin Pregnancies

The changes in the serum concentration of SP$_4$ in *19* twin pregnancies is shown in Fig. 3. Eight of the twin pregnancies showed concentrations higher than, or in the upper part of, the normal range, whereas the SP$_4$ levels in 11 twin pregnancies fell in the middle values of the normal range. As in normal pregnancies, most of the twin pregnancies showed a steeper increase in SP$_4$ concentration in the last few weeks of pregnancy.

Intrauterine Growth Retardation

The SP$_4$ concentrations in pregnant women where the pregnancy was associated with intrauterine growth retardation are shown in Fig. 4. The serum concentrations corresponded to those in the lower half of the normal range, but the gradual rise in concentration did not appear to be different from that of normal pregnancies. In two of these pregnancies intrauterine fetal death occurred, but in only one of these cases was a terminal decrease (10%) of SP$_4$ concentration observed.

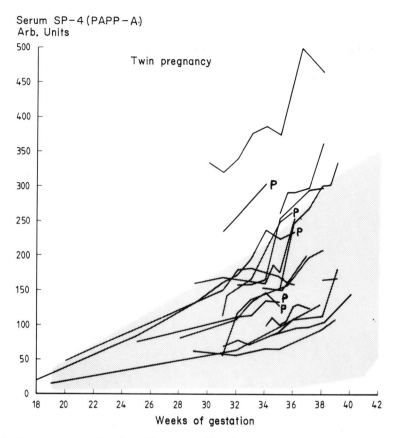

Fig. 3. Serum concentration from 19 women with twin pregnancies (112 samples; 3–9 samples per woman). The shaded area represents the normal range as shown in Fig. 2. P indicates premature birth.

DISCUSSION

The occurrence of PAPP-A in the plasma of pregnant women has been previously described by Lin *et al.* (1974a,b). These authors have also characterized the protein and described its presence in the trophoblast layer in the placenta (Lin and Halbert, 1976). Measurement of circulating PAPP-A was described by Lin *et al.* (1974b), who, by the use of an electroimmunoassay, could detect PAPP-A in plasma of pregnant women from the 20th week of pregnancy.

In the present study, PAPP-A (SP₄) was detected in all pregnant women examined by use of a rocket line radioimmunoassay. Consecutive measurements on a well-defined group of normal pregnancies showed a rise in SP₄ concentration from the 6th week of pregnancy to delivery without great fluctuations. As with other proteins like SP₁ and hPL, which are also derived from the placenta,

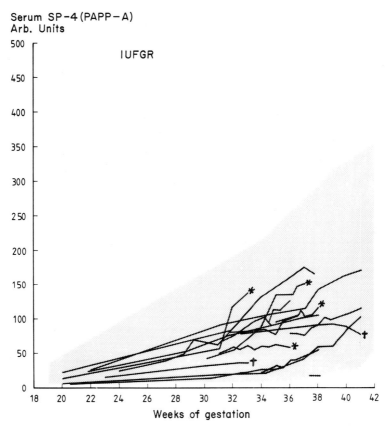

Fig. 4. Serial analyses of serum SP$_4$ concentration from 16 women with pregnancies associated with intrauterine fetal growth retardation (IUFGR) (3–13 samples per woman; total 109 samples). The shaded area indicates the normal range as shown in Fig. 2. x, Severe preeclampsia; +, intrauterine fetal death.

the serum concentrations of SP$_4$ show considerable variation in women with normal pregnancies. However, the serum concentration range is fairly constant from the 20th to the 40th week of pregnancy, which has previously been found to be the case also for SP$_1$ (Gordon *et al.*, 1977) and hPL (Westergaard *et al.*, 1979). In contrast to SP$_1$ and hPL, where the serum concentrations tend to reach a plateau or to decrease slowly after the 36th week of pregnancy, the gradual rise in SP$_4$ concentration was shown to continue up to delivery. In addition, in a considerable number of pregnancies, the increase in SP$_4$ concentration is steeper in the last 1–2 weeks before delivery than in the preceding 10 weeks. This may indicate a difference in the biological function of SP$_4$ as compared to other proteins of placental origin.

This preliminary investigation of the serum concentration of SP$_4$ in pregnancy is based on consecutive blood samples and the material is not adequate for the determination of a normal reference range. Neither can an exact evaluation of the distribution of the concentrations of SP_4 in normal pregnancies versus pathological pregnancies be made.

In the daily clinical examination of pregnant women the biochemical monitoring of patients at risk will often be performed by serial assays where the patient serves as her own control. In the present investigation both twin pregnancies and pregnancies associated with intrauterine growth retardation were selected from a larger material of blood samples due to the well-defined clinical picture in these patients. In spite of this, the serial SP_4 determinations evaluated retrospectively did not give any clear indication of the pathological nature of the pregnancies. The gradual change in the serum concentration of SP_4 for twin pregnancies followed a similar course as for normal pregnancies in the upper part of the normal concentration range. However, the variation in the concentration values was considerable.

When the serum concentrations of SP_4 in women giving birth to growth-retarded children were compared with the concentrations in women with normal pregnancies, no striking differences were observed. The gradual rise in SP_4 was within the same concentration range for both groups. Even intrauterine fetal death caused no dramatic changes in the SP_4 concentration. However, in one patient a terminal fall of 10% in SP_4 concentration was observed between the 38th and 40th weeks. Four patients with a combination of intrauterine fetal growth retardation and serious pre-eclampsia did not differ significantly in SP_4 concentration from other patients in the fetal growth-retarded group. The SP_4 levels were found to vary considerably in the intrauterine fetal growth-retarded group of patients in contrast to what has been reported earlier for SP_1 and hPL concentrations in these patients.

The results of the present study do not allow definite conclusions concerning the possible usefulness of SP_4 determinations as a marker of placental function. However, the results presented here suggest that SP_4 determinations may be of limited value in this respect in spite of the fact that SP_4 measurements show little day-to-day variation and that the SP_4 concentration in serum is relatively high after the 20th week of pregnancy, factors which facilitate the measurement of this protein. It is clear that further investigations are needed to evaluate the potential usefulness of serum SP_4 determinations in screening for specific diseases during pregnancy.

ACKNOWLEDGEMENT

This work was supported by P. Carl Petersens fund and the Danish Medical Research Council (Project no. 512-10202). Thanks are due to Mrs Hanne Clausen and Mrs Jette Brandt for skilful technical assistance.

REFERENCES

Folkersen, J., Westergaard, J. G., Hindersson, P. and Teisner, B. (1979a). *In* "Carcino-Embryonic Proteins" (F. G. Lehman, ed.), Vol. 2, p. 503, Elsevier/ North Holland, Amsterdam.

Folkersen, J., Hindersson, P., Westergaard, J. G. and Teisner, B. (1979b). *Journal of Immunological Methods* in press.

Gordon, Y. B., Grudzinskas, J. G., Lewis, J. D., Jeffrey, D. and Letchworth, A. T. (1977). *British Journal of Obstetrics and Gynaecology* **84**, 642.

Lin, T. M. and Halbert, S. P. (1976). *Science, New York* **193**, 1249.

Lin, T. M., Halbert, S. P. and Spellacy, W. N. (1974b). *Journal of Clinical Investigation* **54**, 576.

Lin, T. M., Halbert, S. P., Kiefer, D., Spellacy, W. N. and Gall, S. (1974a). *American Journal of Obstetrics and Gynecology* **118**, 223.

Ulrich, M. (1979). *Acta paediatrica scandinavica*, Suppl., in press.

Westergaard, J. G. and Gæde, P. (1979). *Acta obstetrica et gynecologia scandinavica* submitted.

PLACENTAL PROTEIN 5: DISTRIBUTION AND PHYSIOLOGICAL VARIATIONS IN LATE PREGNANCY

B. C. Obiekwe, J. G. Grudzinskas and T. Chard

Departments of Obstetrics and Gynaecology, and Reproductive Physiology, St. Bartholomew's Hospital, London, U.K.

INTRODUCTION

Placental protein 5 (PP_5) is one of a new generation of recently identified proteins produced by the human syncytiotrophoblast (Bohn, 1972; Bohn and Winckler, 1977). PP_5 has β_1-electrophoretic mobility, a molecular weight of 36 000 daltons, and a carbohydrate content of 19%. The development of a sensitive and specific radioimmunoassay (RIA) for PP_5 (Obiekwe *et al.*, 1979) has permitted the measurement of circulating levels during pregnancy hitherto not possible using immunodiffusion techniques.

SUBJECTS, MATERIALS AND METHODS

Compartment Study

Maternal blood and urine, amniotic fluid, and fetal umbilical arterial and venous blood were obtained at term delivery in 13 women.

Normal Range Study

Blood samples (752) were obtained from 400 women from 28 to 40 weeks of gestation.

Serono Symposium No. 35, "The Human Placenta", edited by A. Klopper, A. Genazzani and P. G. Crosignani, 1980. Academic Press, London and New York.

Time-to-time Variation Study

A total of 250 blood samples were obtained from five subjects in the third trimester at hourly intervals for 22 h and at 15 min intervals for the remaining 2 h. Each assay included 20 repeat determinations on a single sample to determine within-assay variation. A further 78 blood samples were obtained from 11 subjects on five or more consecutive days.

Half-life Study

Venous blood samples were obtained immediately prior to delivery in eight subjects at term. Further samples were obtained after delivery of the infant's head. Thereafter blood samples were obtained at 5 min intervals for 45 min, at 15 min intervals for 2 h, and hourly for 9 h.

Intrauterine Growth Retardation (IUGR) and Pre-eclampsia (PET) Study

Venous blood was obtained from 20 patients with mild to severe pre-eclampsia (diastolic blood pressure 90–110 mm Hg) and 31 patients with clinical and ultrasonic evidence of intrauterine growth retardation at 36–40 weeks of gestation.

Radioimmunoassay (RIA) of PP_5

Serum was separated within 1 h of blood collection and stored at $-20\,^{\circ}$C until assayed as described previously (Obiekwe *et al.*, 1979).

Statistical Analysis

Normal Range Study
PP_5 levels were listed according to week of gestation, ranked, and the median, 10th and 90th percentile values determined for each week of gestation.

Time-to-time Variation Study
Sample variances were calculated for each subject and compared with assay variance by the 'F' test.

IUGR and PET Study
The birthweights of 360 infants (including 20 patients with PET and 31 patients in whom IUGR had been identified clinically) were ranked and the median, 10th and 90th percentiles determined. Serum PP_5 levels from these women were ranked similarly. The sensitivity, predictive value and specificity of serum PP_5 determinations were calculated according to the equation in Table IV.

RESULTS

Compartment Study

The concentrations of PP_5 in the various fluids studied are shown in Fig. 1. The highest concentrations were found in the maternal blood and there was no

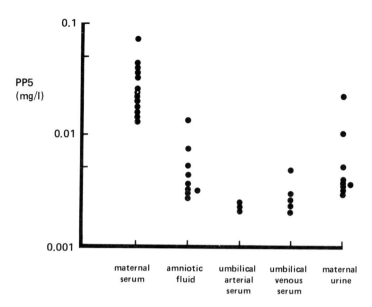

Fig. 1. Concentrations of PP$_5$ in fetal and maternal compartments. (Reproduced by permission of *British Journal of Obstetrics and Gynaecology.*)

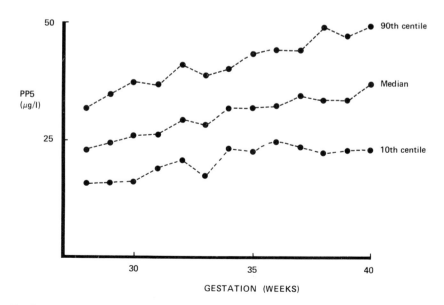

Fig. 2. The median, 10th and 90th percentiles of maternal serum PP$_5$ after 28 weeks gestation during normal pregnancy. (Reproduced by permission of *Clinica chimica acta.*)

Table I. Nyctohemeral variation of maternal serum PP_5 levels in five subjects examined over a 24 h period.

| Patient number | Number of samples | Mean PP_5 (μg/l) | Coefficient of variation (%) | Variance, H | Control sample | | | | |
					Mean PP_5 (μg/l)	Coefficient of variation (%)	Variance, C	'F' value, H/C	Probability, P
1	30	43.7	15.8	47.61	49.7	4.2	4.41	10.79	<0.001
2	31	45.9	12.6	33.64	53.7	4.2	4.84	6.95	<0.001
3	30	22.3	14.1	9.86	24.6	3.58	0.88	12.80	<0.001
4	30	35.9	11.2	16.6	42.0	3.05	1.64	9.85	<0.001
5	30	34.9	12.8	20.07	38.1	4.04	2.37	8.47	<0.001

Table II. Day-to-day variation of maternal serum PP$_5$ levels in 11 subjects studied over a 5 day period.

Patient number	Number of samples	Mean PP$_5$ (μg/l)	Coefficient of variation (%)	Variance, H	Mean PP$_5$ (μg/l)	Coefficient of variation (%)	Variance, C	'F' value, H/C	Probability, P
1	8	27.4	10.8	8.82	30.18	2.9	0.77	11.45	< 0.001
2	5	35.4	12.3	18.66	30.18	2.9	0.77	34.23	< 0.001
3	5	42.6	8.4	12.81	30.18	2.9	0.77	10.90	< 0.001
4	5	28.0	11.0	9.48	30.18	2.9	0.77	12.31	< 0.001
5	5	19.6	15.1	8.82	30.18	2.9	0.77	11.45	< 0.001
6	5	35.8	8.2	8.70	30.18	2.9	0.77	11.29	< 0.001
7	5	27.8	7.8	4.70	30.18	2.9	0.77	6.10	< 0.005
8	5	29.6	5.1	2.31	30.18	2.9	0.77	3.00	< 0.05
9	5	20.8	10.4	4.66	30.18	2.9	0.77	6.05	< 0.005
10	5	26.4	5.8	2.31	30.18	2.9	0.77	3.00	< 0.05
11	5	33.6	10.5	12.32	30.18	2.9	0.77	16.00	< 0.001

correlation between levels in this site and the other fluids examined. PP_5 levels in the various compartments were unrelated to the mode of delivery, the weight or sex of the baby, or to the placental weight.

Normal Range Study

Maternal PP_5 levels rose from a mean of 23 $\mu g/l$ at 28 weeks of gestation to 32 $\mu g/l$ at 35 weeks, and plateaued thereafter. The median and the 10th and 90th percentile values are shown in Fig. 2.

Time-to-time Variation Study

The coefficient of variation of samples obtained over a 24 h period ranged between 11.2 and 15.8% (Table I). In all cases the variation was in excess of that which could be attributed to the assay, though the variation showed no obvious pattern. The coefficient of variation of serial daily samples from 11 subjects ranged from 5.1 to 15.1% (Table II). In all cases the variation was in excess of that which could be attributed to the assay.

Half-life Study

Serum PP_5 levels fell rapidly after the delivery of the placenta, with an estimated half-life ranging from 5 to 39 min in eight patients. In the majority of subjects PP_5 levels were less than 2 $\mu g/l$ after 12 h (Table III).

IUGR and PET Study

The sensitivity and predictive value of PP_5 determinations in the detection of low birthweight babies was 14.3 and 13.9% respectively. The specificity of the determination was 90.3% (Table IV).

DISCUSSION

In common with other placental proteins, placental protein 5 is secreted selectively into the maternal compartment (Josimovich and McLaren, 1962; Grudzinskas et al., 1978). The levels in the maternal blood are one order of magnitude greater than those in the fetal circulation, which is similar to human placental lactogen, but contrasts with *Schwangerschafts* protein 1 (SP_1) in which levels are three orders of magnitude greater (Tatra et al., 1976; Grudzinskas et al., 1978). Levels of PP_5 in the other fluids examined are low, but information on other placental proteins suggests the maternal circulation is likely to be the principal source from whence the protein enters other compartments (Niven et al., 1974; Grudzinskas et al., 1978).

The concentrations of PP_5 in the maternal circulation during late pregnancy is about one-thousandth that of hPL. However, the pattern of levels, with a plateau after the 35th week, is very similar and, in common with all other feto-placental products, the normal range showed a skewed distribution (Chard, 1976). For this reason the results have been presented as a median and percentiles.

Table III. The decline of circulating levels of PP_5 in eight subjects PP_5 levels are expressed as a percentage of the level determined at the delivery of the infant's head (zero time).

Time of delivery of infant's head (min)	1	2	3	4	5	6	7	8
Zero time	100	100	100	100	100	100	100	100
+ 5	71.7	65.0	74.5	50.0	74.0	67.0	74.0	76.0
+ 10	56.5	52.0	54.8	40.4	63.0	50.0	51.4	66.0
+ 15	47.8	52.0	50.0	33.0	66.0	39.0	38.0	56.0
+ 20	51.8	48.0	45.2	31.0	63.0	38.0	35.2	50.0
+ 25	47.8	40.0	38.7	29.0	61.0	30.0	33.5	46.0
+ 30	45.6	37.6	37.0	33.0	56.0	30.0	32.0	41.0
+ 35	45.6	34.0	40.3	28.0	56.0	28.0	32.0	40.0
+ 40	41.1	31.2	35.4	25.0	48.0	29.0	31.0	38.5
+ 45	37.0	29.4	32.2	23.0	48.0	25.0	31.0	37.0
+ 60	34.8	25.2	32.2	21.0	47.0	23.0	26.0	35.0
+ 75	34.8	22.0	29.0	21.0	39.0	–	20.0	8.0
+ 90	26.0	20.8	29.0	19.0	34.0	–	–	8.0
+105	23.9	17.6	29.0	18.0	33.0	–	18.0	<6
+120	19.6	16.0	17.4	14.0	28.0	–	16.0	–
+135	19.6	14.4	19.3	15.0	25.0	–	14.0	<6
+150	17.0	13.4	23.5	14.0	23.0	–	12.0	<6
+165	12.4	10.4	19.3	12.0	20.0	–	15.0	–
+180	12.2	10.0	20.9	13.0	15.0	–	8.0	<6
+240	12.0	10.0	16.1	11.0	–	–	8.0	<6
+300	12.0	10.0	<16	12.0	–	–	8.0	<6
+360	11.0	<8	<16	11.0	–	–	–	<6
+420	10.8	<8	<16	10.4	–	–	8.0	
+480	10.0	<8	<16	7.6	–	–	6	
+540	10.0	<8	<16	–	–	–	<5	
+600	10.0	<8	<16	–	–	–	–	
+660	9.5	<8	<16	–	–	–	–	
+720	8.0	<8	<16	–	–	–	–	

Table IV. Use of maternal serum PP_5 levels at 36–40 weeks gestation in the diagnosis of intrauterine growth retardation.

$$\text{Sensitivity} = \left(\frac{TP}{TP + FN}\right) = \frac{5}{5 + 30} = 14.3\%$$

$$\text{Predictive value} = \left(\frac{TP}{TP + FP}\right) = \frac{5}{5 + 31} = 13.9\%$$

$$\text{Specificity} = \left(\frac{TN}{FP + TN}\right) = \frac{289}{289 + 31} = 90.3\%$$

Abbreviations: TP, true positive; TN, true negative; FP, false positive, FN, false negative

There are both nyctohemeral and day-to-day variations in maternal blood PP_5. However, there is no obvious pattern to the variation and it cannot therefore be described as a rhythm, nor can the variations be related to obvious physiological events such as sleep or meals. The practical implication of these studies is that a single sample from an individual for the estimation of PP_5 may not be representative of all samples taken from the individual.

This is the first description of the half-life of PP_5. An analysis of the data suggested, as with other placental proteins (Pavlou et al., 1972) that each subject has her own characteristic half-life, and that the apparent differences could not be attributed to the assay method. For this reason it is not statistically valid to calculate a mean for all subjects.

The sensitivity and predictive value of serum PP_5 determinations in late pregnancy in the detection of low birthweight babies are low (14.3 and 13.9% respectively). By contrast, SP_1 levels are low in 70-80% of pregnancies complicated by IUGR (Gordon et al., 1977).

Since the precise measurement of low circulating levels of PP_5 is difficult and preliminary clinical studies have been unpromising, there seems to be no reason at this time to suggest that PP_5 measurements present any significant clinical advance as a test of fetal and placental function in late pregnancy.

REFERENCES

Bohn, H. (1972). *Archiv für Gynäkologie* **212**, 165.
Bohn, H. and Winckler, W. (1977). *Archiv für Gynäkologie* **223**, 179.
Chard, T. (1976). *In* "Plasma Hormone Assays in Evaluation of Fetal Wellbeing" (A. Klopper, ed.), pp. 1–19, Churchill-Livingstone, Edinburgh.
Josimovich, J. B. and McLaren, J. A. (1962). *Endocrinology* **71**, 209.
Gordon, Y. B., Grudzinskas, J. G., Lewis, J. D., Jeffrey, D. and Letchworth, A. T. (1977). *British Journal of Obstetrics and Gynaecology* **84**, 642.
Grudzinskas, J. G., Evans, D. G., Gordon, Y. B., Jeffrey, D. and Chard, T. (1978). *Obstetrics and Gynecology* **52**, 43.
Niven, P. A. R., Ward, R. H. T. and Chard, T. (1974). *Journal of Obstetrics and Gynaecology of the British Commonwealth* **81**, 988.
Obiekwe, B. C., Pendlebury, D. J., Gordon, Y. B., Grudzinskas, J. G., Chard, T. and Bohn, H. (1979). *Clinica chimica acta* **95**, 509.
Pavlou, C., Chard, T. and Letchworth, A. T. (1972). *Journal of Obstetrics and Gynaecology of the British Commonwealth* **79**, 629.
Tatra, G., Polak, S. and Placheta, P. (1976). *Archiv für Gynäkologie* **221**, 161.

DAILY VARIATIONS OF HUMAN PLACENTAL LACTOGEN (hPL), PREGNANCY-SPECIFIC β_1-GLYCOPROTEIN (SP$_1$), AND CYSTINE AMINOPEPTIDASE (CAP)

G. Cocilovo, F. Vesce, G. Logallo[1] and L. Pittini

Department of Obstetrics and Gynaecology, University of Ferrara, and [1] Laboratory of Clinical Chemistry and Microbiology, Arcispedale S. Anna, Ferrara, Italy

INTRODUCTION

Several aspects, such as degree of correlation with clinical findings and individual and daily variability, need to be considered in the choice of a reliable indicator of placental function.

Recently it has been demonstrated that measurement of some placental proteins presents the advantage of smaller day-to-day variations by comparison with steroids (Masson *et al.*, 1977).

In this study the daily variability of hPL, SP$_1$ and CAP in late pregnancy has been investigated.

MATERIALS AND METHODS

Plasma levels of hPL, SP$_1$ and CAP were measured over a period of six successive days in seven healthy subjects at 34–35 weeks of gestation.

hPL was estimated by radioimmunoassay, SP$_1$ by radial immunodiffusion, and CAP by the method of Tuppy and Nesvadba as modified by Babuna and Yenen (1966).

Serono Symposium No. 35, "The Human Placenta", edited by A. Klopper, A. Genazzani and P. G. Crosignani, 1980. Academic Press, London and New York.

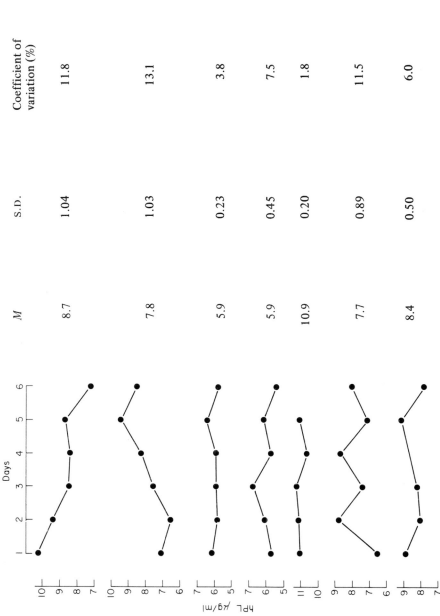

	M	S.D.	Coefficient of variation (%)
	8.7	1.04	11.8
	7.8	1.03	13.1
	5.9	0.23	3.8
	5.9	0.45	7.5
	10.9	0.20	1.8
	7.7	0.89	11.5
	8.4	0.50	6.0

Fig. 1. Day-to-day variations in plasma hPL in seven pregnant women over a period of six successive days. Average coefficient

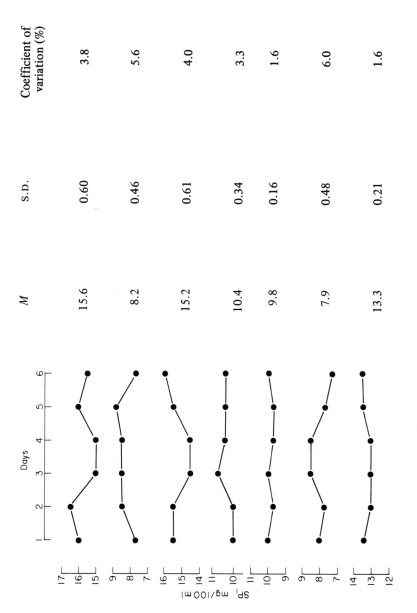

Fig. 2. Day-to-day variations in plasma SP$_1$ in pregnant women over a period of six successive days. Average coefficient of variation: 3.7% (range: 1.6–6%).

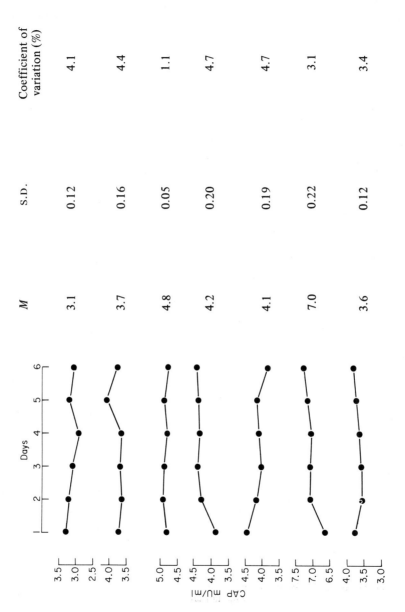

Fig. 3. Day-to-day variations in plasma cystine aminopeptidase (CAP) in seven pregnant women over a period of six successive days. Average coefficient of variation: 3.6% (range: 1.1–4.7%).

RESULTS

The average coefficient of variation was 7.9% (range: 1.8–13.1%) for hPL (Fig. 1), 3.7% (range: 1.6–6%) for SP_1 (Fig. 2), and 3.6% (range: 1.1–4.7%) for CAP (Fig. 3).

DISCUSSION

Few data are available about time-to-time variation of SP_1 and CAP in late pregnancy. More information exists about hPL (Spellacy *et al.*, 1966; Samaan *et al.*, 1966; Grumbach *et al.*, 1968; Teoh *et al.*, 1971; Pavlou *et al.*, 1972; Lindberg and Nilsson, 1973). Recently Masson *et al.* (1977) reported low day-to-day variability for hPL and SP_1 at the 38th week of pregnancy (5.6 and 4.8% respectively). Our findings at 34–35 weeks of gestation agree fairly closely with data of these authors. Small changes were also found by us in the case of CAP, while higher values (17%) had previously been obtained by Carter *et al.* (1974).

It is noteworthy that low variability has been found for all proteins studied, in spite of many methodological and physiological factors which can vary their plasma concentrations. The clinical importance of these findings is that serial assays can be more easily interpreted in the evaluation of placental function.

REFERENCES

Babuna, C. and Yenen, E. (1966). *American Journal of Obstetrics and Gynecology* **95**, 925.

Carter, E. R., Goodman, L. V., DeHaan, R. and Sobota, J. T. (1974). *American Journal of Obstetrics and Gynecology* **119**, 76.

Grumbach, M. M., Kaplan, S. L., Sciarra, J. J. and Burr, I. M. (1968). *Annals of the New York Academy of Sciences* **148**, 501.

Lindberg, S. and Nilsson, A. (1973). *Journal of Obstetrics and Gynaecology of the British Commonwealth* **80**, 619.

Masson, G. M., Klopper, A. I. and Wilson, G. R. (1977). *Obstetrics and Gynaecology* **50**, 435.

Pavlou, C., Chard, T. and Letchworth, A. T. (1972). *Journal of Obstetrics and Gynaecology of the British Commonwealth* **79**, 629.

Samaan, N., Yen, S. S. C., Friesen, H. and Pearson, O. H. (1966). *Journal of Clinical Endocrinology* **26**, 1303.

Spellacy, W. N., Carlson, K. L. and Birk, S. A. (1966). *American Journal of Obstetrics and Gynecology* **96**, 1164.

Teoh, E. S., Spellacy, W. N. and Buhi, W. C. (1971). *Journal of Obstetrics and Gynaecology of the British Commonwealth* **78**, 673.

PREGNANCY PROTEINS AND THE IMMUNE SYSTEM
IN THE RAT

S. Cianci, N. Corbino, G. Palumbo and F. Stivala[1]

*Departments of Obstetrics and Gynaecology, and [1] General Pathology,
University of Catania, Catania, Italy*

INTRODUCTION

Pregnancy has until now been considered a biological paradox since the fetal allograft is not rejected by the maternal host. Many hypotheses have been proposed to explain this problem: (1) the uterus as privileged site; (2) the lack of antigenic and or immunogenic properties of the trophoblast; (3) the peculiar behaviour of the immune competent system of the maternal host toward trophoblastic HI-A antigens, which are foreign to the mother as they are partly of paternal origin. The last hypothesis is commonly accepted, although the mechanisms of this system are not well known.

Chorionic gonadotrophin (hCG) has been advocated by many authors as the main modulator of the maternal immune competent system *in vivo* (Adcock *et al.*, 1973; Jenkins *et al.*, 1972; Stivala *et al.*, 1974). This is confirmed by the abortificient activity of anti-hCG antibodies in the outbred pregnant rat. The same anti-hCG antibodies show a contraceptive action in the early pregnant rat (Stivala *et al.*, 1974; Corbino, 1978).

The observation that a similar effect (full inhibition of lymphocyte response to PHA and MLR) is obtainable *in vitro* only at tremendously high doses of hCG (10 000 IU/ml) (Adcock *et al.*, 1973; Teasdale *et al.*, 1973), and the impossibility of showing lymphocyte surface receptors (F. Stivala and N. Corbino, unpublished data) suggested the need to look for other possible responsible factors. The main

Serono Symposium No. 35, "The Human Placenta", edited by A. Klopper,
A. Genazzani and P. G. Crosignani, 1980. Academic Press, London and New York.

possible factors might be pregnancy-associated proteins such as pregnancy-associated globulins. It seems that α_2-macroglobulin ($\alpha_2 M$) is capable of inhibiting electrophoretic macrophage migration and lymphocyte response to PHA, concanavalin-A (Con-A) and tuberculin (Birkeland, 1977; Stipson, 1976; Straube et al., 1973, 1975).

It has been our aim to check if plasma proteins were able, during pregnancy, to depress lymphocyte response in vitro.

MATERIALS AND METHODS

Wistar Serum Preparation NRS (Normal Rat Serum)

Thirty female Wistar rats with an average weight of 250–300 g were employed to prepare normal Wistar serum. Whole blood (6 ml) was collected directly from the heart from all rats and the sera were centrifuged, mixed in a single pool and then separated into several tubes and stored at $-40\,^\circ$C.

Before use sera were diluted 1:1 with 0.15 M phosphate-buffered saline, pH 7.2.

Anti-hCG Antibody Preparation (Ab hCG)

Fifty male Wistar rats with an average weight of 350–400 g were injected daily for 7 days with 50 IU lyophilized, highly purified hCG in 2 ml physiological saline and 1 ml of complete Freund's adjuvant added before intraperitoneal administration.

After 4 days the animals received a booster with 50 IU of highly purified hCG. Three days after the booster, 6 ml of whole blood were collected directly from the heart from all rats and the sera were centrifuged, mixed in a single pool and separated into several tubes.

An agglutination reaction was performed by using hCG adsorbed on latex particles, and after dialysis in cold polyethylene glycol up to one-third of the starting volume, the agglutinating strength of the serum was standardized at 1 ml/3500 IU.

Normal Pregnant Rat Serum (PRS)

Ten female Wistar rats with an average weight of 250–280 g were mated with syngenic males. Pregnancy was timed according to Kalter, presuming that pregnancy started on the first day after spermatozoa were found in vaginal fluid (Kalter, 1968).

Whole blood (1.5 ml) was collected from the caudal vein from all rats on days 7, 10, 13, 16, 19. The sera were mixed in a single pool, separated in several tubes and stored at $-40\,^\circ$C.

Pregnant Rat Rabbit Antiserum Preparation (ARRS)

PRS (1 ml) was added to 1 ml of Freund's complete adjuvant and was injected in syngenic male rabbits daily for 5 days. After 15 days a booster was performed with 0.5 ml of serum. Three days after the booster, 10 ml of whole blood were collected directly from the hearts of all rabbits and the sera were centrifuged, mixed into a single pool and then separated in several tubes.

Amounts decreasing progressively from 5 ml to 0.1 ml of ARRS in 10 tubes were mixed with 0.5 ml of female rat serum and incubated for 1 h at 37 °C.

The tubes in which the Ag–Ab reaction was equivalent were centrifuged for 10 min at 3000 r.p.m. and the clear supernatant was mixed in a single pool and dialysed in cold polyethylene glycol up to one-third of the starting volume.

The proteins were measured by the Lowry method and the sera were diluted with phosphate buffer at pH 7.2 to a concentration of 1000 mg/ml.

A precipitation reaction was performed with amounts decreasing progressively from 5 ml to 0.1 ml of PRS and constant amounts (0.5 ml) of ARRS. The area of equivalence included serum concentrations between 1 and 2.5 ml.

Lymphocyte Cultures

Splenocytes of rat obtained by squeezing the spleen in sterile Hanks medium at 4 °C were centrifuged in a density gradient according to Boyum (1968) and placed at 37 °C in a sterile petri dish. After 30 min the lymphocytes were recovered and exposed to a dye test with trypan blue; the cells obtained were regulated to a concentration of 3×10^6 for cell culture.

Cultures were performed in triplicate on plates 5 cm in diameter, containing 4 ml of RPMI 1640 added to 10% of fetal calf serum (FCS), and 2 M L-glutamine at pH 7.2. They were stimulated with mitogens (PHA, 0.75 μg/culture; PWM, 7 μg/culture). Afterwards 2 ml of PRS or NRS were added to each culture and 0.5 ml of ARRS to all cultures. To some cultures 3500 IU of hCG were also added.

Cultures incubated for 72 h at 37 °C under air and CO_2 (5%) were centrifuged, and the percentage blast cells were calculated according to Moorhead *et al.* (1960).

RESULTS

Cultures Stimulated with Addition of PHA

Cultures stimulated with PHA caused a blast transformation in over 72% of lymphocytes. The addition of NRS alone (74%), or added to ARRS (75%), or the addition of ARRS alone (73%) does not affect lymphocyte response. On the other hand, the addition of PRS alone (45%) or mixed with hCG (40%) strongly depressed lymphocyte response.

The addition of specific antisera to the cultures previously treated causes a normal lymphocyte response (PRS plus ARRS, 75%; PRS plus hCG plus anti-hCG serum, 52%). The hCG alone (63%) or mixed with specific antiserum (68%), or anti-hCG serum alone (70%), did not affect lymphocyte response. The results are shown in Fig. 1.

Cultures Stimulated with Addition of PW

Cultures stimulated with PWM produced a response in over 58% of lymphocytes. The addition of NRS alone (60%), or added to ARRS (64%), or the addition of

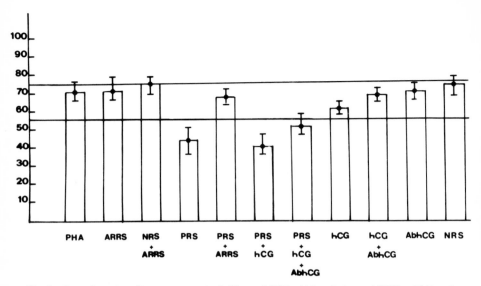

Fig. 1. Lymphocyte culture response to 0.75 μg of PHA. Abbreviations: ARRS, rabbit anti-rat serum; NRS, normal rat serum; PRS, pregnant rat serum; hCG, profasi hp 3500 IU (Serono); Ab hCG, anti-hCG antibodies.

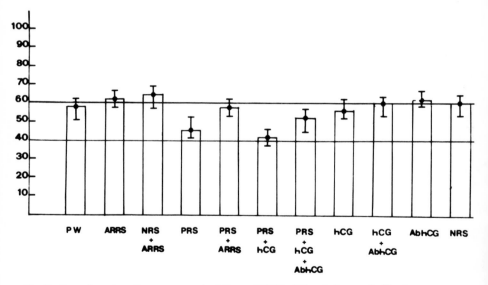

Fig. 2. Lymphocyte culture response to 7.0 μg of PWM. Abbreviations as in Fig. 1.

ARRS alone (61%) did not affect the lymphocyte response. Once again, however, the addition of PRS alone (45%) or mixed with hCG (42%) strongly depressed lymphocyte response.

The addition of specifica antisera to the previously heated cultures causes a normal lymphocyte response (PRS plus ARRS, 58%; PRS plus hCG plus anti-hCG serum, 56%). The hCG alone (57%) or mixed with specific anti-hCG serum (60%) or anti-hCG serum alone (62%) did not affect lymphocyte response. The results are shown in Fig. 2.

DISCUSSION

Our results give rise to a number of conclusions:

1. The response of PHA-treated lymphocytes added to pregnant rat serum is markedly depressed as compared to controls. This is particularly evident for T line cells. B line lymphocytes show less depression.
2. The addition of pregnant rat serum and of hCG (3500 IU/culture) causes a further depression of lymphocyte response.
3. The lymphocyte response returns to normal when anti-hCG antibodies are added to the culture.

These results, together with our experimental protocol—necessarily rather complicated because of strict adherence to the *in vivo* ecology—shows that pregnancy-associated proteins (or some protein-coupled factor present in pregnant rat serum) are capable of inhibiting lymphocyte response to mitogens at normal serum concentration. The additional depression caused by hCG leads to the conclusion that hCG is somehow involved in the regulation of lymphocyte activity.

Suppression of this phenomenon by anti-hCG antibodies might suggest that, *in vivo*, hCG might act as an intermediate messenger on a plasma factor whose synthesis might be modulated by hCG itself.

Our material is not sufficeint for definitive conclusions and our data have to be confirmed by *in vivo* experiments; such experiments are in progress both in rats and in humans.

ACKNOWLEDGEMENT

The authors are indebted to Mrs A. Fusco for help in translation.

REFERENCES

Adcock, E. W., Teasdale, F., August, C. S., Cox, S., Meschia, G., Battaglia, F. C. and Naughton, M. A. (1973). *Science, New York* **181**, 845.

Birkeland, S. A. (1977). *Danish Medical Bulletin* **24**, 42.

Boyum, A. (1968). *Scandinavian Journal of Clinical and Laboratory Investigation* **21**, Suppl. 97, 77.

Corbino, N. (1978). *Acta Eur. fert.* **12**, 38.

Jenkins, T., Acres, J., Riley, K. T. and Peter, W. D. (1972). *American Journal of Obstetrics and Gynecology* **114**, 56.

Kalter, H. (1968). *Teratology* **1**, 231.

Moorhead, P. S., Nowell, P. C., Hungeford, D. A. (1960). *Experimental Cell Research* **20**, 613.

Stipson, W. H. (1976). *Clinical and Experimental Immunology* **25**, 199.
Stivala, F., Corbino, N., Russo, I., Palumbo, G., Bernardini, A. (1974). *Clinica ginecologia* **16**, 51.
Straube, W., Suchodoletz, W. V., Hofmann, R. and Klausch, B. (1973). *Zentralblatt für Gynäkologie* **94**, 1462.
Straube, W., Klausch, B. and Hofmann, R.: *Archiv für Gynäkologie* **218**, 313.
Teasdale, F., Adcock, E. W., August, C. S., Cox, S., Battaglia, F. C. and Naughton, M. A. (1973). *Gynecological Investigations* **4**, 263.

Section Two
NEW PLACENTAL PROTEINS AND OESTRIOL IN THE
ASSESSMENT OF PLACENTAL FUNCTION

RADIOIMMUNOLOGICAL MEASUREMENTS OF SP$_1$ IN COMPARISON TO hPL AND OESTRIOL IN NORMAL AND PATHOLOGICAL PREGNANCIES

M. Pluta, W. Hardt and M. Schmidt-Gollwitzer

Klinikum Charlottenburg der Freien Universität Berlin, German Federal Republic

In addition to their use in supervising high risk pregnancies, biochemical parameters are used to complete the clinical findings. At the Universitäts Frauenklinik Charlottenburg, placental lactogen (hPL) and oestriol are regularly determined during the second half of pregnancy at intervals of 1–2 weeks. The pregnancy-specific β_1-glycoprotein (SP$_1$) was also determined in the samples collected. We were interested to see if measurements of this placental protein would give reliable information on fetal well-being or risk.

Highly purified SP$_1$ and the corresponding antisera were kindly donated by Dr Bohn, Behringwerke AG. After establishing a radioimmunoassay for SP$_1$ we set up our own normal range for SP$_1$ from 372 serum samples obtained from 40 women in the second half of a normal singleton pregnancy. Figure 1 shows the normal range of serum concentration for SP$_1$ with the 10th and 90th percentile limits. The mean value rises from 40 μg/ml in the 22nd week of pregnancy to 168 μg/ml in the 36th week, and reached a plateau thereafter. A comparison of the mean value of our normal curve with the mean values of other authors shows similarly shaped curves but some clear differences in the absolute values (Tatra *et al.*, 1974; Gordon *et al.*, 1977; Sorensen, 1978).

Eighty-nine serum samples were obtained from 9 twin pregnancies. The birthweights of all the twins lay within the normal range of the growth curves for twins (Basso *et al.*, 1970). Figure 2 shows serial values of SP$_1$, hPL and oestriol

Serono Symposium No. 35, "The Human Placenta", edited by A. Klopper, A. Genazzani and P. G. Crosignani, 1980. Academic Press, London and New York.

M. Pluta et al.

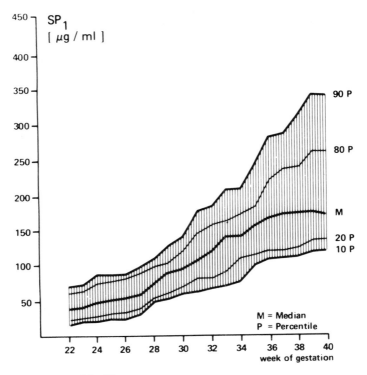

Fig. 1. Reference interval for SP_1.

for the twins as compared to the normal singleton range. The twin values for all three parameters lay mostly above the 90th percentile.

In cases with mild EPH gestosis (International Gestosis Society classification; *see* Rippmann and Rippert, 1972) there was no difference in comparison to undisturbed pregnancies (Fig. 3). Only a few serial curves were partially or completely outside the normal range. These pregnancies had a normal fetal outcome and placental weight.

In 10 pregnancies with intrauterine growth retardation an average of 10 serum samples per patient were obtained. Those infants having a birthweight below the 10th percentile of Nickl's growth curves were considered to be growth retarded (Nickl, 1972). The serial values for slight intrauterine growth retardation lay between the 10th and 50th percentiles of the normal range for the most part (Fig. 4). In cases 8, 9 and 10, with severe growth retardation, however, the curves lay well below the 10th percentile during the whole time.

The last figure shows the mean values of each parameter in the three different risk groups. Figure 5 shows that there were no significant differences to be found between SP_1, hPL and oestriol in twin pregnancies and pregnancies with mild EPH gestosis.

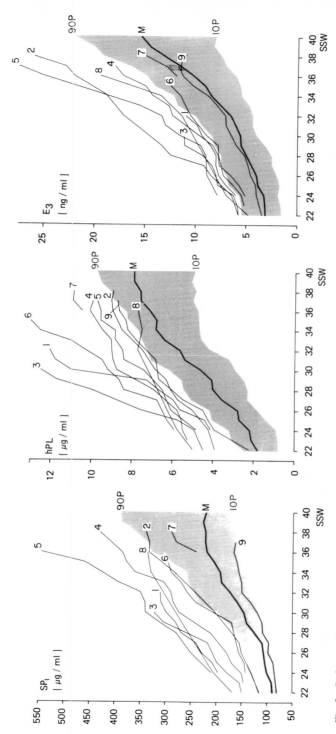

Fig. 2. Reference intervals for SP₁, hPL and oestriol with serial estimations from nine twin pregnancies.

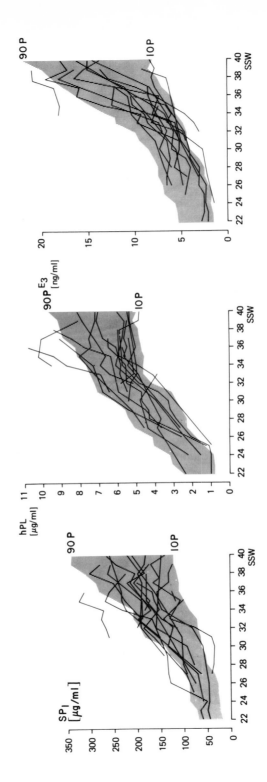

Fig. 3. Serum concentrations for SP$_1$, hPL and oestriol from 17 patients with mild EPH gestosis.

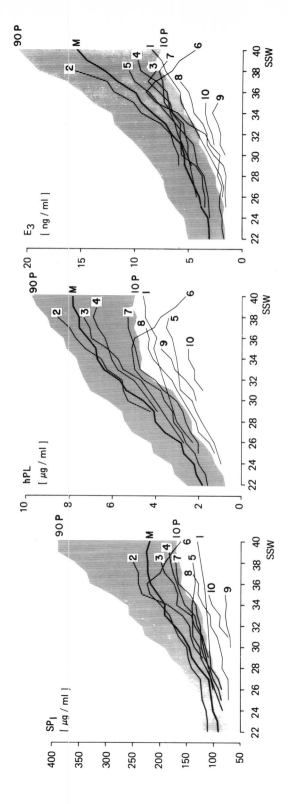

Fig. 4. Serum concentrations for SP_1, hPL and oestriol from 10 pregnancies with intrauterine growth retardation.

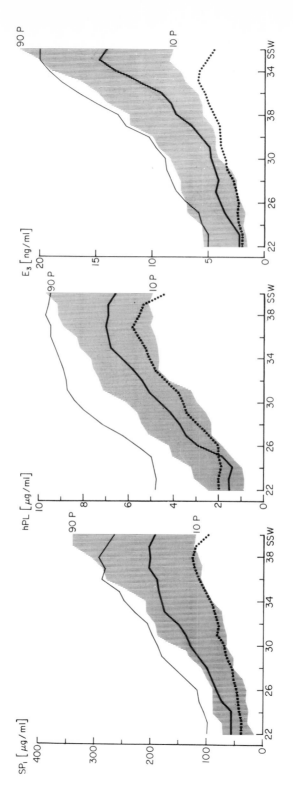

Fig. 5. Mean value evaluation of risk pregnancies. ———, Twins; ——, EPH gestosis; · · · · · · , intrauterine growth retardation.

In pregnancies with intrauterine growth retardation, both placental proteins were equally useful in the prediction of chronic placental insufficiency, but oestriol assays showed the beginning of intrauterine growth retardation at an earlier date and with more reliability.

REFERENCES

Basso, J., Dolhay, B. and Pohanka, O. (1970). *Zentralblatt für Gynäkologie* **92**, 628.

Gordon, Y. B., Grudzinskas, J. G., Jeffrey, D. and Chard, T. (1977). *Lancet* i, 331.

Nickl, R. (1972). Inaugural Dissertation.

Rippmann, E. T. and Rippert, C. (1972). EPH Gestosis, Diagnose und Resultäte. 3. Meeting der Organisation Gestose, 4. Meeting der Organisation Gestose. Walter de Gruyter, Berlin.

Sorensen, S. (1978). *Acta obstetrica et gynecologia Scandinavia* **57**, 193.

Tatra, G., Breitenecker, G. and Gruber, W. (1974). *Archiv für Gynäkologie* **217**, 283.

PLACENTAL LACTOGEN AND TOTAL OESTRIOL IN THE SMALL FOR DATE SYNDROME. A REVIEW OF 31 PREGNANCIES WITH HYPERTENSION

F. Calcagnile, C. Varagnolo, P. L. Ceccarello, A. Fazzino and F. Destro

Department of Obstetrics and Gynaecology, City Hospital, Gorizia, Italy

INTRODUCTION

Hypertension is a major factor in placental deficiency. It is a general opinion that, in these situations, the small for date (SFD) syndrome is the expression of a fetal adaption to an unfavourable environment. The early recognition of this syndrome is of primary importance in the reduction of perinatal morbidity and mortality. For this purpose measurements of placental lactogen (hPL) and of oestriol have been widely used, albeit with conflicting results. We considered it a matter of interest to review both tests in a group of patients with hypertension who delivered SFD babies.

MATERIALS AND METHODS

Plasma hPL and total oestriol (E_3) were measured in 31 pregnancies affected by hypertension at 32–41 weeks of gestation. Four patients were hypertensive before pregnancy; the remainder developed it during pregnancy. In arriving at the diagnosis of SFD we confined ourselves to the fetal parameters, using a weight correction for sex and parity according to Brenner *et al.* (1976) and the criteria laid down by Thomson *et al.* (1968). The distribution of our cases is shown in Fig. 1.

Serono Symposium No. 35, "The Human Placenta", edited by A. Klopper,
A. Genazzani and P. G. Crosignani, 1980. Academic Press, London and New York.

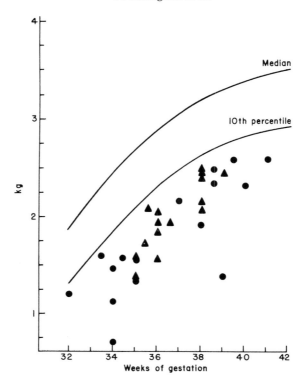

Fig. 1. Birthweight of babies as compared to median and 10th percentile of normal distribution according to Thomson *et al.* (1968). ●, Asymmetrical small for date; ▲, symmetrical small for date.

Gestational age at birth was checked against neurological and somatic findings.

Radioimmunoassay kits were used for the estimation of hPL (Lepetit, Milano) and total E_3 (Radiochemical Centre, Amersham, U.K.). Values more than two standard deviations below the mean were defined as low; those between −2 s.d. and −1 s.d. were called doubtful, and those between −1 s.d. and +1 s.d. were regarded as normal. The ratio of cephalic to abdominal circumference was measured at birth and recorded on a graph of normal values as determined by ultrasound (Ceccarello *et al.*, 1978). We have arbitrarily assumed that values more than two standard deviations above the mean represent a pathological disproportion. With this criterion, the newborns have been classified as follows: symmetrical small for date (SSFD), 15 out of 31 (48.38%); asymmetrical small for date (ASFD), 16 out of 31 (51.6%) (Fig. 2).

Two neonatal deaths and three respiratory distress syndromes were recorded; 18 cases ended in caesarean section. (In all cases pulmonary maturity was verified by foam test, according to the technique of Ianniruberto *et al.* (1975).) In nine cases a pathological fetal heart rate was found by external cardiotocography. Five patients had a positive oxytocin test, in two cases decelerations of fetal heart rate

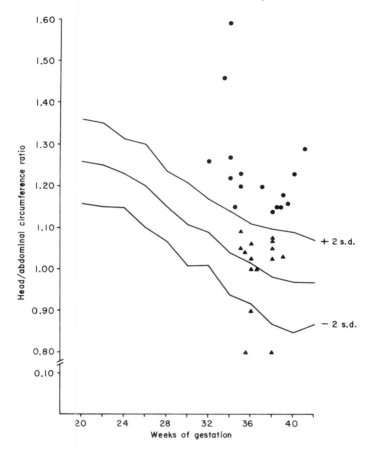

Fig. 2. The ratio of cephalic to abdominal circumference in 31 newborn. The normal distribution was determined by Ceccarello *et al.* (1978). ●, Asymmetrical small for date; ▲, symmetrical small for date.

occurred between the first and second stages of labour. In addition, two cases showed decelerations which were unclassifiable because no contractions were present. The results are summarized in Table I (hormonal levels refer to a maximum interval of 5 days before delivery).

RESULTS AND DISCUSSION

hPL and Neonatal Weight

hPL is correlated with neonatal weight both corrected (Fig. 3) and uncorrected for sex and parity ($r = 0.44$, $a = 3.05$, $b = 0.09$, $p < 0.05$).

Table I. Hormonal levels.

Patient	Weeks	hPL	E_3	Fetal heart rate (by cardiotocography)	Delivery	Weight[a] (g)	Type of SFD	Perinatal course
1	32	N	LN	P	CS	1200	A	Alive
2	$33\frac{3}{7}$	L	N	N	CS	1600	A	Alive
3	34	L	L	P	V	710[b]	A	Dead
4	34	L	LN	P	CS	1480	A	Alive[c]
5	34	L	LN	P	CS	1130	A	Alive[c]
6	$34\frac{3}{7}$	L	LN	N	CS	1600	A	Alive
7	35	L	L	N	CS	1400	S	Alive
8	35	L	LN	N	CS	1600	S	Alive
9	35	LN	LN	N	V	1570	A	Alive[c]
10	35	LN	LN	N	V	1350	A	Alive[c]
11	$35\frac{3}{7}$	N	N	N	CS	1730	S	Alive
12	$35\frac{4}{7}$	L	N	N	CS	2100	S	Alive
13	36	LN	N	N	CS	2050	S	Alive
14	36	LN	LN	N	V	1850	S	Alive
15	36	LN	LN	N	CS	1570	S	Alive
16	36	L	HN	N	CS	1950	S	Alive
17	$36\frac{4}{7}$	L	H	N	V	1950	S	Alive

18	N	N	N	2180	A	V	Alive
19	L	LN	P	2170[b]	S	CS	Alive
20	N	H	P	1930[b]	A	CS	Alive[d]
21	L	L	P	2080[b]	S	CS	Alive
22	L	N	N	2470	S	V	Alive
23	N	N	N	2500	S	V	Alive
24	N	LN	N	2400	A	V	Alive
25	L	LN	N	2360	A	V	Alive
26	N	N	N	2500	A	V	Alive
27	L	L	P	1400[b]	A	CS	Dead
28	LN	N	N	2460	S	V	Alive
29	L	L	P	2600	A	CS	Alive
30	L	L	N	2340[b]	A	CS	Alive
31	L	N	N	2610	A	V	Alive

Hormonal level abbreviations: H, high ($\geq$ +2 S.D.); HN, high normal (between +1 and +2 S.D.); N, normal (between +1 and −1 S.D.) LN, low normal–doubtful (between −1 and −2 S.D. under normal mean); L, low ($\leq$ −2 S.D.).

Fetal heart rate abbreviations: P, pathological: N, normal.

Delivery abbreviations: CS, caesarian section; V, normal.

[a] Weight at birth correct for sex and parity.

[b] Weight $\leq$ −2 S.D.

[c] Moderate respiratory distress syndrome.

[d] Hyperthyroidism.

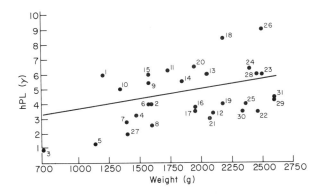

Fig. 3. hPL and weight at birth corrected for sex and parity (linear regression). For numbers *see* Table I. $r = 0.412$, $a = 3.17$, $b = 0.09$; $p < 0.05$.

Table II shows a comparison between hPL in normal and SFD subjects week by week from 31 to 41 weeks of gestation. At each week the patients carrying an SFD baby had significantly lower hPL levels (Student t-test).

We then compared the hPL values of 31 cases affected by hypertension with the hPL concentrations in a group of SFD mothers without hypertension. As can be seen in Table III, hPL levels tended to be lower in patients with hypertension, but only on a few occasions did this reach statistical significance.

hPL and the Prenatal Diagnosis of SFD

hPL values were more than two standard deviations below the normal mean in 18 subjects (58.6%); in seven cases they were in the doubtful zone and in six patients the hPL value was in the normal range.

hPL and Fetal Distress

A pathological fetal heart rate was recorded in seven out of 18 cases (38.8%) with low hPL (61.1%, false positives) and in two cases out of 13 with normal hPL (15.38%, false negatives). These results agree with previous findings and confirm the general opinion that hPL is much more effective in the diagnosis of fetal growth retardation than in the diagnosis of fetal distress.

Oestriol and Birthweight

There is a positive correlation between E_3 values before delivery and neonatal weight both corrected (Fig. 4) and uncorrected for sex and parity ($r = 0.38$, $a = 41.14$, $b = 2.74$, $p < 0.05$).

Table II. hPL concentrations (in micrograms per millilitre) in normal and SFD patients.

						Weeks					
	31	32	33	34	35	36	37	38	39	40	41
Normal	6.35 ± 1.49 (25)	7.13 ± 1.62 (29)	7.16 ± 1.46 (23)	7.60 ± 1.45 (28)	7.88 ± 2.15 (32)	8.37 ± 1.96 (30)	7.80 ± 1.72 (34)	8.36 ± 1.84 (24)	9.04 ± 2.35 (30)	7.32 ± 1.05 (17)	7.95 ± 2.84 (24)
SFD	4.31 ± 0.30 (4)	4.77 ± 0.91 (6)	4.06 ± 2.09 (9)	3.56 ± 1.98 (9)	4.32 ± 1.31 (9)	5.78 ± 1.33 (9)	5.17 ± 1.60 (8)	5.53 ± 2.31 (8)	4.83 ± 2.34 (6)	3.83 ± 0.35 (3)	4.4 (1)
p	< 0.01	< 0.0025	< 0.0005	< 0.0005	< 0.0005	< 0.0005	< 0.0005	< 0.0025	< 0.0005	–	–

Table III. Comparison of hPL concentrations (in micrograms per millilitre) in normal SFD pregnancies and SFD pregnancies with hypertension.

					Weeks					
	31	32	33	34	35	36	37	38	39	40
Normal SFD pregnancy	6.02 ± 2.28 (5)	7.13 ± 2.41 (4)	6.5 ± 2.19 (5)	7.62 ± 1.76 (5)	5.83 ± 1.24 (9)	6.5 ± 2.55 (5)	6.26 ± 1.35 (10)	6.55 ± 2.12 (17)	5.76 ± 1.81 (8)	7.36 ± 2.38 (5)
SFD pregnancy with hypertension	4.31 ± 0.30 (4)	4.77 ± 0.91 (6)	4.06 ± 2.09 (9)	3.56 ± 1.98 (9)	4.32 ± 1.31 (9)	5.78 ± 1.33 (9)	5.17 ± 1.60 (8)	5.53 ± 2.31 (8)	4.83 ± 2.34 (6)	3.83 ± 0.35 (3)
p	n.s.	< 0.05	< 0.05	< 0.0025	< 0.0125	n.s.	n.s.	n.s.	n.s.	

n.s., not significant.

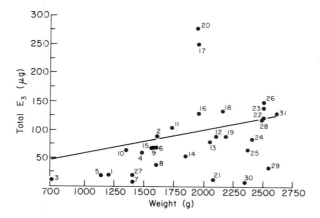

Fig. 4. Total E_3 and weight at birth corrected for sex and parity (linear regression). For number *see* Table I. $r = 0.38; a = 40.99; b = 2.75; p < 0.05$.

Mean Oestriol Values

Weekly E_3 mean values in 31 SFD cases tended to be lower than the normal mean, but statistically the difference is significant only at 31, 34, 35 and 39 weeks (Table IV).

Oestriol and the Prenatal Diagnosis of SFD

Low E_3 values were found in six out of 31 cases (19.35%).

Oestriol and Fetal Distress

Of six cases with low E_3 values, four cases (66.6%) showed a pathological fetal heart rate (FHR); in one case with normal E_3, pathological FHR was recorded (8.3%, false negatives).

Types of SFD

As mentioned above, neonates have been classified into symmetrical and asymmetrical. According to the Gruenwald (1970) classification, six newborns (four asymmetrical and two symmetrical) with weight < -2 s.d. were also recorded. In Table V the correlation between types of SFD, hormonal levels and fetal heart rate is shown. The results confirm that asymmetry is a severe fetal hazard, particularly in neonates with a birthweight more than two standard deviations below the mean. The perinatal deaths occurred in this group. Therefore the population considered includes three different types of SFD, each with well-differentiated clinical problems. It is quite possible that the conflicting results are due to the different proportions of these types of SFD in different study populations.

Table IV. Weekly mean E_3 values (in micrograms per millilitre).

						Weeks					
	31	32	33	34	35	36	37	38	39	40	41
Normal	76.85 ± 39.91 (27)	81.50 ± 35.99 (28)	88.31 ± 54.54 (26)	99.50 ± 41.06 (28)	114.73 ± 44.94 (37)	128 ± 54.77 (34)	138.46 ± 49.65 (37)	153.63 ± 59.10 (24)	137.37 ± 41.19 (27)	150 ± 57.25 (17)	147 ± 48.6 (25)
SFD	38.50 ± 27.93 (4)	56.93 ± 40.11 (6)	60 ± 45.74 (9)	56 ± 36.04 (9)	69.44 ± 29.63 (9)	100.33 ± 47.08 (9)	143.25 ± 63.91 (8)	119.88 ± 81.29 (8)	76.67 ± 55.67 (6)	60.33 ± 66.71 (3)	130 (1)
p	< 0.05	n.s.	n.s.	< 0.0125	< 0.005	n.s.	n.s.	n.s.	< 0.0025	—	—

n.s., not significant.

Table V. Type of SFD hormonal levels and risk of fetal distress (FHR).

Types of SFD	N	hPL (%)			Total E$_3$ (%)			Pathological FHR (%)
		Normal	Doubtful	Low	Normal	Doubtful	Low	
Total								
SFD	31	19.35	22.58	58.06	41.93	38.70	19.35	29.00
SSFD	15	20.00	26.66	53.00	53.30	33.33	13.33	13.33
ASFD	16	18.75	12.50	68.00	31.25	43.75	25.00	43.75
SFD								
< -2 s.d.	6	16.66	—	83.33	16.66	16.66	66.66	83.33

CONCLUSIONS

Our experience indicates quite clearly that plasma levels of total E_3 and hPL are related to both fetal weight and placental function.

hPL is of value in the early recognition of this syndrome, but, from a clinical point of view, overlapping values of this test are compatible with uncomplicated vaginal delivery (cases 17, 22, 25 and 31; Table I) or, on the other hand, precede pathological FHR (cases 5, 19, 29; Table I). Therefore to rely on this test for the active management of pregnancy may result in unnecessary caesarean sections. Nevertheless, as doubt is now cast on the safety of the oxytocin challenge test (Kundu *et al.*, 1978), and metabolic acidosis due to late decelerations (Kubli *et al.*, 1973) may compromise the synthesis of surfactant, we think that a low hPL is sufficient for active management of pregnancy. In our experience total E_3 is poor in prenatal diagnosis of SFD. Although a low total E_3 may be a relative indicator of fetal distress, E_3 changes may be too late when fetal viability is already compromised.

REFERENCES

Brenner, E. W., Edelman, D. A. and Hendrieks, C. H. (1976). *American Journal of Obstetrics and Gynecology* **126**, 555.

Ceccarello, P. L., Morgan, G., Perini, G., Calcagnile, F., Castello, C., Varagnolo, C., Fazzino, A., Capozzi, A. and Destro, F. (1978). *In* "Recent Advances in Ultrasound Diagnosis" (A. Kurjak, ed.), Excerpta Medica, Amsterdam.

Gruenwald, P. (1970). *In* "Physiology of the Perinatal Period". (U. Stave, ed.). New York.

Ianniruberto, A., Destro, F., Capozzi, A., Zisa, F., Cubesi, G. and Parisi, S. (1975). *Journal of Medical Perinatology* **3**, 105.

Kubli, F., Hon, E. H., Khezin, A. F., Tahemura, H. (1969). *American Journal of Obstetrics and Gynecology* **104**, 1190.

Kundu, N., Carmody, P. J., Didolkar, S. M. and Petersen, L. P. (1978). *Obstetrics and Gynecology* **52**, 513.

Thomson, A. M., Billewicz, W. Z. and Hytten, F. E. (1968). *Journal of Obstetrics and Gynaecology of the British Commonwealth* **75**, 903.

PLACENTAL PERFUSION AND PLACENTAL HORMONES AS AN INDEX OF PLACENTAL FUNCTION IN EPH GESTOSIS AND PLACENTAL INSUFFICIENCY

H. Janisch and J. Spona

First Department of Obstetrics and Gynaecology, University of Vienna, A 1090 Vienna, Austria

INTRODUCTION

Estimations of urinary oestrogens have been used in the supervision of high risk pregnancies for many years (Beling, 1971). During the past few years, however, determination of oestrogen urinary excretion has been replaced by radio-immunoassay of oestriol serum levels. Much progress has been achieved by using antisera with high specificity against oestriol, which allowed a more rapid estimation of oestriol serum levels. In addition, human placental lactogen (hPL) has become an important diagnostic aid in the management of high risk pregnancies since the first report on this placental hormone (Josimovich and MacLaren, 1962). Serum levels of hPL and oestriol have been measured in a variety of complications of pregnancy. As production of hPL is related to placental mass, several authors have suggested that it should be of value in pregnancies complicated by retarded fetal growth (Lindberg and Nilsson, 1973; Spencer, 1971). Oestriol was also reported to be a valuable indicator of intrauterine growth retardation (Melchert, 1978). Several other workers have stated that both oestriol and hPL are valuable predictors of fetal distress and neonatal asphyxia in otherwise normal pregnancies (England *et al.*, 1974; Letchworth and Chard, 1972; Kundu *et al.*, 1978; Trolle *et al.*, 1976). Furthermore, hPL has been well documented as an index of placental function (Spona and Janisch, 1971, 1972; Gitsch *et al.*, 1973; Melchert, 1978).

Serono Symposium No. 35, "The Human Placenta", edited by A. Klopper,
A. Genazzani and P. G. Crosignani, 1980. Academic Press, London and New York.

171

However, conflicting reports accumulated on hPL and oestriol estimations as predictors of fetal distress as well as of retarded fetal growth. The aim of the present investigation was to assess placental function more precisely by a simultaneous assay of hPL and oestriol serum levels and determination of uterine blood flow.

PATIENTS AND METHODS

A total of 3317 births were registered (Table I) during 1977–78, and 215 patients (6.48%) of this group suffered from EPH gestosis. There were 62 patients out of the 215 subjects with EPH gestosis who were completely monitored for placental blood flow and serum hormone levels. In addition, 64 subjects with placental insufficiencies were included in this study. Only those patients in whom data on placental blood flow estimations and serial hormone determinations were available are included in this study.

Table I. Total number of subjects in each group.

Total birth rate (1977 – 1978)	EPH gestosis		Placental insuff.	i.u. fetal death
	total number	completely monitored		
3317	215 (6.48%)	62	64	8

Radioimmunoassay of hPL was carried out using a solid-phase coated tube procedure, which was described in detail previously (Spona, 1972). Estimation of serum oestriol levels was performed by a radioimmunoassay method reported recently (Gitsch *et al.*, 1977).

The uteroplacental blood flow was measured by quick intravenous administration ("bolus technique") of 250 μCi to 1 mCi of ^{113}In, and the radioactivity uptake curve of the placenta was recorded by a gamma scintillation camera after localization of the placenta by means of ultrasound. Radioactivity was recorded as a function of time, and the curve obtained is approximated to $A_t = A_0(\text{I-e}^{-kt})$ by a Newton iteration (Janisch and Leodolter, 1977; Janisch *et al.*, 1977). Previous studies showed that the curves could be classified into three types, which were designated as types I, II and III. Perfusion type I indicates unimpaired uteroplacental blood flow, and type II is considered as being of intermediary nature. The delay in radioactivity uptake as found in type III curves results from impairment of blood flow (Janisch *et al.*, 1977).

RESULTS

EPH Gestosis

Good correlation between perfusion type and hPL serum levels was noted in patients with EPH gestosis (Table II). Thus 65% of patients who presented with perfusion type I had normal hPL serum levels, and in 31% of subjects with blood

Table II. Correlation of hPL and E_3 serum levels with type of placental perfusion in patients suffering from EPH gestosis.

Perfusion type	n	HPL serum levels			E_3 serum levels		
		normal	decreased	elevated	normal	decreased	elevated
I	40	26 (65%)	12 (30%)	2 (5%)	18 (45%)	14 (35%)	8 (20%)
II	9	8 (89%)	1 (11%)	0	4 (44%)	2 (22%)	2 (22%)*
III	13	9 (69%)	4 (31%)	0	5 (38%)	8 (62%)	0

* E_3 serum levels not determined in one patient

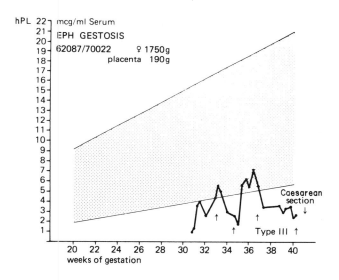

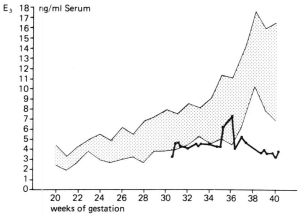

Fig. 1. Serum hPL and oestriol in a patient with EPH gestosis.

Table III. Correlation of type of placental perfusion with serum levels of hPL and E_3 in placental insufficiencies.

Perfusion type	n	HPL serum levels			E_3 serum levels		
		normal	decreased	elevated	normal	decreased	elevated
I	44	38 (86%)	5 (12%)	1 (2%)	26 (59%)	8 (18%)	10 (23%)
II	13	11 (85%)	2 (15%)	0	4 (30%)	1 (8%)	8 (62%)
III	7	4 (57%)	3 (43%)	0	3 (14%)	1 (14%)	3 (43%)

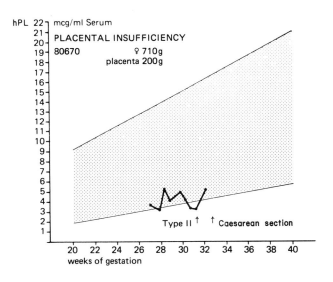

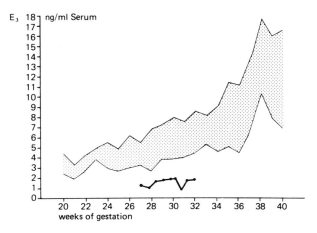

Fig. 2. Serum hPL and oestriol in a patient with placental insufficiency.

flow type III decreased hPL values were observed. Similar results were noted for oestriol serum levels. A typical example of hPL and oestriol patterns of a patient with EPH gestosis is presented in Fig. 1. The patient was also frequently monitored by blood flow measurements, and type III was recorded four times. A dystrophic child was delivered by caesarean section. A placental weight of 190 g and a fetal weight of 1750 g was registered. The baby died 4 days after delivery from respiratory insufficiency.

Placental Insufficiency

A total of 64 patients were included in this group (Table III). Perfusion type I patterns were recorded in 44 subjects, and 38 subjects (86%) presented with normal hPL serum levels. Similarly, 59% of patients with type I blood flow were

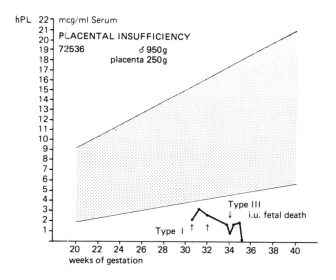

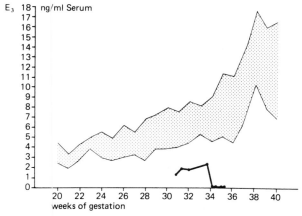

Fig. 3. Serum hPL and oestriol in a patient with deteriorating placental blood flow.

found to have normal oestriol values. On the other hand, 43% of subjects with perfusion type III presented with pathological hPL serum levels.

hPL and oestriol patterns in a patient with placental insufficiency suggested fetal distress, and placental perfusion was of type II, indicating slight impairment of blood flow (Fig. 2). A caesarean section was performed at 33 weeks of gestation due to the high degree of fetal distress, and a highly dystrophic baby was delivered. A fetal weight of 710 g and a placental weight of 200 g were recorded.

Similarly, decreased hPL and oestriol levels were noted in another subject (Fig. 3). Type I placental perfusion was recorded twice at times at which pathological hormone levels were already seen. Type III of placental perfusion was registered when oestriol levels had dropped to undetectable values and intrauterine death had occurred. Placental weight of 150 g and fetal weight of 950 g were recorded.

CONCLUSIONS

The early detection of fetal distress is of importance in order to reduce the rate of morbidity and mortality. Previous experiences suggested that one single clinical or one isolated laboratory parameter is inadequate for deciding treatment. On the other hand, a great many reports have indicated the value of hPL estimation as a prognostic and diagnostic tool (Spona and Janisch, 1971, 1972; Janisch *et al.*, 1973; Janisch and Spona, 1973; Gitsch *et al.*, 1977). An improved interpretation of data is possible by the simultaneous determination of oestriol serum levels (Altmann *et al.*, 1978), since acute fetal distress can be detected by oestriol estimations during the course of chronic placental insufficiency as noted by hPL assays.

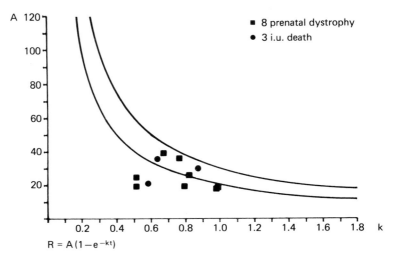

Fig. 4. Placental blood flow in patients with prenatal dystrophy or intrauterine death.

Determination of hPL and oestriol has been used not only as a diagnostic tool (Josimovich *et al.*, 1969; Josimovich, 1977; Letchworth and Chard, 1972) but also to assess the prognosis (Spellacy *et al.*, 1966; Sandstedt, 1979; Höpker and Ohlendorf, 1979). The routine evaluation of placental blood flow adds another valuable predictive parameter to present diagnostic and prognostic tools. In patients with dystrophies and intrauterine fetal death types II or III, placental perfusion was noted (Fig. 4). Impaired placental blood flow may cause decreased placental hormone synthesis, since perfusion types II and III are closely correlated with pathological serum levels of hPL and oestriol. Impaired blood flow was recorded in severe EPH gestosis and in placental insufficiencies, in which fetal growth retardation was also noted. Disturbances of the intervillous blood flow are mainly provoked by maternal factors located in uterine vessels. Prostaglandins were thought to regulate uterine blood flow during pregnancy (Lauersen *et al.*, 1974). Whether hPL biosynthesis is under direct control of prostaglandins cannot be deduced from recent experiments (Spona and Reinold, 1978).

The higher risk of fetal intrauterine death in fetal growth retardation justifies the introduction of another parameter specifically to assess placental function. Repeated estimations of placental blood flow starting at 27 weeks of gestation are possible since whole-body radiation exposure of the fetus is in the order of 2.5-10 mrem. The data presented combine to suggest that simultaneous estimations of placental blood flow and serial determinations of hPL and oestriol are a valuable diagnostic and prognostic aid.

ACKNOWLEDGEMENTS

We greatly appreciate a gift of highly purified hPL from the National Institutes of Arthritis, Metabolism and Digestive Diseases, Bethesda, Md, U.S.A., which was used in the RIA of hPL. We thank Mrs J. Adolph for her excellent secretarial work.

REFERENCES

Altmann, P., Janisch, H., Müller-Tyl, E., Reinold, E., Spona, J. and Havelec, L. (1978). *Wiener klinische Wochenschrift* **90**, 121.

Beling, C. G. (1971). *In* "Endocrinology of Pregnancy" (F. Fuchs and A. Klopper, eds), pp. 32–65, Harper and Row, New York.

England, P., Lorrimer, D., Fergusson, J. C., Moffat, A. M. and Kelly, A. M. (1974). *Lancet i*, 5.

Gitsch, E., Janisch, H. and Spona, J. (1973). *Wiener klinische Wochenschrift* **85**, 585.

Gitsch, E., Janisch, H., Leodolter, S., Schneider, W. H. F. and Spona, J. (1977). *In* "Radioisotope in Geburtshilfe und Gynäkologie" (E. Gitsch, ed.), pp. 373–420, Walter de Gruyter, Berlin.

Höpker, W.-W. and Ohlendorf, B. (1979). *In* "Perinatal Pathology" (E. Grundmann, ed.), p. 57, Springer, Berlin.

Janisch, H. and Leodolter, S. (1977). *In* "Radiosotope Geburtshilfe und Gynä-kologie" (E. Gitsch, ed.), pp. 169–204, Walter de Gruyter, Berlin.

Janisch, H. and Spona, J. (1973). *Zeitschrift für Geburtshilfe und Perinatologie* **177**, 349.

Janisch, H., Leodolter, S. and Philipp, K. (1977). *In* "Poor Intrauterine Fetal Growth" (B. Salvadori and A. B. Modena, eds), Edizioni Minerva Medica Centro.

Janisch, H., Leodolter, S. and Spona, J. (1973). *Wiener klinische Wochenschrift* **85**, Suppl. 6.

Josimovich, J. B. (1977). *In* "Endocrinology of Pregnancy" (F. Fuchs and A. Klopper, eds), p. 191, Harper and Row, New York.

Josimovich, J. B. and MacLaren, J. A. (1962). *Endocrinology* **71**, 209.

Josimovich, J. B., Kosor, B., Mintz, D. H. (1969). *In* "Ciba Foundation Symposium on Foetal Autonomy" (G. E. W. Wolstenholm, and M. O'Connor, eds), p. 117, Churchill, London.

Kundu, N., Carmody, P. J., Didolkar, S. M. and Petersen, L. P. (1978). *Obstetrics and Gynecology* **52**, 513.

Lauersen, N. H., Wilson, K. H., Beling, C. G. and Fuchs, F. (1974). *American Journal of Obstetrics and Gynecology* **120**, 875.

Letchworth, A. T. and Chard, T. (1972). *Lancet i*, 704.

Lindberg, B. S. and Nilsson, B. A. (1973). *Journal of Obstetrics and Gynaecology of the British Commonwealth* **80**, 1046.

Melchert, F. (1978). *In* "Biochemisch-immunologische Möglichkeiten der Schwangerschaftsüberwachung", Georg Thieme Verlag, Stuttgart.

Sandstedt, B. (1979). *In* "Perinatal Pathology" (E. Grundmann ed.), p. 1, Springer, Berlin.

Spellacy, W. N., Carlson, K. L. and Birk, S. A. (1966). *American Journal of Obstetrics and Gynecology* **95**, 118.

Spencer, T. S. (1971). *Journal of Obstetrics and Gynaecology of the British Commonwealth* **78**, 232.

Spona, J. (1972). *Zeitschrift für immunologische Forschung* **143**, 192.

Spona, J. and Janisch, H. (1971). *Acta endocrinologia, Copenhagen* **68**, 401.

Spona, J. and Janisch, H. (1972). *Wiener klinische Wochenschrift* **84**, 385.

Spona, J. and Reinold, E. (1978). *In* "Proceedings of Sulpostone Symposium", Vienna.

Trolle, D., Bock, J. E. and Gaede, P. (1976). *American Journal of Obstetrics and Gynecology* **126**, 834.

Section Three
TESTS OF PLACENTAL FUNCTION

INTEGRATED USE OF PHYSICAL AND ENDOCRINE
PARAMETERS IN PERINATAL MEDICINE

A. Scommegna and J. Bieniarz

Department of Obstetrics and Gynecology, Michael Reese Hospital and Medical Center and the Pritzker School of Medicine of the University of Chicago, Chicago, Illinois U.S.A.

INTRODUCTION

The recent decline in perinatal mortality is attributable mainly to a fall in neonatal deaths, whereas intrauterine fetal demise still accounts for 40% of perinatal losses occurring after the 32nd week of pregnancy (Westin, 1977). Such high losses at a stage of fetal development compatible with extrauterine survival presents a formidable challenge to the obstetrician. The detection of placental insufficiency developing slowly over a period of weeks taxes the skills of the most astute obstetrician. Moreover, assessment of its severity and its effect on the growing fetus poses an acute dilemma which can be intellectually challenging but therapeutically frustrating. The decision to allow a pregnancy to continue rather than to interrupt it might very well spell the difference between life and death of the fetus (Scommegna and Chattoraji, 1967).

In order to decrease perinatal mortality and morbidity the high risk pregnancy must be first identified so that available preventive and corrective measures can be appropriately applied. During routine prenatal care physical examination of the mother, clinical measurements of maternal weight, uterine size and blood pressure, the use of certain laboratory tests and recognition of diseases during pregnancy will permit the identification of one-fourth to one-third of high risk pregnancies which account for the majority of perinatal deaths and morbidity (Fig. 1).

Serono Symposium No. 35, "The Human Placenta", edited by A. Klopper, A. Genazzani and P. G. Crosignani, 1980. Academic Press, London and New York.

Physical factors	*Endocrine factors*
Weight gain	E_3 determination
Uterine height	24 h urine
Blood pressure changes	Plasma free E_3
Ultrasound	Plasma total E_3
Antenatal FHR monitoring	hPL

Fig. 1. Fetal risk assessment.

Our aim is to outline those physical and endocrine tests which can be used to assess the dangers of the high risk pregnancy for the fetus in a hostile intrauterine environment, and to balance these risks against the dangers of early prematurity for the newborn (Crane *et al.*, 1976; Salvadori, 1977).

MONITORING FETAL GROWTH

Normal *maternal weight gain* is a simple but important indicator of normal fetal growth and development. Perinatal morbidity and mortality is highest when maternal weight gain during pregnancy is far from normal: 1 lb (0.45 kg) per week during the second and third trimesters, or 27.5 lb (12.5 kg) for the whole pregnancy. Lack of maternal weight gain may be the first indication of small for gestational age (SGA) babies, as well as of increased tendency to prematurity. Conversely, excessive weight gain (more than 2.5 lb (1.1 kg) per week) suggests either development of pre-eclampsia with fluid retention, multiple pregnancy, polyhydramnios or large for gestational age (LGA) babies which occur in diabetes, or Rh incompatibilities with their respective, well-known risks.

Sequential charting of *weight gain*, uterine height and blood pressure changes in a given pregnant woman may alert the obstetrician to the development of gestational abnormalities. According to Westin (1977) uterine height has the smallest coefficient of variation and was therefore selected as an indirect indicator of fetal growth. When *uterine growth* was clearly below normal (mean -1 S.D.), 75% of all SGA babies were correctly predicted. Fetuses whose birthweight is more than one standard deviation below the mean weight for gestational age account for two-thirds of mentally retarded and cerebral palsy infants. When uterine growth was greater than mean $+1$ S.D., 65% of LGA babies were correctly predicted. When the mean $+2$ S.D. were considered as suspicious of twin pregnancy this was confirmed in all but one case (polyhydramnios).

Repeated *blood pressure* measurements of 135/85 mm Hg or higher indicate hypertensive disturbances of pregnancy. Recently a clinical test has been used to identify the liability to develop hypertension (Gant and Worley, 1977). At 28–32 weeks of gestation the patient is placed in the lateral recumbent position and diastolic blood pressures are recorded for a minimum of 15 min, or until it has become stable. At this point the patient is "rolled over" on her back and the pressure is taken again at 1 and 5 min. An increase in diastolic blood pressure of 20 mm Hg or more is regarded as a positive roll-over test. In a prospective study on 700 women, those patients who exhibited a positive roll-over response ultimately developed pregnancy-induced hypertension in 76% of cases. Conversely,

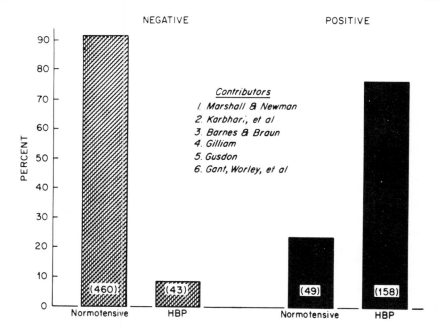

NEGATIVE   POSITIVE

Contributors

1. *Marshall & Newman*
2. *Karbhari, et al*
3. *Barnes & Braun*
4. *Gilliam*
5. *Gusdon*
6. *Gant, Worley, et al*

Fig. 2. The predictive ability of the roll-over test. In a prospective study on 710 women, those patients who exhibited a positive roll-over response ultimately developed pregnancy-induced hypertension in 76% of cases. Conversely, 92% of patients with a negative roll-over test remained normotensive throughout pregnancy (Reproduced from Gant and Worley (1977) with the permission of the authors.)

92% of patients with a negative roll-over test remained normotensive throughout pregnancy (Fig. 2).

Reliable determination of *gestational age* is a major diagnostic problem because it affects the correct interpretation of all tests, as well as all decision making processes in high risk pregnancy. Without accurate gestational age, timing of delivery cannot be optimized.

Menstrual history is often inaccurate and therefore unreliable. In addition to a detailed menstrual history, early pregnancy test, date of first uterine size estimation, date of quickening, and whether oral contraceptives were used immediately prior to conception, represent additional information necessary to estimate gestational age correctly (Fig. 3).

Ausculation of fetal heart rate (FHR) with a non-electronic fetoscope around 20 weeks of gestation is a simple but reliable method of physical diagnosis. This

History	*Examination*
LNMP	Early uterine size
PNMP	Early pregnancy test
Quickening	First FH tones heard
Oral contraceptive use	First ultrasound measurement

Fig. 3. Gestational age determination.

Measurement of	at
Gestational sac	5–6 weeks
Crown-rump length	7–14 weeks
Serial BPD	20–30 weeks
Head/abdomen circumference ratio	32–40 weeks

Fig. 4. Use of ultrasound for gestational age and fetal growth assessment.

establishes the gestational age at 20–21 weeks. Although FHR can be detected by ultrasound (US) earlier, the time is less precise, varying between 8 and 12 weeks. However, measuring the crown–rump length by beta-scan image is a most reliable index of fetal age before 12 weeks of gestation (Robinson, 1973). Similarly, serial biparietal diameter (BPD) measurements are utilized between the 20th and 30th weeks of pregnancy when its weekly growth reaches 3 mm. A slower rate of increase would suggest fetal growth retardation, while a small BPD with normal weekly growth suggests misdating (Sabbagha, 1977). In advanced pregnancy the changing ratio between fetal head and abdominal circumferences facilitates the diagnosis of SGA babies (Campbell and Wilkin, 1975). In this condition the liver is reduced in size more than the head because of the preferential cerebral circulation in the fetus (Fig. 4).

Once the fetus of a pregnancy at risk reaches viability (26–30 weeks) its condition must be closely supervised by sequential endocrine tests monitoring fetoplacental function and by FHR tests monitoring the fetal status. The purpose now is to assure the fetus the benefits of intrauterine growth and development as long as possible, and to save the viable fetus from the possible harm when the intrauterine environment may deplete its reserves and affect its survival (Fig. 5).

ANTENATAL MONITORING: ENDOCRINE AND ELECTRONIC

Because of their convenience and their relatively low cost, *endocrine tests* lend themselves to the routine screening of high risk pregnancies. Among the endocrine tests the measurement of estriol (E_3), either in the urine or in the plasma, and of human placental lactogen (hPL) in the blood are accepted by many but not all American obstetricians as being of value in the assessment of fetal well-being. Each test reflects a different aspect of fetoplacental physiology. Estriol production is related to the integrated ability of the fetus to produce estrogen precursors and to the functional capability of the placenta to convert them into estriol. Human placental lactogen, on the other hand, is the product of the syncytiotrophoblast only.

Both substances increase progressively with advancing gestation, reflecting, presumably, the growth of the fetus. However, as pointed out by Klopper *et al.* (1977), neither correlated closely with fetal or placental size in a group of normal pregnant women.

In pathologic pregnancies, on the other hand, the production of both the fetoplacental steroid and the placental protein hormones are clearly affected. It is tempting to speculate that the pathologic entity is responsible for the decrease in the estriol and placental lactogen values as well as the impairment in fetal growth and placental functions independently. For the perinatologist the critical question is which test best detects fetoplacental problems such as intrauterine growth retardation (IUGR) and fetal distress.

Although some studies have shown that hPL may have a higher predictive accuracy (Chard, 1974), the combination of the two tests gives more specific information than either test alone.

hPL measurements are useful in conditions that compromise placental function (e.g. hypertensive disturbances of pregnancy, IUGR, postmaturity) so as to cause hPL values to fall to less than 4 mg/ml after 30 weeks. The test fails in fetal disorders in which placental function is adequate (e.g. class A diabetes mellitus, fetal anomalies, erythroblastosis) (Genazzani *et al.*, 1972; Spellacy *et al.*, 1975).

A great deal of controversy exists as to the use of urinary estriol versus plasma estriol and plasma total estriol versus plasma free estriol. Those who prefer urinary estriol assays point to the advantages of the integration of the fetoplacental function over the time by the urinary collection. Those who prefer the plasma assays point to the inconvenience of the 24 h urine collection and to the problems with their interpretation when the sample is incomplete. Plasma assays also avoid the delay associated with the urinary collection, the problems associated with diurnal and postural variations, or impaired renal function.

Free plasma estriol levels are thought by some people to be likely to reflect placental estriol production more directly than total estriol as the concentration of free estriol depends mainly on rates of placental secretion and its hepatic conjugation. Total estriol, on the other hand, depends also on excretion by the liver and intestinal reabsorption and on the efficiency of renal excretion.

In practice, the preference of one assay over the other depends on the ease with which the laboratory can perform that assay, on the degree of scatter of values in a normal population, on the lack of variability from moment to moment in normal patients and on the speed and degree of change in the presence of fetal jeopardy. Seen in this light, no one assay is clearly superior to the others.

In general, tests that have the least variability respond least quickly to changes in the fetal status. Therefore, the choice may be dictated by the particular clinical situation. As a screening test, plasma total estriol and placental lactogen may be preferred in an ambulatory setting because it is easy to get a blood sample. With a hospitalized patient, urinary estriol and plasma free estriol may be preferable.

Although both urinary and plasma estriol assays present a wide range of normal values and large daily variations even in normal pregnancy, there is a reassuring rising trend with the normal progress of pregnancy, recognizable in serial estriol determinations. However, a fall of 40% or more below the previous peak as well as continuous low values after the 34th week of pregnancy raise serious concern for the fate of the fetus.

Antenatal fetal heart rate (FHR) monitoring is a simple, easily available physical method which may give important insight into the condition of the fetus of quite high reliability if the results are normal, although abnormal results are less reliable. The non-stress test (NST) (Hammacher *et al.*, 1969) consists of 30 min of spontaneous electronic FHR recording: a normal fetal reactivity is recognized by a baseline FHR level between 120–160 beats/min, with a variability of 10–25 beats/min and at least two or three transient FHR accelerations (usually related to fetal movements or external stimuli). A non-reactive test suggests fetal hypoxia and includes a fetal heart rate that has no transient accelerations, reduced baseline FHR variability of less than 5 beats/min, is unresponsive to external stimuli and has reduced long-term variations, less than three per minute (sinusoidal rhythm). Late decelerations with the occasional spontaneous contractions confirm severe fetal compromise (Kubli *et al.*, 1977).

The oxytocin challenge test (OCT) (Pose *et al.*, 1969) consists of inducing uterine contractions by oxytocin infusion until three contractions are produced in 10 min. Each uterine contraction transiently reduces uteroplacental blood flow and may gradually slow down the FHR if the oxygen reserves of the fetus and placenta are already depleted due to vasoconstriction or sclerotic or atheromatic changes in the spiral arteries. Combined with reduced baseline variability, tachycardia or bradycardia, consistent late decelerations suggest severe fetal compromise and inability of the fetus to sustain the stress of labor. Unlike the non-stress test, which is simple to perform and without risk, the oxytocin challenge test is more time consuming and therefore more expensive; thus its use is restricted to the further investigation of fetal hypoxia in patients who have shown abnormal endocrine tests or a non-reactive NST (Fig. 5).

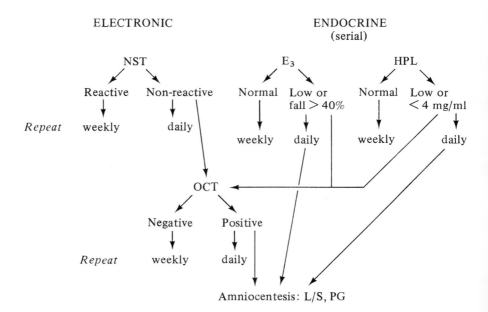

Fig. 5. High risk fetal screening and monitoring. Weekly FHR non-stress tests (NST), as well as hormonal estriol (E_3) and human placental lactogen (hPL) determinations, are used for screening of fetuses at risk. If such a fetus is found, oxytocin challenge test (OCT) is performed to assess the degree of fetal oxygen reserve. If positive, amniocentesis for measurement of lecitin–sphingomyelin ratio (L/S) and phosphatidyl glycerol (PG) is performed to assess the risk of respiratory distress syndrome if interruption of pregnancy is carried out. Amniocentesis may also be indicated if E_3 and/or hPL assays are consistently low.

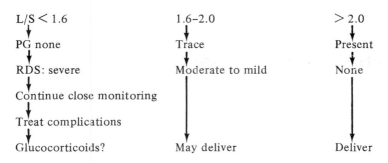

Fig. 6. The prognosis of respiratory distress syndrome (RDS) in an identified perinate at risk is based on L/S ratio and on the presence of phosphatidyl glycerol in an amniotic fluid sample obtained under ultrasound guidance. The results determine either conservative treatment under close fetal monitoring or termination of pregnancy.

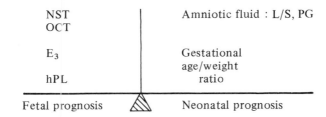

Fig. 7. Integrated indices of perinatal prognosis. The optimal time for delivery is established when integrated fetal risks outweigh neonatal risks.

Once the intrauterine environment no longer assures fetal growth and development, further prolongation of pregnancy may result in fetal damage or death. Now is the time to integrate the assessment based on clinical and laboratory tests and weigh fetal prognosis against the prognosis for the premature baby.

Amniocentesis and fluid sampling for assessing fetal lung maturation is carried out under US control. A lecitin to sphingomyelin ratio (L/S) less than or equal to 1.5 indicates that the baby will almost certainly develop a severe respiratory distress syndrome (RDS) with poor prognosis for the baby's survival: pregnancy should therefore be continued. An L/S ratio of 1.6–1.9 suggests mild to moderate RDS for the newborn, with a good prognosis, especially if phosphatidyl glycerol (PG) is present in the amniotic fluid: pregnancy may be terminated if the integrated tests suggest possible fetal damage caused by prolongation of intrauterine life (Fig. 6). An L/S ratio greater than or equal to 2.0 and presence of PG in amniotic fluid give a good prognosis for the newborn's survival: there is no aim in further prolongation of pregnancy (Fig. 7). On the other hand, a most useful tool in assessing neonatal mortality risks by birthweight and gestational age is the table worked out by Lubchenco *et al.* (1972) (Fig. 8).

In dramatic situations of early pregnancy, 26–32 weeks with low L/S ratio where the integrated fetal evaluation suggests dangers of further intrauterine life,

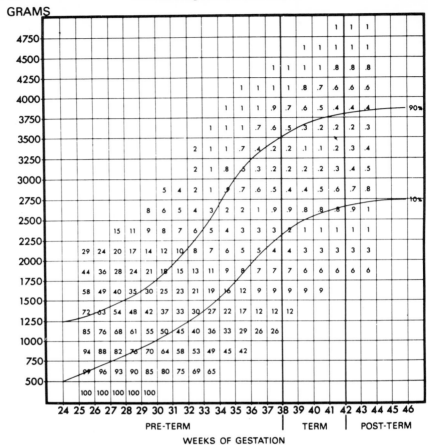

Fig. 8. Neonatal mortality risk by birthweight and gestational age. Integrated data based on mathematical fit from 10 000 deliveries at the University of Colorado Medical Center, 1958–69. The highest mortality rates were reached in SGA (small for gestational age) premature babies (left lower quadrant) while the lowest mortality was found in the AGA (appropriate for gestational age) full-term babies. (Reproduced from Lubchenco *et al.* (1972) with the permission of the authors.)

administration of *glucocorticoids* 24–48 h before delivery may accelerate maturation of fetal lungs and improve neonatal prognosis (Liggins and Howie, 1974). This treatment used in Europe is still considered controversial in the USA as long as possible harm to the baby's central nervous system and other organs cannot be excluded.

CONCLUSIONS

In summary, simple physical measurements as well as sequential ultrasound studies reveal abnormal fetal growth and help to determine exact gestational age. This information is of basic importance in decision making processes in perinatology. Estriol determinations are valuable screening procedures to determine the endocrine function of the fetoplacental unit, while hPL plasma levels assess the functional trophoblastic area of the placenta itself.

The antenatal FHR NST is used as a tool for screening patients with high risk pregnancy while OCT is performed to assess depleted fetal oxygen reserves if the NST is non-reactive or equivocal, or endocrine indices are compromised.

Once the perinate at risk is identified, the dangers of further intrauterine life integrated from the above tests are weighed against the dangers of prematurity. We hope that most appropriate timing of delivery thus attained will reduce perinatal morbidity and mortality and improve the quality of the human being at the time of its birth.

REFERENCES

Campbell, S. and Wilkin, D. (1975). *British Journal of Obstetrics and Gynaecology* **82**, 689.

Chard, T. (1974). *Clinical Obstetrics and Gynecology* **1**, 85.

Crane, J. P., Sauvage, J. P. and Arias, F. (1976). *American Journal of Obstetrics and Gynecology* **125**, 227.

Gant, N. F. and Worley, R. J. (1977). *In* "Perinatal Medicine" (R. J. Bolognese and R. H. Schwarz, eds), pp. 228–245, The Williams & Wilkins Co, Baltimore.

Genazzani, A. R., Cocola, F., Neri, P. and Fioretti, P. (1972). *Acta endocrinologica, Copenhagen* Supplement **167**, 71.

Hammacher, K., Hüter, K. A., Bokelman, J., *et al.* (1969). *Gynaecologia* **166**, 349.

Klopper, A., Masson, G. and Wilson, G. (1977). *British Journal of Obstetrics and Gynaecology* **84**, 648.

Kubli, F., Boos, R., Rüttgers, H., *et al.* (1977). *In* "Proceedings of the Sixth Study Group, Royal College of Obstetricians and Gynaecologists, London", p. 28.

Liggins, G. C. and Howie, R. N. (1974). *In* "Modern Perinatal Medicine" L. Gluck, ed.), p. 415. Yearbook Medical Publishers, Chicago.

Lubchenco, L. O., Searls, D. T. and Brasie, J. V. (1972). *Journal of Pediatrics* **81**, 814.

Pose, S. V., Castillo, J. B., Mora-Rojas, E. D., *et al.* (1969). Pan American Health Organization, Washington, D.C. p. 96.

Robinson, H. P. (1973). *British Medical Journal* iv, 28.

Sabbagha, R. E. (1977). *Clinical Obstetrics and Gynecology* **20**, 297.

Salvadori, B. (1977). *Acta obstetrica et gynaecologica scandinavica* **56**, 267.

Scommegna, A. and Chattoraji, S. C. (1967). *American Journal of Obstetrics and Gynecology* **99**, 1087.

Spellacy, W. N., Buhi, W. C. and Birk, S. A. (1975). *American Journal of Obstetrics and Gynecology* **121**, 835.

Westin, B. (1977). *Acta obstetrica et gynaecologica scandinavica* **56**, 273.

PLACENTAL PROVOCATIVE TESTS

P. J. Keller

*Department of Obstetrics and Gynaecology, University of Zürich, Zürich,
Switzerland*

INTRODUCTION

The benefits of the biochemical assessment of fetal well-being have been a matter of controversy for many years. At the present time it is generally accepted that several methods such as the estimation of oestrogens or of human placental lactogen (hPL) are of considerable value in the management of high risk pregnancies. However, due to the number of variables affecting the serum concentration of these hormones, fetal jeopardy may not be detected early enough. As in other fields of reproductive endocrinology, attempts have therefore been made to overcome some of the inherent problems by dynamic rather than static measurements.

One of the first placental function tests was introduced in 1967 by Lauritzen, who measured the total urinary oestrogen excretion after intravenous injection of dehydroepiandrosterone sulphate (DHA-S) to the mother. Subsequently more sophisticated procedures have been developed, all of which measure the conversion of steroid precursors. While some of these methods have been accepted with great enthusiasm, further evaluation revealed a number of significant problems.

THEORETICAL ASPECTS

Placental steroidogenesis, which involves the conversion of fetal C_{19} steroids, depends on the activity of a number of enzyme systems, which are believed to reflect placental perfusion and oxygenation. A detailed analysis of the kinetics

Serono Symposium No. 35, "The Human Placenta", edited by A. Klopper,
A. Genazzani and P. G. Crosignani, 1980. Academic Press, London and New York.

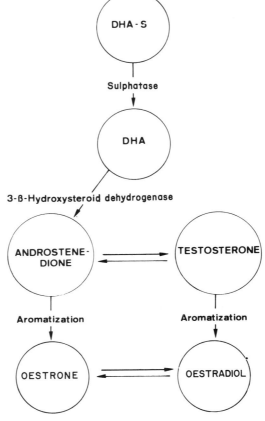

Fig. 1. Principal routes of placental steroidogenesis.

of placental metabolism is therefore indispensable to the interpretation of any dynamic function tests.

The main route involves the conversion of DHA-S to unconjugated dehydro-epiandrosterone (DHA) by placental sulphatase, which is transformed subsequently into androstenedione by 3-β-hydroxysteroid dehydrogenase and 1,4-isomerase and partly reduced to testosterone. Androstenedione and testosterone are easily converted into oestrone and oestradiol respectively by aromatizing enzymes (Fig. 1). Formation of oestriol by 16-hydroxylation depends primarily on the fetal and maternal liver function; it therefore does not necessarily reflect placental conditions.

Considering these metabolic pathways, the most attractive principle for any dynamic system should be the measurement of the appearance of androstenedione or oestrone or oestradiol after administration of DHA-S or the estimation of the disappearance of the substrate from the maternal blood.

The effect of intravenous injection of 50 mg of DHA-S on the plasma levels of

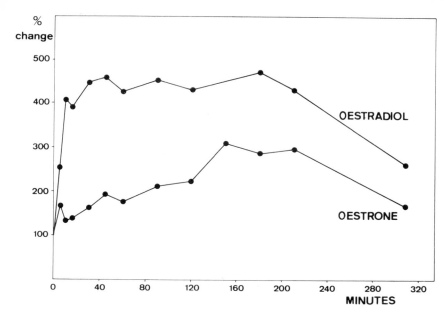

Fig. 2. Percentage increase in plasma oestrone and oestradiol after intravenous injection of 50 mg DHA-S (Klopper and Varela-Torres, 1976).

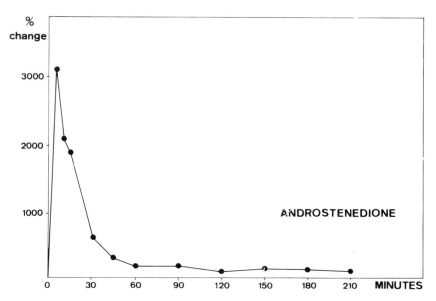

Fig. 3. Percentage increase in plasma androstenedione after intravenous injection of 50 mg DHA-S (Klopper and Varela-Torres, 1976).

androstenedione, testosterone, oestrone and oestradiol was studied by various
groups (Buster *et al.*, 1974; Künzig *et al.*, 1974; Klopper and Varela-Torres, 1976;
Strecker *et al.*, 1978). Buster *et al.* (1974) showed in midtrimester pregnancies a
two- to eightfold increase of the baseline levels of plasma oestrone and a four- to
eightfold increase of plasma oestradiol within 2–4 h after an infusion of DHA-S at
a rate of 2.5 mg/kg body weight. There was no significant alteration in plasma
oestriol levels. Klopper and Varela-Torres (1976) demonstrated a rather moderate
and slow rise of plasma oestrone following the injection of 50 mg DHA-S. This
increase did not exceed 300% of the pre-injection value. On the other hand, the
oestradiol levels showed a much steeper rise in the first 30 min (Fig. 2). The
concentration of plasma androstenedione increased very impressively with a peak
value of more than 3000% 5–10 min after the administration of DHA-S. However,
as is evident from Fig. 3, there was an immediate fall and a return to near baseline
values within 30 min. These findings are easily comprehensible when the pathways
of placental steroid formation are considered. Similar results were published by
Strecker *et al.* (1978): after an injection of 50 mg of DHA-S the highest and
most rapid increase was obtained for unconjugated oestradiol (482%), the lowest
for unconjugated oestriol (76%).

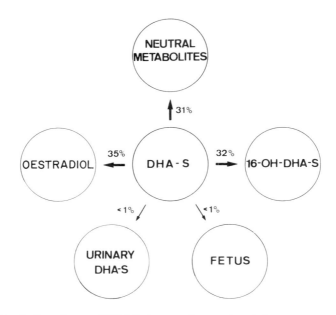

Fig. 4. Metabolic pathways of DHA-S clearance from maternal plasma.

It should be pointed out that the reported individual variations are rather high.
Klopper and Varela-Torres' mean peak value of plasma oestradiol was 366.6 nmol/l
with a standard deviation of 235.8 nmol/l; the mean androstenedione peak value
was 1191.2 nmol/l with a standard deviation of 1117.2 nmol/l ($n = 10$). These
facts should be considered whenever the clinical value of a dynamic placental
loading test is discussed.

The rate of disappearance was most extensively studied by Gant *et al.* (1971) and by Buster *et al.* (1974). As shown in Fig. 4 about 35% of DHA-S is converted to oestradiol, 31% is modified to neutral metabolites and 32% is 16-hydroxylated. Less than 1% is excreted in the urine (Madden *et al.*, 1976). The mean circulatory half-life of intravenously infused DHA-S in five normally pregnant women was calculated to be 2.99 ± 0.62 h (Buster *et al.*, 1974). In non-pregnant women the half-life was much longer (4.76 ± 1.44 h), since the precursor is not removed by the placenta.

CLINICAL APPLICATION

The basic principle of any dynamic test is a well-defined conversion rate of the precursor by the normal placenta. It is assumed that this mechanism becomes impeded early in the course of an obstetric disorder with impaired placental function (Fig. 5). Although a number of clinical studies have been performed and various modifications have been proposed, results are still conflicting (Lauritzen, 1967, 1969, 1973; Crabben *et al.*, 1970; Keller and Schreiner, 1970; Künzig *et al.*, 1974; Korda *et al.*, 1975; Klopper and Varela-Torres, 1976; Strecker *et al.*, 1978). Some of the most important findings, however, will briefly be summarized.

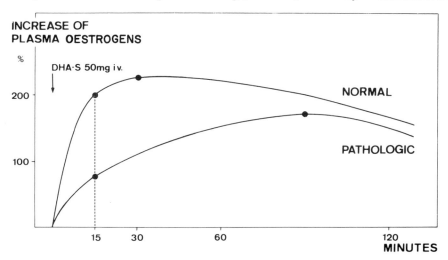

Fig. 5. Percentage increase in plasma oestrogens in normal and pathologic pregnancies (*n* = 35) (Strecker and Lauritzen, 1974).

While there is a general agreement that DHA-S is the precursor to be used, there is no unanimity about the end-point of the test. From the theoretical point of view the estimation of plasma oestradiol should be most useful for this purpose. However, Strecker *et al.* (1978), who investigated the plasma levels of unconjugated oestrone, oestradiol and oestriol as well as total oestrone and oestriol in normal and pathologic pregnancies, concluded that oestrone was the most sensitive indicator of fetal jeopardy (Fig. 6). By using a special scoring system (Table I), which evaluates the maximal and the percentage increase as well as the net and the percentage increase 15 min after DHA-S injection, the authors claimed to predict the fetoplacental state with an accuracy of 82% compared to only 66% using single plasma oestriol assays.

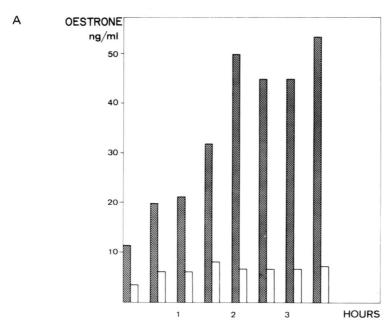

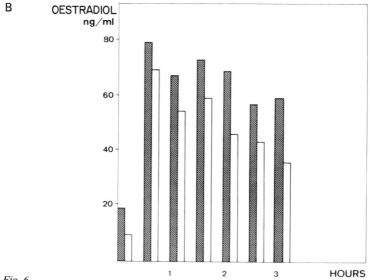

Fig. 6

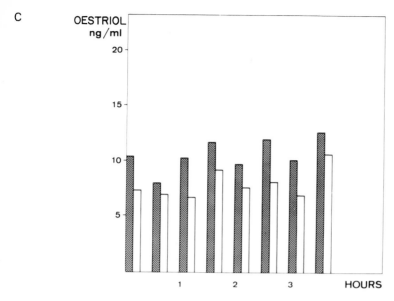

Fig. 6. Plasma oestrone (A), oestradiol (B) and oestriol (C) after intravenous injection of 50 mg DHA-S in normal ($n = 6$) and toxaemic ($n = 7$) pregnancies (Künzig *et al.*, 1974).

Table I. Score system for the evaluation of the DHA-S loading test (Strecker *et al.*, 1978).

E_1 (ng/ml)	Maximal increase (ng/ml)	Increase after 15 min (ng/ml)	Percentage increase	Percentage after 15 min	Score
0.1–2.5	0.1–5.0	< 4.0	0 or > 150	0 or > 100	0
2.6–5.0	5.1–7.5	4.1–6.0	101–150	61–100	1
5.1–7.5	7.6–10.0	6.1–10.0	51–100	51–60	2
7.6–10.0	10.1–20.0	–	1–50	–	3
> 10.0	> 20.0	> 10.0	–	1–50	4

These promising results are not undisputed. Controversial findings have been reported by Keller and Schreiner (1970), Korda *et al.* (1975) and Klopper and Varela-Torres (1976), who could not distinguish the variable response in normal pregnancy from that in patients with growth-retarded fetus, severe hypertension or even impending fetal death (Fig. 7). Their findings are supported by the data of Buster *et al.* (1974), who failed to demonstrate a significant difference in the rate of disappearance of intravenously administered DHA-S in pregnancies with live (mean half-life 2.99 h) and with dead fetus (mean half-life 2.66 h) (Fig. 8).

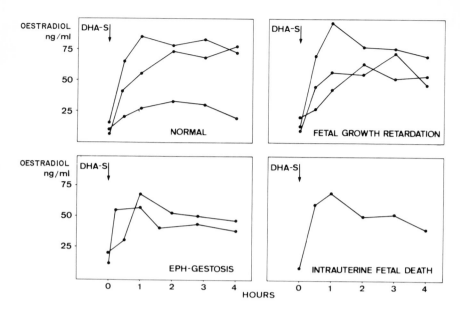

Fig. 7. Placental loading test with 50 mg DHA-S in normal and pathologic pregnancies.

CONCLUSIONS AND PERSPECTIVES

While there is no doubt about the theoretical interest of dynamic placental function tests, the clinical value is not yet fully elucidated. The best modification for the time being seems to be the assessment of unconjugated plasma oestrone and oestradiol following an injection of 50 mg DHA-S. The shape of the dose-response curve should be established since in some cases placental dysfunction might be reflected by prolongation of the conversion time rather than by an absolute increment, a fact which is also considered by the Strecker score (Strecker *et al.*, 1978). Because there is a great variety of results from one individual to the other, it is doubtful whether serial estimations of plasma oestriol or hPL are inferior to dynamic function tests.

Although physical methods compete strongly with the presently available hormonal methods for the monitoring of high risk pregnancies, there is no doubt that further efforts will be made to explore the biochemical capacity of the placenta. Suppression of the fetal C_{19} steroids with betamethasone might provide a more specific test for the placental function and progress in radio-immunoassay may enable us to investigate a number of various enzyme systems *in vivo*, e.g. the sulphatase, the 3-β-hydroxysteroid dehydrogenase or the aromatase activity by administration of the appropriate precursor (Fig. 9). Whether or not such tests will provide additional information to the clinician remains open.

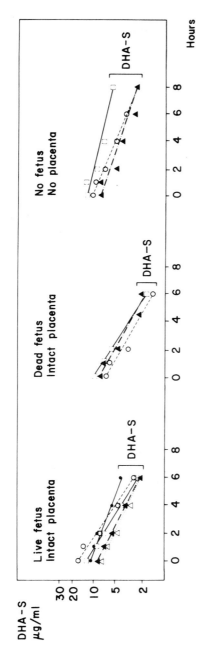

Fig. 8. Plasma levels of DHA-S after intravenous infusion of 2.5 mg DHA-S/kg body weight in various conditions (Buster *et al.*, 1974).

DYNAMIC PLACENTAL FUNCTION TESTS

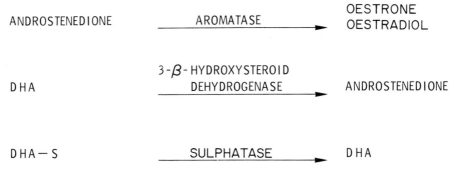

Fig. 9. Suggested dynamic evaluation of placental enzyme activity in risk pregnancies.

REFERENCES

Buster, J. E., Abraham, G. E., Kyle, F. W. and Marshal, J. R. (1974). *Journal of Clinical Endocrinology and Metabolism* **38**, 1031.

Crabben, H. van der, Hammacher, K., Werner, Ch. and Kaiser, E. (1970). *Geburtshilfe und Frauenheilkunde* **30**, 71.

Gant, N. F., Hutchinson, H. T., Siiteri, P. K. and MacDonald, P. C. (1971). *American Journal of Obstetrics and Gynecology* **111**, 555.

Keller, P. J. and Schreiner, W. E. (1970). *Schweizerische Zeitschrift für Gynäkologie und Geburtshilfe* **1**, 327.

Klopper, A. and Varela-Torres, R. (1976). *British Journal of Obstetrics and Gynaecology* **83**, 478.

Korda, A. R., Challis, J. J., Anderson, A. B. and Turnbull, A. C. (1975). *British Journal of Obstetrics and Gynaecology* **82**, 656.

Künzig, H. J., Geiger, P. and Gwuzdz, P. (1974). *Zeitschrift für Geburtshilfe und Perinatologie* **178**, 245.

Lauritzen, Ch. (1967). *Acta Endocrinologica, Copenhagen* Suppl. 119, 188.

Lauritzen, Ch. (1969). *Hormone and Metabolic Research* **1**, 96.

Lauritzen, Ch. (1973). *Geburtshilfe und Frauenheilkunde* **33**, 238.

Madden, J. D., Siiteri, P. K., MacDonald, P. C. and Gant, N. F. (1976). *American Journal of Obstetrics and Gynecology* **125**, 915.

Strecker, J. R. and Lauritzen, Ch. (1974). *Zeitschrift für Geburtshilfe und Perinatologie* **178**, 254.

Strecker, J. R., Killus, M., Lauritzen, Ch. and Neumann, G. K. (1978). *American Journal of Obstetrics and Gynecology* **131**, 239.

PHYSIOLOGY OF STEROID HORMONES IN MOTHER AND FETUS

G. R. Wilson and A. I. Klopper

Department of Obstetrics and Gynaecology, Royal Infirmary, Aberdeen, Scotland

INTRODUCTION

As in so many other areas of reproductive endocrinology we are in debt to the work of Diczfalusy and his group in Stockholm on the physiology of oestrogens in pregnancy. In a recent publication by Diczfalusy (1978) the author stated that during the period 1963–72 a systematic exploration of the fetal, placental and maternal interrelations in the formation of sterols and steroids produced 80 full publications; however, the original concept of the "feto-placental unit" (as described in Diczfalusy, 1964) was only slightly modified (e.g. Diczfalusy, 1974). Despite this exponential increase in knowledge, many of the regulatory mechanisms governing changes in oestrogen metabolism in pregnancy are not fully understood. There is still no rational explanation, for example, for the enormous amounts of oestriol produced in late pregnancy, most of which is gone within 24 h of delivery. It is the purpose of this article to examine some of the differences between maternal and fetal handling of an oestrogen precursor, dehydroepiandrosterone sulphate (DHAS) and to present some recent evidence on the compartmental distribution of oestradiol and oestriol in late pregnancy.

Serono Symposium No. 35, "The Human Placenta", edited by A. Klopper,
A. Genazzani and P. G. Crosignani, 1980. Academic Press, London and New York.

BIOSYNTHESIS OF OESTRONE, OESTRADIOL AND OESTRIOL

Most of the pathways describing the formation of these oestrogens are well documented and only a brief resume is necessary. In 1963, Siiteri and MacDonald showed that about 90% of the oestriol produced in the fetoplacental unit is derived from fetal DHAS and only 10% originates from the maternal side. In early pregnancy the percentage conversion of DHAS to oestradiol is about 2% whereas the conversion is about 40% at term (Siiteri and MacDonald, 1966). DHAS is therefore an important precursor for the formation of oestradiol. The production rate was calculated to be about 10–16 mg/day at term. Similar studies were reported by Tulchinsky and Korenman (1971), who found that about 60% of the oestradiol originated from maternal DHAS. In view of this important contribution by the maternal precursor to the formation of oestradiol it is now assumed that the use of oestradiol assays in the assessment of fetal well-being is not as informative as was originally thought by many investigators.

DHAS CONVERSION TO OESTROGENS *IN VIVO*

The conversion of administered DHAS to oestrogens and, in particular, oestradiol might be useful as a means of testing the steroidogenic capacity of the placenta. The idea was originally explored by Lauritzen (1967), who gave 10 mg DHAS by intravenous injection to women in late pregnancy. He measured the increase in total urinary oestrogens and under the conditions of the experiment this was almost entirely an increase in urinary oestriol. The contribution which 10 mg DHAS can make to a 24 h urinary output of oestriol is so small as to be swallowed up in the normal day-to-day variation in oestriol levels. The dose was soon raised to 50 mg and many publications began to appear on this so-called dynamic test of placental function (e.g. Lauritzen *et al.*, 1976).

Table I. Mean oestradiol concentration after intravenous DHAS.

Time (min)	No. of subjects	Mean oestradiol (nmol/l)	Standard deviation (nmol/l)
0	19	80.6	31.1
5	11	200.8	137.7
10	12	324.4	319.5
15	19	312.1	211.8
30	19	361.1	301.1
45	16	366.6	235.8
60	16	343.5	241.5
90	16	363.6	220.4
120	15	344.9	201.0
180	6	373.5	235.8
210	6	343.5	240.2
310	2	205.2	—

Korda *et al.* (1975) measured the change in maternal peripheral oestradiol levels after the injection of DHAS and concluded that the test was not a useful addition to the armamentarium of tests of fetoplacental function. These authors suggested that its main defect was that the response was too variable to allow a confident interpretation of the results in a compromised pregnancy. In an attempt to examine the steps by which the placenta converts DHAS to oestrogens, Klopper *et al.* (1976) studied the test critically. These authors measured the plasma levels of androstenedione, testosterone, oestrone and oestradiol in normal late pregnancy after intravenous injection of 50 mg DHAS.

The change in oestradiol concentration is shown in Table I. This table shows that the oestradiol concentration changed from a mean pre-injection value of 80.6 nmol/l to a maximum value of 373.5 nmol/l following DHAS injection.

Table II.   Mean oestrone concentration after intravenous DHAS.

Time (min)	No. of subjects	Mean oestradiol (nmol/l)	Standard deviation (nmol/l)
0	19	42.6	18.6
5	11	72.0	18.3
10	12	54.1	24.0
15	19	57.9	22.6
30	19	67.1	31.7
45	16	80.2	43.2
60	16	74.3	37.3
90	16	89.2	48.8
120	15	95.4	63.8
150	5	129.7	67.4
180	6	121.2	59.2
210	6	124.4	66.5
310	4	66.7	31.4

Table III.   Mean testosterone concentration after intravenous DHAS.

Time (min)	No. of subjects	Mean oestradiol (nmol/l)	Standard deviation (nmol/l)
0	19	5.7	2.3
5	11	22.5	9.1
10	12	13.1	8.2
15	19	15.0	9.9
30	18	9.8	7.4
45	16	9.0	7.0
60	17	7.1	3.0
90	16	6.2	2.9

Although the values at every point are significantly above the baseline and every subject showed an increase over her baseline values, the large standard deviations show that there was a big scatter in individual responses. At about 30 min the oestradiol level is about 4.5 times the baseline value. It is maintained at this level for about $3\frac{1}{2}$ h and then slowly declines. In the two subjects studied at 5 h the value was still twice the baseline.

The response of plasma oestrone to the injection of DHAS is shown in Table II. The oestrone concentration rose from a baseline value of 42.6 nmol/l to a peak of 129.7 nmol/l. By 5 min the concentration had already risen significantly; however, there was a large variation in response from one patient to another. Oestrone concentration rises more slowly than does oestradiol; it does not reach a peak value until 150 min−$2\frac{1}{2}$ h later than the oestradiol peak.

The changes in testosterone after injection of DHAS are shown in Table III. The mean testosterone concentration rises from 5.7 nmol/l to 22.5 nmol/l but the rise is not sustained−the value at 1 h is not significantly raised. The peak value is reached much sooner−after 5 min compared to 30 min for oestradiol. There is no plateau−the fall to baseline starts after 5 min.

Table IV. Mean androstenedione concentration after intravenous DHAS.

Time (min)	No. of subjects	Mean androstenedione (nmol/l)	Standard deviation (nmol/l)
0	17	38.5	15.2
5	10	1191.2	1117.2
10	12	807.3	734.2
15	17	733.1	834.5
30	17	255.3	299.6
45	15	136.0	79.2
60	15	105.0	53.5
90	13	105.0	68.5
120	12	73.1	54.6

The effect of DHAS injection on maternal plasma androstenedione levels is recorded in Table IV. The change in androstenedione is proportionately larger. The concentration rises from a baseline level of 38.5 nmol/l to a peak value of 1191 nmol/l 5 min after injection. The large standard deviations show that the scatter from one subject to another is very large and the mean figure has little meaning. The large differences between individuals is due not to a difference in the pattern of response but to the large range in baseline values and in the absolute values of the subsequent response. In terms of proportionate increase over the baseline the rise in androstenedione is most marked; 10 times that of any other steroid.

FETAL HANDLING OF DHAS

In 1977 Gamissans *et al.* studied the fate of DHAS injected directly into the fetus. This group postulated that the extent to which maternal oestrogens rose after intrafetal injection might give some indication as to whether the fetoplacental unit is capable of manipulating maternal oestrogen concentration by utilizing fetal as compared to maternal DHAS as substrate.

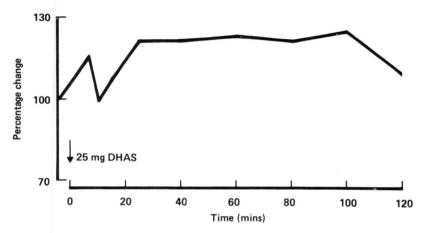

Fig. 1. The percentage change in oestrone concentration after injection of 25 mg DHAS into the fetus (*n* = 10). The pre-injection value is taken as 100%.

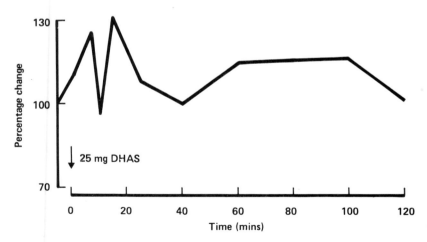

Fig. 2. The percentage change in oestradiol concentration after injection of 25 mg DHAS into the fetus (*n* = 10). The pre-injection value is taken as 100%.

G. R. Wilson and A. I. Klopper

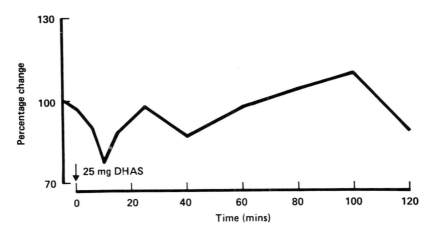

Fig. 3. The percentage change in oestriol concentration after injection of 25 mg DHAS into the fetus (*n* = 11). The pre-injection value is taken as 100%.

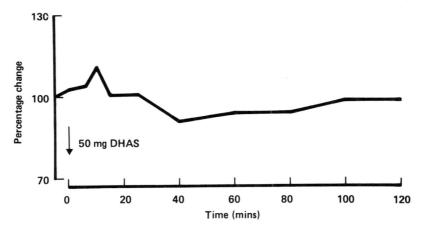

Fig. 4. The percentage change in oestrone concentration after injection of 50 mg DHAS into the fetus (*n* = 11). The pre-injection value is taken as 100%.

The subjects studied were 21 normal pregnancies between 36 and 41 weeks of gestation. The placenta was localized by ultrasonagraphy and the injection carried out only if it did not overlie the breech. DHAS was injected into the fetal breech through the abdominal wall of the mother. In 10 cases 25 mg was injected and the remaining 11 patients received 50 mg. None of the patients went into labour within 48 h of the procedure and all the patients subsequently delivered normal babies. The results for the group of patients who received 25 mg substrate are shown in Figs 1–3. The pre-injection value was taken as 100% and the percentage

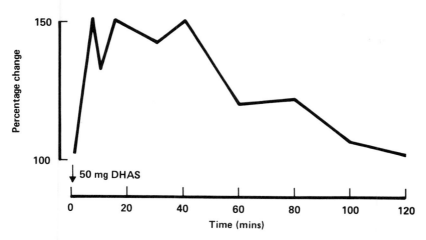

Fig. 5. The percentage change in oestradiol concentration after injection of 50 mg DHAS into the fetus (*n* = 11). The pre-injection value is taken as 100%.

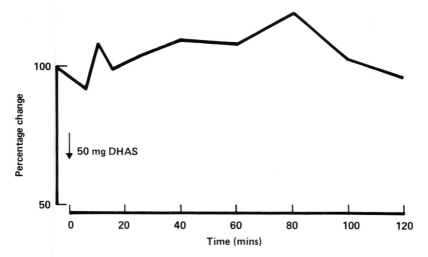

Fig. 6. The percentage change in oestriol concentration after injection of 50 mg DHAS into the fetus (*n* = 11). The pre-injection value is taken as 100%.

increase is shown for oestrone, oestradiol and oestriol. The curves shown are the mean responses and once more, as with the experiments on maternal handling of the substrate, there was a wide scatter in individual responses. The experiments were continued for 2 h post-injection and there was no significant rise in oestrone, oestradiol or oestriol levels. When the dose of DHAS was raised to 50 mg again, there was no significant rise in the levels of the three oestrogens. The results are illustrated as mean responses in Figs 4–6.

MATERNAL AND FETAL COMPARTMENTALIZATION OF OESTROGENS

In a recent study designed to examine the distribution of oestrogens through the fetal and maternal compartments, Smith *et al.* (1979) measured unconjugated oestriol, total oestriol and unconjugated oestradiol in a variety of compartments in normal late pregnancy. Parallel measurements were made in maternal tissue fluid, cerebrospinal fluid and uterine vein blood; or in retroplacental blood, umbilical cord blood (artery and vein) and amniotic fluid. In a further group of 16 women, uterine vein samples were collected at caesarean section and the samples analysed for unconjugated oestriol and oestradiol.

The results for the uterine vein samples are shown in Fig. 7. The values for each steroid are expressed as percentages of the corresponding peripheral vein values. There is no pattern from patient to patient and in most cases the percentage of oestriol and oestradiol in the uterine veins are different.

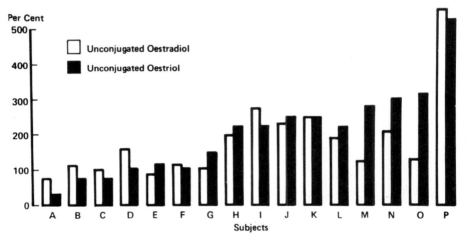

Fig. 7. Unconjugated oestradiol and oestriol in 16 uterine vein samples expressed as percentages of the corresponding peripheral vein values.

Although the final step in the biosynthesis of oestriol and oestradiol probably takes place in the placenta, it seemed relevant in a study of compartmentalization to examine separately the distribution of the fetoplacental oestrogen, oestriol, and of the purely placental oestrogen, oestradiol. The molecular sizes of oestriol and its various conjugates such as oestriol-3-sulphate and oestriol-16-glucosiduronate are not greatly different, but their lipophilic characteristics, and hence their likely transmission rates across the membrane barriers between compartments, differ greatly. It was hoped that this comparison of the compartmental distribution of various placental and fetal products would give some insight into the site and nature of their physiological action in pregnancy. The results are shown in Table V.

The highest mean value of total oestriol was found in umbilical arterial plasma. Smaller mean values were found in cord vein and amniotic fluid. The mean values

Table V. Oestrogens in maternal and fetal compartments.

		Interstitial fluid	Cerebrospinal fluid	Peritoneal fluid	Peripheral vein	Uterine vein	Retroplacental blood	Cord vein	Cord artery	Amniotic fluid
Total oestriol nmol/l	Range	–	30, 38	256–1223	417–1584	330–1965	800–5356	3337–9295	5460–14 370	1057–6336
	Mean	717	34	773,1	879.1	993.6	3229.2	6572.7	7774.2	4045.8
	S.D.	–	–	364.9	350.0	426.4	1294.5	1572	3003.8	1772.2
	No.	1	2	13	22	18	20	16	7	5
Unconjugated oestriol (nmol/l)	Range	–	6, 17	17–18	18–109	29–285	306–2576	125–449	48–176	24–166
	Mean	70	11.5	38.1	57.1	107.1	840.5	260.1	100.4	75.83
	S.D.	–	–	15.2	26.3	74.6	557.9	99.0	38.1	48.33
	No.	1	2	13	22	19	20	16	7	6
Oestradiol (nmol/l)	Range	–	–	13–79	33–156	53–385	54–510	12–67	5–21	2.2–5.0
	Mean	4.1	0.53	46.5	98.5	163.1	245.4	35.7	14.3	3.45
	S.D.	–	–	19.54	37.6	99.6	140.4	14.4	5.5	0.93
	No.	1	1	10	21	19	19	16	9	5

in retroplacental blood were smaller than in cord blood, although they represented the highest concentration found in the maternal compartments. Values fell in order from retroplacental blood to uterine vein, peripheral vein, and peritoneal fluid.

Retroplacental blood had the highest mean value of unconjugated oestriol with a progressive reduction in level to cord vein, cord artery and amniotic fluid. On the maternal side the order was uterine vein, peripheral vein, and peritoneal fluid.

Oestradiol was also found in highest concentration in retroplacental blood, and the pattern of diminution seen on either side of the placenta was similar to that seen with unconjugated oestriol, although the gradients were more acute.

As the parameters measured do not have a normal distribution Spearman's rank order correlation was used to relate values in one compartment with another. In maternal peripheral blood a positive correlation was found between unconjugated oestriol and oestradiol ($P = 0.55, p < 0.05, n = 17$). There was no significant correlation between peritoneal fluid and uterine vein or retroplacental blood. Peripheral vein levels correlated significantly with the values in the following compartments:

1. Peritoneal fluid ($P = 0.64, p < 0.05, n = 12$).
2. Uterine vein ($P = 0.44, p < 0.05, n = 17$).
3. Retroplacental blood ($P = 0.5, p < 0.05, n = 14$).
4. Cord vein ($P = 0.07, p < 0.01, n = 14$).
5. Cord artery ($P = 0.09, p < 0.05, n = 5$).

Retroplacental blood showed a significant correlation with both uterine vein values ($P = 0.9, p < 0.01, n = 16$) and cord vein values ($P = 0.9, p < 0.01, n = 13$). Amongst the fetal compartments the numbers of results were too few for useful comparison.

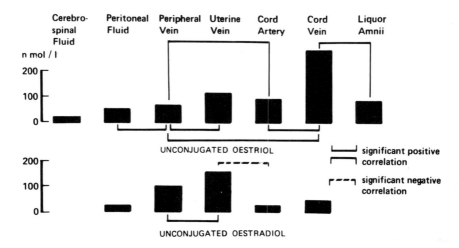

Fig. 8. The distribution of unconjugated oestriol and oestradiol between maternal and fetal compartments.

Significant correlations for oestradiol were found only between peripheral vein and uterine vein ($P = 0.56$, $p < 0.05$, $n = 16$) and retroplacental blood ($P = 0.41$, $p < 0.05$, $n = 16$). A significant negative correlation was found between uterine vein and cord artery ($P = 0.9$, $p < 0.02$), but only six paired results were available for calculation. These significant correlations for unconjugated oestriol and oestradiol are represented diagrammatically in Fig. 8.

DISCUSSION

In the experiments described by Klopper *et al.* (1976) the maternal concentration of testosterone was raised for 5 to 10 min but there was no evidence of untoward effect on the infants. The possibility of more subtle damage to the nervous control of reproductive function in adult life is remote. Even if the transient rise in androgens was reflected in a similar rise in fetal concentration, testosterone would be carried in a biologically inactive state bound to sex hormone binding globulin. It has been shown by Simmer *et al.* (1972) that large doses of testosterone causing maternal levels much higher than those reported in this study do not cause any rise in fetal testosterone levels.

The fact that androstenedione rose more sharply was not surprising in view of the established pathways for oestrogen biosynthesis from DHAS. The fact that the androgen peak precedes the oestrogen peak fits with the precursor role of the former; however, the short duration of the androgen rise is less easy to explain. Since oestrone rises more slowly than oestradiol, it is probable that the latter is the primary product. The main pathway is likely to be via testosterone to oestradiol, and possibly the main bulk of the oestrone is produced by oxidation of oestradiol. If a sizeable proportion of the oestrone was made from androstenedione it would rise earlier since androstenedione rises at the same time as testosterone. It is generally assumed that 17β-dehydrogenase activity is widely distributed and that interconversion between oestrone and oestradiol is rapid. It would appear from our results that when the equilibrium is disturbed by rapid formation of excess oestradiol it takes several hours for it to be restored.

Recently, Wolf *et al.* (1978) found higher concentrations of oestrone in placental perfusion studies with DHAS. These findings suggest that oestrone and not oestradiol, as found *in vivo*, is the main placental oestrogen metabolized from DHAS. It adds to the speculation as to whether the relatively high levels of oestradiol detectable in the *in vivo* test are a secondary product of the widely distributed 17β-dehydrogenases in the maternal organism. It may be that these experiments are misleading in that only the fetal compartment was perfused, and the authors demonstrated by the use of [99]Te-labelled macroparticles that only 40–55% of the organ participated adequately in the fetal circulation. There are many technical problems to be overcome in dual perfusion systems, but it may be that such a system is necessary to shed light on this interesting contradiction.

The extent of the fetal contribution to the levels of oestrone, oestradiol and oestriol in maternal plasma can be assessed from the work of Gamissans *et al.* (1977). It can be concluded that fetal DHAS plays little or no part in the biosynthesis. Almost all the experiments on which our present concept of the importance of fetal DHAS in the biogenesis of oestrogens is based were done in early pregnancy (before 20 weeks of gestation). Sixteen years ago Klopper and Billewicz (1963) suggested that changes in oestrogen, and in particular oestriol, biosynthesis were a feature of fetal maturation after 34 weeks of gestation. Perhaps that salient observation should now be resurrected. There are many reasons why no rise in maternal peripheral oestrogens was observed after injection of DHAS into the fetus. Not the least of these is that adsorption from fetal tissues might be too slow to produce any change in the maternal circulation. These findings suggest that studies on the termination of pregnancy or hydatidiform moles may not be suitable models for the study of steroidogenesis in late pregnancy.

The results on the compartmentalization studies on oestriol and oestradiol are important in that they may help in our understanding and interpretation of hormone assays for the assessment of fetoplacental function. The highest concentration of oestradiol is found in the retroplacental blood, supporting in part the hypothesis that this is its main point of entry. By the time it reaches the uterine vein it has been diluted and the peripheral venous level is still lower. An impeded outflow from the vascular compartment is reflected in the low concentration in the peritoneal fluid. Although only a few samples could be obtained, oestradiol is clearly present in the cerebrospinal fluid and it is possible that this steroid may exert some physiological action in the nervous system during pregnancy. Oestradiol levels are low in the fetal compartments and there are few correlations between the various compartments. The fact that peripheral vein and peritoneal fluid levels are not related suggests that outflow from the vascular compartment is limited by the protein binding of oestradiol, presumably to sex hormone binding globulin.

Diczfalusy and Mancuso (1969) showed that part of the biogenesis of oestriol takes place in the fetus. It is not surprising, therefore, to find higher concentrations of this steroid in the fetal compartment as compared to the purely placental steroid such as oestradiol. The large number of correlations between oestriol concentrations in various compartments, even across the placenta, is taken as evidence of its poor affinity for binding protein as compared to oestradiol.

The results for total oestriol, a mixture of molecular species, are very different from the unconjugated moiety. The highest concentration occurs in the fetal circulation, presumably as sulphate. It is not surprising that the concentration of total oestriol falls after leaving the retroplacental circulation; surprisingly, however, there is no gradient from uterine vein to peripheral vein. Again, total oestriol concentration in the peritoneal fluid is high, presumably reflecting the relatively easy flow of this mixture of oestriol moieties from the vascular compartment.

The distribution of the steroids studied would fit the following model. Oestradiol and unconjugated oestriol are secreted by the placenta into *both* maternal and fetal compartments, although passage across intercompartmental barriers is impeded, more so with oestradiol than oestriol. Sulphate conjugates of oestriol are carried to the placenta in the fetal circulation. They are further hydrolysed in their passage through the placenta. A further flow of oestriol conjugates, mainly glucosiduronates, takes place by conjugation of the steroid in the gut. In the light of these findings perhaps some of our tests of fetoplacental function are really only as good as our understanding of the physiology of the compounds routinely measured. It was recently suggested by Diczfalusy (1978) that one of the weaknesses of the work by the Stockholm group was that they did not measure the absolute mass of the many products detected, only the amount of *radioactive* product isolated in each experiment. He put forward the very interesting speculation: "What might have happened if steroid radioimmunoassays had become available some 10 years before the introduction of prostaglandins? Probably we would have had today a more complete view of the fetoplacental unit and in much more quantitative terms."

REFERENCES

Diczfalusy, E. (1964). *Federation Proceedings. Federation of American Societies for Experimental Biology* **23**, 791.

Diczfalusy, E. (1974). *American Journal of Obstetrics and Gynecology* **119**, 419.

Diczfalusy, E. (1978). *Journal of Endocrinology* **79**, 3p.

Diczfaluzy, E. and Mancuso, S. (1969). *In* "Foetus and Placenta" (A. Klopper and E. Diczfalusy, eds), p. 191, Blackwell Scientific Publications, Oxford.

Gamissans, O., Wilson, G. R., Cuyas, J., Davi, E. and Pujol-Amat, P. (1977). *Obstetrics and Gynecology* **50**, 439.

Klopper, A. and Billewicz, W. (1963). *Journal of Obstetrics and Gynaecology of the British Commonwealth* **70**, 1024.

Klopper, A., Varela-Torres, R. and Jandial, V. (1976). *British Journal of Obstetrics and Gynaecology* **83**, 479.

Korda, A. R., Challis, J. J., Anderson, A. B. and Turnbull, A. C. (1975). *British Journal of Obstetrics and Gynaecology* **82**, 656.

Lauritzen, Ch. (1967). *Acta endocrinologica, Copenhagen* Suppl. 119, 188.

Lauritzen, Ch., Strecker, J. and Lehmann, W. D. (1976). *In* "Plasma Hormone Assays in Evaluation of Fetal Wellbeing" (A. Klopper, ed.), pp. 113–135, Churchill Livingstone, Edinburgh.

Panigel, M. (1962). *American Journal of Obstetrics and Gynecology* **84**, 1664.

Schneider, H., Panigel, M. and Dancis, J. (1972). *American Journal of Obstetrics and Gynecology* **114**, 822.

Siiteri, P. K. and MacDonald, P. C. (1963). *Steroids* **2**, 713.

Siiteri, P. K. and MacDonald, P. C. (1966). *Journal of Clinical Endocrinology and Metabolism* **26**, 571.

Simmer, H. H., Frankland, M. V. and Griepel, M. (1972). *Steroids* **19**, 229.

Smith, R., Klopper, A., Hughes, G. and Wilson, G. (1979). *British Journal of Obstetrics and Gynaecology* **86**, 119.

Strecker, J. R., Killus, C. M., Lauritzen, Ch. and Neumann, G. K. (1978). *American Journal of Obstetrics and Gynecology* **131**, 239.

Tulchinsky, D. and Korenman, S. G. (1971). *Journal of Clinical Investigation* **50**, 1490.

Wolf, A. S., Musch, K. A., Spiedel, W., Strecker, J. R. and Lauritzen, Ch. (1978). *Acta endocrinologica, Copenhagen* **87**, 181.

METABOLISM OF THE PHYSIOLOGICAL PRECURSOR STEROID DEHYDROEPIANDROSTERONE (DHA) IN THE PERFUSED HUMAN PLACENTA

A. S. Wolf, K. Musch and C. Lauritzen

*Department of Obstetrics and Gynaecology,
University of Ulm, Ulm, German Federal Republic*

INTRODUCTION

The human placenta is an incomplete endocrine gland, since precursor substances such as dehydroepiandrosterone (DHA), dehydroepiandrosterone sulphate (DHA-S) and 16α-hydroxydehydroepiandrosterone (16α-OH-DHA) from the fetal adrenals are needed for oestrogen biogenesis. Difficulties in the evaluation of endocrine parameters in pregnancy as parameters of fetoplacental well-being arise from the problem that the available information always reflects the overall activity of the three compartments of mother, fetus and placenta. Determinations of oestrogens in plasma and urine, or results from the DHA-S loading test (Lauritzen, 1967), therefore express the activity of the entire unit. Tests for placental function alone are not yet available. Therefore it seemed desirable to analyse parts of this system separately to get a better understanding of the integrated system. Since the placenta is the only easily available part of this system, a perfusion system for the study of placental endocrine capacity has been developed.

Serono Symposium No. 35, "The Human Placenta", edited by A. Klopper,
A. Genazzani and P. G. Crosignani, 1980. Academic Press, London and New York.

MATERIALS AND METHODS

Perfusion Technique

A system for the perfusion of a single placental cotyledon was developed according to Cedard 1971) (see Fig. 1). The placental chamber (PC) is kept in a waterbath (WB) at 37 °C. The perfusate is circulated by a motor roller pump (MP) into the

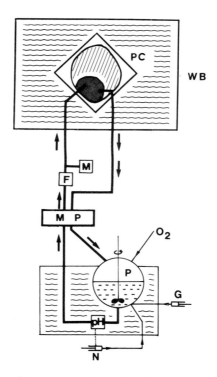

Fig. 1. Diagram of the perfusion system. For explanations see the text.

artery of the cotyledon. Flow and pressure are recorded by an electromagnetic flowmeter (F) and a manometer (M). The venous return of perfusion medium is collected in a pool (P), where NaHCO₃ solution (N), oxygen (O₂), and glucose (G) are added and mixed. The pH of the medium is automatically adjusted to 7.25–7.30. The perfusate consists of a buffered isotonic Ringer solution, containing 1.5 g glucose, 10 000 IU heparine (Roche), and 30 g Dextran T40 (Pharmacia) per 1000 ml. The use of blood or protein solutions (Biotest) resulted in haemolysis, clotting, and foaming of proteins and was therefore rejected.

Only fresh placentae obtained after spontaneous delivery or caesarean section were used.

Viability Criteria

The following criteria were used for the assessment of placental vitality (mean ± S.D.):

1. Vascular resistance (1.88 ± 0.77);
2. Oxygen consumption (0.17 ± 0.07 ml O_2 (100 g placenta)$^{-1}$ min^{-1});
3. Glucose consumption (3.43 ± 1.24 g (kg placenta)$^{-1}$ h^{-1});
4. Lactate/pyruvate ratio;
5. Determination of lactate dehydrogenase (LDH);
6. Morphological evaluation by transmission electronmicroscopy and regional perfusion control.

Experimental Design

For studies of the metabolism of the physiological precursor steroid DHA in mature ($n = 34$), immature ($n = 8$) and pathological placentae ($n = 6$), the same procedure was followed. Samples of perfusate were taken at 15, 30, 60, 90 and 120 min after addition of the precursor steroid and stored frozen until analysis. Different amounts (0.2–100.0 mg) of precursor steroids (DHA) were injected altogether with 2.5 μCi of the ^{14}C-labelled compound.

Samples for determination of glucose, pO_2, pCO_2, lactate, pyruvate and LDH were taken every hour.

Steroid Analysis

Ether-extracted steroids from the perfusate and homogenate were separated by thin layer chromatography using chloroform and ethyl acetate at a 110:15 ratio as solvents. The TLC plates with separated steroids were scanned by a thin layer scanner (Berthold), the impulses were computed by a multichannel scaling analyser to values of radioactive peaks of each steroid. Subsequently the silica gel was scraped off and determination by β-scintillation counting was performed as a control. All values obtained were calculated by means of an experimental standard of DHA and expressed as picomoles of steroid per millilitre of perfusate per gram of placenta.

By this procedure the placental steroids 4-androstene-3,17-dione (A), dehydro-epiandrosterone (DHA), testosterone (T), oestrone (Oe$_1$), 17β-oestradiol (Oe$_2$) and polar androgens (pA) were sufficiently separated.

RESULTS

Aromatization of DHA to Oestrogens in Mature, Normal Placentas

According to previous investigations and to data from the DHA-S loading test the following parameters were chosen as indicators of the steroidogenesis of the placenta: Oe$_1$(15′) = oestrone at 15 min; Oe$_{tot}$(90′) = Oe$_1$ + Oe$_2$ at 90 min;

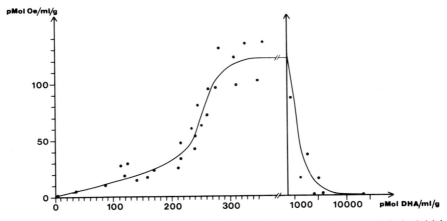

Fig. 2. Correlation of total oestrogens (Oe$_{tot}$(90')) after 90 min of perfusion with the initial concentration of DHA.

Oe$_{tot}$(P + H) = total Oe in perfusate and homogenate; *aromatization rate* = percentage of aromatized products in the perfusate and homogenate in relation to the amount of DHA added; *aromatization ratio* = Oe/DHA and Oe/androgens.

In the following analysis (Fig. 2), the concentrations of aromatized steroids, Oe$_{tot}$(90'), were compared to initial concentrations of DHA. A small aromatization rate is found at low basal DHA concentrations of 10–250 pmol ml^{-1} g^{-1}, with a slight linear increase. A marked increase in aromatization with a plateau is found at 250–350 pmol ml^{-1} g^{-1}, reflecting a substrate saturation of the placental enzymes. Concentrations of more than 500 ⨍mol ml^{-1} g^{-1} DHA lead to a drop of aromatization. Therefore, the aromatization rate is characterized by the basal concentration of DHA.

Oestrone (Oe$_1$) is the main oestrogenic placental compound, as compared with 17β-oestradiol (Oe$_2$). As can be deduced from Fig. 3, the concentration of Oe$_1$ is 3.5–4.1 times higher than that of Oe$_2$.

Aromatization Ratios Oe/DHA and Oe/Androgens

The introduction of "aromatization ratios" as a mathematical simplification seemed to be a valuable description of the aromatization as a function of consumption and transport of DHA (Oe/DHA), and also as a function of the enzyme system (Oe/androgens).

Metabolism of DHA in Immature Placentas

The aromatizing capacity of immature placentas (*n* = 8) from week 19 to week 38 increased with the age of gestation. The Oe/DHA ratio was found within the higher (mean value = 27.4), the Oe/androgen ratio within the lower range (mean value = 14.9). In the immature placental tissue more Oe$_2$ than Oe$_1$ was found (week 19: Oe$_2$/Oe$_1$ = 18), decreasing with the age of gestation (week 38: Oe$_2$/Oe$_1$ = 1).

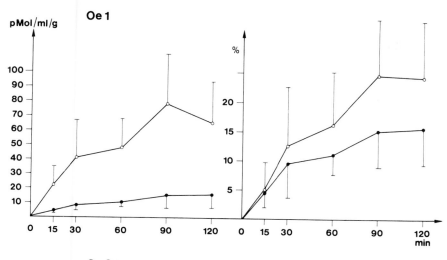

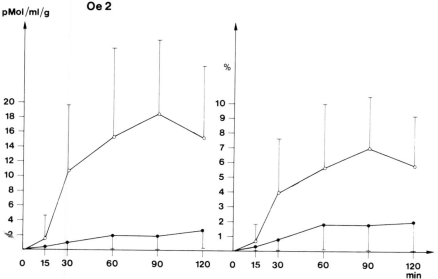

Fig. 3. Concentrations of Oe$_1$ and Oe$_2$ over 2 h of perfusion (mean ± S.D.) using two different basal concentrations of DHA. o, Basal DHA concentration 250–350 pmol ml^{-1} g^{-1} (n = 9); •, basal DHA concentration < 250 pmol ml^{-1} g^{-1} (n = 18). (*Left* panel in picomoles per millilitre per gram; *right* panel in per cent of the DHA concentration.)

Metabolism of DHA in Pathological Placentae

Severe EPH Gestosis

Oe$_{tot}$(90′) was reduced in placentae from severe EPH gestosis to 3–10% of basal DHA concentrations compared to 20–30% in normal placentae. In addition,

Table 1. Perfusion data of pathological placentae from severe EPH gestosis ($n = 3$).

Week	Basal DHA (pmol ml^{-1} g^{-1})	Oe$_1$(15') (pmol ml^{-1} g^{-1})	Oe$_{tot}$(90') (pmol ml^{-1} g^{-1})	Oe$_{tot}$(P + H) (%)	Oe/DHA	Oe/androgens
32	173.4	3.1	6.1	5.3	2.5	0.5
38	201	2.4	10.0	7.4	1.7	0.3
34	157	4.0	7	10.0	2.0	0.7

the total aromatization rate was 5.3–10% compared to 30% in normal placentae. The Oe/DHA ratio was less impaired (2–2.5) than the Oe/androgen ratio (0.3–0.5), which might be a sign of placental pathology (Table I).

Placental Insufficiency of Different Origin

Placentae were obtained from pregnancies with "idiopathic intrauterine growth retardation" of the fetus. The endocrine analyses during pregnancy showed pathologic values. Assays between weeks 30 and 38 showed subnormal values for placental lactogen (hPL), unconjugated plasma oestriol, total oestrogens in the 24 h urine and a pathological result in the DHA-S loading test (Fig. 4).

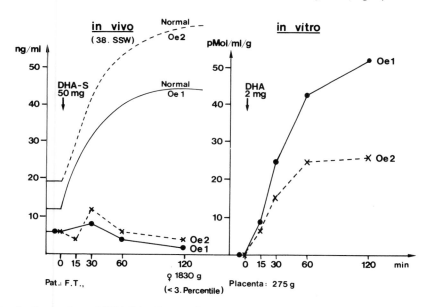

Fig. 4. Comparison of DHA-S loading test *in vivo* (left panel) and DHA perfusion *in vitro* (right panel) in one case. The normal expected values of Oe_1 and Oe_2 in the DHA-S loading test are indicated. In spite of a grossly deficient DHA-S loading test (left panel) the *in vitro* aromatization to oestrogens is normal (right panel).

The newborn babies delivered by caesarean section were hypotrophic; however, the placentae seemed macro- and microscopically normal. The data obtained from perfusion of the placenta showed normal aromatization of DHA to oestrogens.

DISCUSSION

The investigation of the metabolism of DHA in normal and pathological placentae is important with regard to the DHA-S loading test. When 50 mg DHA-S is injected into the antecubital vein of the mother, high concentrations of Oe_2 and lower levels of Oe_1 are found in the maternal plasma. Extracorporal experiments, however, on mature placentas (Varangot *et al.*, 1965; Wolf *et al.*, 1978) demonstrated oestrone and not oestradiol to be the main oestrogen metabolite from DHA in the placenta, in contrast to the *in vivo* situation. From this experience, the DHA-S test was modified using the net increase of oestrone as the main parameter for evaluation (Strecker *et al.*, 1978).

Incubation studies by Ryan (1959) and Yates and Oakey (1972) demonstrated that the metabolism of DHA shows a stable aromatization rate after 90 min. For this reason, the total oestrogen concentrations in the perfusate at 90 min was chosen as one parameter for oestrogen biogenesis. When $Oe_{tot}(90')$ is correlated with different basal DHA concentrations, three groups can be differentiated. At low basal DHA concentrations (250 pmol ml^{-1} g^{-1}) weak aromatization is found, probably due to lack of substrate. For DHA concentration of 250–350 pmol ml^{-1} g^{-1} optimal saturation of enzyme results in a high yield of oestrogens. At basal DHA concentrations of more than 500 pmol ml^{-1} g^{-1}, the aromatization decreases again probably due to competitive inhibition of transport, or direct influence of DHA on glucose-6-phosphate dehydrogenase, which provides co-enzymes for hydroxylation (Bergheim and Oertel, 1976). At these high concentrations, inhibition by the substrate may be the reason for decreasing aromatization. These characteristics have not yet been applied to the DHA-S loading test, where the placental trophoblast is exposed to low DHA concentrations of 30–100 pmol ml^{-1} g^{-1}. The aromatization ratios were calculated from steroid concentrations in the perfusate and chosen as artificial parameters to describe special functions, e.g. transport of DHA (Oe/DHA) or enzyme reaction of the aromatase system (Oe/androgens). In immature placentae Oe/DHA was found in a range comparable to that observed in mature placentae, whereas the lower Oe/androgen ratio might serve as an indicator of an inadequate enzyme array. Pathological placentae from EPH gestosis have a low normal Oe/DHA ratio, but an abnormally low Oe/androgen ratio, probably due to damage of the enzyme systems.

According to Cedard *et al.* (1966) and also Lehmann *et al.* (1973), the immature placentae show a moderate increase of aromatization with the age of gestation. While more Oe_1 is found in the perfusate, Oe_2 was the predominant steroid in the homogenate up to the 35th week of gestation. This may be caused by increasing differentiation. The decreased steroidogenesis in placentae from severe EPH gestosis is mainly caused by a defective enzyme system (Laumas *et al.*, 1968; Menini and Menini, 1970; Lehmann *et al.*, 1973), with a concomitant decrease of the microsomal protein content. This damage of intracellular enzymes is obviously the consequence of reduced uteroplacental blood flow, with consequent damage to the trophoblast cell (MacLennan *et al.*, 1972). In contrast to EPH gestosis or diabetes, where the trophoblast cells are damaged, normal aromatization of DHA can be found in cases of "idiopathic intrauterine fetal growth retardation". In such cases, a haemodynamic disorder results in decreased supply of the fetus, with consequent abnormal endocrine parameters *in vivo*. However, in the extracorporal perfusion of the placenta with DHA, normal test results were obtained. In these cases, the aromatization ratios Oe/DHA and Oe/androgens were of help in defining the derangement of the DHA transport and not the defective enzyme system as the main pathogenic mechanism. Although considerable differences exist between the conditions *in vivo*, where DHA-S is supplied from the maternal circulation and perfusion of the fetal circulation with DHA, placental perfusion experiments seem to be an interesting tool to elucidate isolated placental functions.

REFERENCES

Bergheim, E. and Oertel, G. W. (1976). *Journal of Endocrinology* **70**, 11.

Cedard, L. (1971). In "Karolinska Symposia on Research Methods in Reproductive Endocrinology. 4th Symposium. Perfusion Techniques" (E. Diczfalusy, ed.), p. 331, Karolinska Institutet, Stockholm.

Cedard, L., Varangot, J. and Yanotti, S. (1966). *European Journal of Steroids* **1**, 287.

Laumas, K. R., Malkani, P. K., Koshti, G. S. and Hingorani, V. (1968). *American Journal of Obstetrics and Gynecology* **101**, 1062.

Lauritzen, Ch. (1967). *Acta endocrinologia, Copenhagen* Suppl. 119, 88.

Lehmann, W. D., Lauritzen, Ch. and Schuhmann, R. (1973). *Acta endocrinologia, Copenhagen* **73**, 771.

MacLennan, A. H., Sharp, F. and Shaw-Dunn, J. (1972). *Journal of Obstetrics and Gynaecology of the British Commonwealth* **79**, 113.

Menini, E. and Menini, P. V. (1970). In *International Congress Series No. 210*, p. 191, Excerpta Medica, Amsterdam.

Ryan, K. (1959). *Journal of Biological Chemistry* **234**, 268.

Strecker, J. R., Killus, C. M., Lauritzen, C. and Neumann, G. K. (1978). *American Journal of Obstetrics and Gynecology* **131**, 239.

Varangot, J., Cedard, L. and Yanotti, S. (1965). *American Journal of Obstetrics and Gynecology* **92**, 534.

Wolf, A. S., Musch, K., Speidel, W., Strecker, J. R. and Lauritzen, Ch. (1978). *Acta endocrinologia, Copenhagen* **87**, 18i.

Yates, J. and Oakey, R. (1972). *Steroids* **19**, 119.

CLINICAL VALUE OF DHA-S HALF-LIFE DURING LOADING TESTS IN CASES OF INTRAUTERINE GROWTH RETARDATION

G. Tanguy, H. Thoumsin, J. R. Zorn and L. Cedard

Laboratoire de Chimie Hormonale des Maternités Cochin-Port-Royal, U. 166 INSERM, Paris 75014, France

The determination of maternal oestrogens formerly in 24 h urine and more recently in plasma, has been well established as a reliable method for monitoring the fetoplacental function. But large individual variations, diurnal and random fluctuations, have obscured the value of these methods as an aid in the managment of complicated pregnancy.

Several publications indicate that the efficiency with which the human placenta extracts circulating maternal dehydroepiandrosterone sulphate (DHA-S) and converts it to oestrogens is decreased early in cases of impaired placental function (Gant *et al.*, 1971). The oestrogen increase in urine and plasma was taken by Lauritzen (1969) as a measure of the placental capacity for oestrogen biosynthesis, which was assumed to run parallel to other placental functions of vital importance for fetal well-being (Lauritzen, 1969; Strecker *et al.*, 1978).

In practice, several modifications of this loading test have been proposed, including the metabolic clearance rate of DHA-S (Gant *et al.*, 1971) and its metabolic conversion into plasma E_2 (Madden *et al.*, 1976) (these two determinations need the use of radioactive tracer) which reflect uteroplacental perfusions and enzymatic placental activity.

The same type of information can be obtained by measuring the half-life of DHA-S by radioimmunology (Cohen and Cohen, 1977), which as such may provide an assessment of the placental function in a variety of clinical conditions.

Serono Symposium No. 35, "The Human Placenta", edited by A. Klopper, A. Genazzani and P. G. Crosignani, 1980. Academic Press, London and New York.

We have been particularly interested by the determination of the best criteria of intrauterine growth retardation (IUGR). The diagnosis of IUGR is difficult. In our recent experience (Cedard *et al.*, 1979), from a group of clinically suspected IUGR patients, only 30% of the babies have a birthweight less than the 10th percentile of Lubchenco *et al.* (1963).

These small for gestational age (SGA) babies are also sometimes not predicted before birth. A further improvement in this evaluation could be expected from ultrasound echotomography (biparietal and/or umbilical diameter less than the 10th percentile of our chart) and by hormone assay in plasma of the pregnant mother (low values of chorionic somatotrophin, unconjugated E_2, E_3 and total E_3) and low urinary oestrogens. But after this selection SGA babies still constitute only 67% of the population. It is in this group that the DHA-S loading test may be of clinical interest.

Tests were performed in 102 consenting pregnant women between 30 and 41 weeks pregnant (mean 35) who were then classified as follows: "control group", 43 pregnant women hospitalized for pathology unrelated to IUGR (mainly threatened premature labour) and finally delivered of a normal baby; "suspected IUGR", 59 women hospitalized for IUGR diagnosed clinically and by ultrasound echotomography. The latter group was subsequently divided in two subgroups: 39 cases where the babies were of appropriate birthweight for gestational age (AGA); 20 cases in which the babies were small for gestational age (SGA).

We have compared in these cases the predictive values of plasma total E_3 and, after intravenous injection of 50 mg DHA-S, the maximal increase of unconjugated E_2 (ΔE_2), its rate of increase per minute during the first 15 min (VE_2) (Thoumsin, 1977) and the DHA-S half-life. After direct radioimmunoassay of DHA-S on

Table I.

	Control	AGA	SGA
Number of cases	43	39	20
Birthweight (g) (mean ± S.E.M.)	3066 ± 65	2730 ± 68	1881 ± 89
Maximal E_2 increase (ng/ml) (mean ± S.E.M.)	34.4 ± 2.45 (36)[a]	33.7 ± 2.9 (26)	19.5 ± 1.92 (17), $p < 0.001$[b]
Rate of increase of E_2 (ng/ml) (mean ± S.E.M.)	1.86 ± 0.21 (30)	1.73 ± 0.20 (26)	1.08 ± 0.15 (16), $p < 0.02$
DHA-S half-life (h) (mean ± S.E.M.)	2.90 ± 0.12 (43)	3.24 ± 0.12 (39)	5.05 ± 0.20 (20), $p < 0.001$

[a] The numbers of assays in each category are given in parentheses.
[b] Student's *t*-tests were used to compute the significance of the difference between the AGA and SGA group.

diluted plasma, a least squares analysis was performed on the plot of log DHA-S concentration versus time to calculate the half-life of this compound (DHA-S $t_{1/2}$).

The results obtained by these different measurements are summarized in Table I.

It is first interesting to note that the mean birthweight of the babies classified in the AGA group ($>$ 10th percentile for gestational age) is smaller than in the control group, the heaviest newborn weighing 3160 g. This phenomenon explains why the hormonal measurements are often low in cases when IUGR is suspected (Cedard *et al.*, 1978, 1979).

The maximal ΔE_2 is similar in the control and the AGA groups, the mean values being respectively 34.4 and 33.7 ng/ml, but is lower in SGA infants (19.5). The difference between AGA and SGA is highly significant ($p < 0.001$).

The rate of E_2 increase during the first 15 min after DHA-S injection is also similar in control and AGA groups (respectively 1.86 and 1.73 ng ml^{-1} min^{-1}) and significantly lower in SGA infants (1.08 ng ml^{-1} min^{-1}) ($p < 0.02$).

The mean value of DHA-S half-life is similar in control and AGA groups (2.90 and 3.27 h) and corresponds to the published results (Cohen and Cohen, 1977).

In the case of SGA infants the DHA-S $t_{1/2}$ is longer (5.05 h) and the difference between AGA and SGA is highly significant ($p < 0.001$).

Figure 1 shows clearly that all the SGA babies, except one, have DHA-S $t_{1/2} \geqslant 4.29$ and that most of the normal babies exhibit values lower than this.

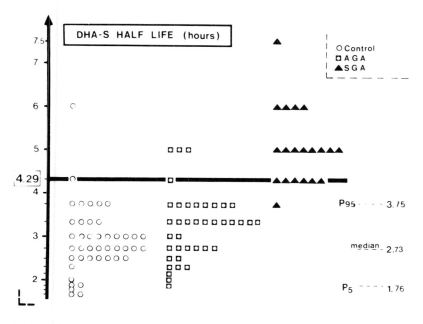

Fig. 1. The half-life of DHA-S in normal pregnancy and in women suspected of carrying a growth-retarded fetus. AGA, appropriate for gestational age; SGA, small for gestational age.

The lowest value observed in any case of SGA was 3.75 (one case), a value which corresponds to the 95th percentile of the control group.

The assessment of the exogenous DHA-S $t_{1/2}$ is very useful for the determination of the outcome of pregnancy, as shown in Table II where the predictive values of the different biochemical parameters are compared.

Table II.

DHA-S loading test	Control	AGA	SGA
Total basal E_3			
$\geqslant 50\%$ of the normal mean value	23	17	6
$< 50\%$ of the normal mean value	17	18	12
Maximal E_2 increase			
$\geqslant 25$ ng/ml	25	19	2
< 25 ng/ml	11	7	15
Rate of E_2 increase during the first 15 min			
$\geqslant 1.50$ ng ml^{-1} min^{-1}	12	13	3
< 1.50 ng ml^{-1} min^{-1}	18	13	13
DHA-S half-life			
< 4.29 h	41	35	1
$\geqslant 4.29$ h	2	4	19

The total basal E_3 value is not a good criterion because in cases with a normal birthweight a level $< 50\%$ of the normal mean value is often observed. The maximal E_2 increase is a better parameter, most of the normal birthweights gave an increase $\geqslant 25$ ng/ml, and on the other hand 15 out of 17 values were < 25 ng/ml in cases of SGA. Despite the fact that the rate of E_2 increase during the first 15 min is lower than 1.50 ng ml^{-1} min^{-1} in 13 out of 16 SGA, this parameter is not very useful because a slow increase is observed in 50% of the AGA.

The evaluation of the birthweight was correct with DHA-S $t_{1/2}$ in 95 cases out of 102 (76 babies with normal birthweight < 4.29 h and 19 SGA $\geqslant 4.29$ h), showed false positive results in six cases, and showed a false negative in one case. A value lower than 3.75 always corresponds to a normal birthweight for gestational age, and a DHA-S $t_{1/2} \geqslant 4.29$ h resulted in SGA in 82% of the cases.

To know if exogenous DHA-S metabolism reflects variations in the placental blood flow and/or enzymatic activity, we have perfused 25 corresponding placentae *in vitro* immediately after delivery (Cedard and Alsat, 1975). We performed radioimmunological assays of DHA-S, E_1 and E_2 in the perfusion fluid collected at different times after a load of 10mg DHA-S in the cord.

Preliminary results seem to indicate a good correlation between *in vivo* and *in vitro* DHA-S half-life except in two cases of severe hypertension where *in vivo* values are higher than *in vitro*. But the E_2 increase during the first 15 min after DHA-S addition does not seem to be correlated *in vivo* and *in vitro*, suggesting that the influence of other factors, such as uteroplacental blood flow or protein binding, are involved *in vivo*.

REFERENCES

Cedard, L. and Alsat, E. (1975). *Methods in Enzymology* **39 D**, 244–252.

Cedard, L., Bedin, M., Le Blond, L. and Tanguy, G. (1979). *Journal of Steroid Biochemistry* in press.

Cedard, L., Tanguy, G., Le Blond, L. and Kaminsky, M. (1978). *Colloques INSERM "Endocrinologie Prénatale et Parturition"* **77**, 149–168.

Cohen, H. and Cohen, M. (1977). *Journal of Steroid Biochemistry* **8**, 381–383.

Gant, N. F., Hutchinson, H. T., Siiteri, P. K. and MacDonald, P. C. (1971). *American Journal of Obstetrics and Gynecology* **111**, 555–569.

Lauritzen, Ch. (1969). *Hormone Metabolism Research*, **1969**, 1–96.

Lubchenco, M., Hansman, C., Dressler, M. and Boyd, E. (1963). *Journal of Pediatrics* **32**, 793–800.

Madden, J. D., Siiteri, P. K., MacDonald, P. C. and Gant, N. F. (1976). *American Journal of Obstetrics and Gynecology* 125, 915–920.

Strecker, J. R., Killus, C. M., Lauritzen, C. and Neumann, G. K. (1978). *American Journal of Obstetrics and Gynecology* **131**, 239–249.

Thoumsin, H. J. (1977). Thèse de Doctorat des Sciences Cliniques, University of Liège.

THE USE OF HIGHLY SPECIFIC ANTISERA IN LATEX AGGLUTINATION TESTS FOR THE DETECTION OF HUMAN CHORIONIC GONADOTROPHIN (hCG)

A. R. Ayala, Ma. A. Guzmán and C. Fernandez del Castillo

*Centro Materno Infantil "Gral. Maximino Avila Camacho",
S.S.A., Mexico City, Mexico*

INTRODUCTION

Human chorionic gonadotrophin (hCG) is a glycoprotein normally synthesized and secreted by the cytotrophoblast and syncytiotrophoblast of the placenta (Dreskin *et al.*, 1970; Yoshimoto *et al.*, 1977). It is composed of two dissimilar non-covalently bound polypeptide subunits designated *a* and *β* (Morgan *et al.*, 1975; Donini *et al.*, 1975).

The primary structure of the *a*-subunit closely resembles that of the glyco-protein hormones of pituitary origin, namely human luteinizing hormone (hLH), follicle stimulating hormone (hFSH) and thyroid stimulating hormone (hTSH) (Vaitukaitis and Ross, 1974; Louvet *et al.*, 1974); whereas the *β*-subunit is only similar to that of hLH. However, hCG-*β* has an additional 30 amino acid residue carboxyl-terminal sequence which is distinctive (Carlsen *et al.*, 1973; Chen *et al.*, 1976). This molecular resemblance between hCG and hLH seemingly reduces the specific detection of hCG in agglutinating tests where antibodies against the intact molecule of hCG are generally utilized (Vaitukaitis *et al* 1972b; Paul and Ross, 1964).

Since hCG was discovered (Ascheim and Zondek, 1927), several immunoprecipitation methods have been designed to measure the protein (Albert and Berkson, 1951; Brody and Carlstrom, 1960; Keele *et al.*, 1962; Tietz, 1965; Lau *et al.*, 1977), but they lack the capacity to discriminate between subunits.

Serono Symposium No. 35, "The Human Placenta", edited by A. Klopper,
A. Genazzani and P. G. Crosignani, 1980. Academic Press, London and New York.

A. R. Ayala et al.

The first agglutination reaction assay for detection of hCG was reported by Wide and Gemzell (1960). This time-honoured technique has undergone several modifications and is widely applied at present. Nonetheless, there seems to be no data available upon the utilization of highly specific antisera under the same conditions.

In the present study observations are reported on the interaction of antibodies either against the whole β-subunit of hCG or against the terminal amino acid residues of hCG, either free or linked to latex particles.

MATERIAL AND METHODS

The antiserum to β-hCG (anti-β-hCG) and to the terminal fraction of β-hCG (anti-COOH-β-hCG) have been previously characterized (Donini *et al.*, 1975; Chen *et al.*, 1976; Ayala *et al.*, 1978). Chorionic gonadotropin bound to latex particles was donated by Organon Mexicana S. A., Organan Division Teknika. Purified hCG (CR-119) used as reference preparation was a gift from the National Pituitary Agency, National Institutes of Health, U.S.A. Its biological potency was 13 500 IU/mg relative to the Second International Standard hCG by the ventral prostate weight bioassay (Louvet *et al.*, 1976). Different doses of crude hCG (Pregnyl, Organon Mexicana S.A.) were also included for study.

The antisera were diluted in a logarithmic progression ranging from 1:100 up to 1:100 000. Antibodies as well as hormonal preparations were diluted in a phosphate buffer solution (0.01 M PO_4^{3-}, 0.15 M NaCl, pH 7.8, 2.5% normal rabbit serum). In order to examine the precipitating activity of anti-β-hCG and anti-COOH-β-hCG antisera in the presence of pituitary hormones with gonadotrophic activity, various concentrations of Pergonal (Cutter S.A.) which contains 75 IU of FSH and 75 IU of LH were also added. The methodology of the agglutination reaction tests was the same as that suggested for commercial kits for the diagnosis of early pregnancy.

RESULTS

Results were compared with those obtained by control samples containing buffer phosphate solution, and the sensitivity with that of a commercial preparation (Pregnosticon planotest, 2500 IU/l, Organon).

Table I. hCG immunoprecipitation levels (in international units per litre) obtained with different antisera.

Antiserum	hCG immunoprecipitation (IU/l)
Anti-hCG (intact)	2000
Anti-COOH-β-hCG	500–1000
Anti-β-hCG	50–500

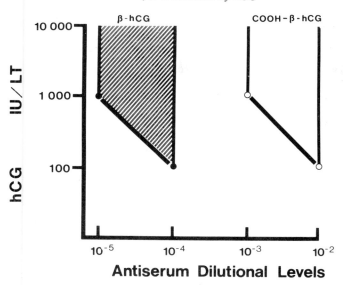

Fig. 1. Highest margin of dilution required by anti-β-hCG and anti-COOH-β-hCG antisera to precipitate low concentrations of choriogonadotrophin.

Table II. FSH/LH cross-reactivity observed with highly specific antisera to hCG.

Antiserum	FSH/LH (IU/l)			
	150	300	3000	30 000
β-hCG	—	—	+	+
COOH-β-hCG	—	—	+	+

The antiserum against β-hCG (anti-β-hCG) exhibited higher precipitating activity at dilutions of 1:10 000 and 1:100 000. The minimum detectable dose of hCG ranged from 50 to 500 IU/l, respectively. The anti-COOH-β-hCG antiserum showed less sensitivity than anti-β-hCG (500-1000 IU/l) (*see* Table I). Its use in higher concentrations than anti-β-hCG was also required since a better performance was achieved at dilutions of 1:100 and 1:1000 (*see* Fig. 1). Pergonal concentrations under 300 IU/l did not have any cross-reactions with the antisera studied (*see* Table 2).

DISCUSSION

The improvement in sensitivity achieved by our agglutination reaction tests depended on the capacity of both antisera to precipitate hCG. Anti-β-hCG and anti-COOH-β-hCG proved to be highly specific since no cross-reactivity with LH-FSH was shown above the dose of 300 IU/l. This is of particular interest if

IU/LT

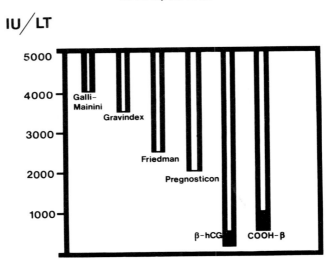

Fig. 2. Sensitivity of various methods of measuring hCG. The use of antibodies with increased specificity enhanced the performance of agglutination reaction tests for hCG.

it is taken into account that during a normal menstrual cycle the maximal values registered for LH and FSH are 100 and 50 IU/l, respectively (Vaitukaitis *et al.*, 1972a), which at times give false positive reactions in some commercial kits.

The sensitivity (50 IU/l) of immunoprecipitation tests using highly specific antisera was much better than tests where antibodies to the intact molecule of hCG are employed. Figure 2 shows the sensitivity of various procedures widely applied for detection of hCG. It can be seen that with anti-β-hCG and anti-COOH-β-hCG antibodies, the sensitivity was 50 times better than one of the most recent methods used to measure hCG. This constitutes a considerable improvement for hCG agglutination reaction tests without changing the method, while in its qualitative aspect hCG agglutination gets closer to radioligand methods for hCG measurement in serum (Vaitukaitis *et al.*, 1972b). The time taken to do the assay is the same as with other immunoprecipitation techniques.

The use of highly specific antisera in agglutinating tests for hCG should give a more reliable diagnosis of pregnancy and a more efficient treatment of tropho-blastic neoplasms.

REFERENCES

Albert, A. and Berkson, J. (1951). *Journal of Clinical Endocrinology and Metabolism* **11**, 805.
Ascheim, S. and Zondek, B. (1927). *Klinische Wochenschrift* **6**, 1321.
Ayala, A.R., Nisula, B.C., Chen, H.C., Hodgen, G.D. and Ross, G.T. (1978). *Journal of Clinical Endocrinology and Metabolism* **47**, 767.
Brody, S. and Carlstrom, G. (1960). *Lancet* ii, 99.
Carlsen, R.B., Bahl, O.P. and Swaminathan, N. (1973). *Journal of Biological Chemistry* **248**, 6796.

Chen, H.C., Hodgen, G.D., Matsuura, S., Lin, L.J., Gross, E., Reichert, L.E., Birken, S., Canfield, R.E. and Ross, G.T. (1976). *Proceedings of the National Academy of Sciences of the U.S.A.* **73**, 2885.

Donini, S., D'Alessio, I. and Donini, P. (1975). *Acta Endocrinologica, Copenhagen* **79**, 749.

Dreskin, R.B., Spicer, S.S. and Greene, W.B. (1970). *The Journal of Histochemistry and Cytochemistry* **18**, 862.

Keele, D.K., Remple, J., Bean, J. and Webster, J. (1962). *Journal of Clinical Endocrinology and Metabolism* **22**, 287.

Lau, H.L., Limkins, S.E. and King, T.M. (1977). *American Journal of Obstetrics and Gynecology* **127**, 394.

Louvet, J.P., Ross, G.T., Birken, S. and Canfield, R.E. (1974). *Journal of Clinical Endocrinology and Metabolism* **39**, 1155.

Louvet, J.P., Harman, S.M., Nisula, B.C., Ross, G.T., Birken, S. and Canfield, R.E. (1976). *Endocrinology* **99**, 1126.

Morgan, F.J., Birken, S. and Canfield, R.E. (1975). *Journal of Biological Chemistry* **250**, 5247.

Paul, W.E. and Ross, G.T. (1964). *Endocrinology* **75**, 352.

Tietz, N.W. (1965). *Obstetrics and Gynecology* **25**, 197.

Vaitukaitis, J.L. and Ross, G.T. (1974). *Israel Journal of Medical Sciences* **10**, 1280.

Vaitukaitis, J.L., Braunstein, G.D. and Ross, G.T. (1972a). *American Journal of Obstetrics and Gynecology* **113**, 751.

Vaitukaitis, J.L., Ross, G.T., Reichert, L.E. and Ward, D.N. (1972b). *Endocrinology* **91**, 1337.

Wide, L. and Gemzell, C.A. (1960). *Acta Endocrinologica, Copenhagen* **35**, 261.

Yoshimoto, Y., Wolfsen, A.R. and Odell, W.D. (1977). *Science, New York* **197**, 575.

THE VALUE OF SIMULTANEOUSLY APPLIED HORMONAL AND ULTRASONIC METHODS IN TWIN PREGNANCIES

C. A. Brugnoli, R. Russo, R. Argelà, R. Triacca, A. Sciarra, G. Elena, G. Biso, E. Righi, A. Pellegrini, G. Ciuffi, P. Poggi, A. Zacutti and A. Coli

Department of Obstetrics and Gynaecology and Nuclear Medicine Service, City Hospital, La Spezia, Italy

INTRODUCTION

Hormonal tests of placental function certainly represent an important diagnostic tool in the evaluation of chronic fetal distress. However their use in the assessment of multiple pregnancies has severe drawbacks, as hormonal levels cannot discriminate between fetuses. The predictive value of hormone assays in twin pregnancy becomes, therefore, significantly lessened, due to the high incidence of intrauterine fetal growth retardation (IUGR) and correlated risk of antepartum fetal death in each member of the pair (Houlton, 1976; Klammer *et al.*, 1977).

Ultrasound methods seem to offer the combined possibilities of both diagnosing the condition of twin pregnancy and monitoring the growth rates of the individual twins (Scheer, 1974; Dorros, 1976; Bessis *et al.*, 1977; Bleker *et al.*, 1977; Sarramon *et al.*, 1977; Argelà *et al.*, 1978; Elena *et al.*, 1978). The relative value of hormonal and ultrasonic parameters and their integrated use, which at present appears to be the most reliable approach in the management of IUGR in singleton gestation, are retrospectively evaluated in 24 twin pregnancies.

Serono Symposium No. 35, "The Human Placenta", edited by A. Klopper,
A. Genazzani and P. G. Crosignani, 1980. Academic Press, London and New York.

MATERIAL AND METHODS

Serial estimations of human placental lactogen (hPL) and total oestriol (E_3) in maternal serum, along with weekly ultrasound measurements of the biparietal diameters (BPD) of the individual twins, were obtained between 30 weeks of gestation, or earlier, and delivery from 24 women, certain of their last menstrual period.

The diagnosis of a twin pregnancy was always ascertained by ultrasound before 30 weeks of gestation. Once a twin pregnancy was diagnosed, antenatal care was continued along conventional lines for at risk pregnancy.

Nineteen pregnancies were classified as normal, while the remaining five patients suffered from minor obstetric complications.

Patients were grouped on the basis of the birthweight of each member of the pair. When the birthweight was below the 10th percentile for single pregnancy, the infant was assumed to be small for gestational age (SGA).

Serum hPL and E_3 were estimated using commercially available RIA kits (Radiochemical Centre, Amersham). A total of 145 hPL and 126 E_3 assays were performed in 23 and 20 cases, respectively.

In all patients weekly ultrasound assessments of the individual BPD were carried out (216 single measurements) using a KretzTechnik compound A and B scanner with a 2 MHz transducer.

Hormone and ultrasound estimations were grouped according to fetal birthweight, and related mean and standard deviation (s.d.) values were compared with each other for corresponding gestational ages. The data were plotted against the normal hPL, E_3 and BPD ranges (means and s.d.) obtained in a group of normal single pregnancies, from which the mothers were delivered of healthy babies between the 10th and 90th percentiles in weight (appropriate for gestational age, AGA).

Statistical significance was assessed by Student's t-test.

RESULTS

Perinatal Loss, Birthweight and Placenta

In our population there was a total of four perinatal deaths (8.3%): a stillbirth occurred at nearly the 37th week of gestation; one pair, born at 33 weeks of gestation, died in the immediate neonatal period of respiratory distress syndrome; the remaining neonatal death was due to gross congenital abnormality.

With respect to birthweight, 10 women delivered babies who were all in the AGA range (mean gestational age 260.1 days): in eight cases one member of the pair was SGA (mean gestational age 264.5 days), while in the remaining six cases both infants were SGA (mean gestational age 268.3 days). A birthweight lower than 2500 g occurred in 58.3% of the infants and it was below the 10th percentile for gestational age in 20 infants (41.7%). A statistically significant difference in birthweight was not observed in twins which were both SGA ($p < 0.25$) and nearly the same figure was observed in twins which were both AGA ($p < 0.10$).

When one member of the pair was SGA, the mean birthweight of smaller and larger twins were significantly different (1.87 kg and 2.81 kg, respectively; $p <$ 0.025).

A monochorial or fused bichorial placenta was found in 50% of the cases. In the group with one SGA twin the incidence of these types of placenta was significantly higher (75%).

Hormone Assays

Almost all hPL values exceeded 1 S.D. above the normal mean for single pregnancy after 30 weeks of gestation. The distribution of values week by week is shown in Fig. 1. Although the mean value of hPL in twins of which one was SGA was higher than the singleton mean, it was lower than when both babies were AGA (Table I). There was, however, no statistically significant difference between the AGA group and the group with one SGA from 33 to 39 weeks ($p < 0.3$). In the patients who were delivered of two SGA babies, hPL concentrations were significantly lower than those observed in the former two groups ($p < 0.0025$), although mostly situated in the upper zone of the normal range for singletons (Figs 1 and 2).

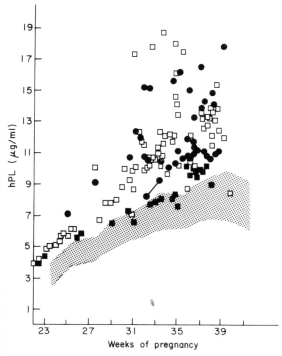

Fig. 1. The distribution of serum hPL from 23 twin pregnancies is plotted against the normal range (1 S.D.) for singleton pregnancies. □, ●, ■ indicate both AGA, one SGA and both SGA twins, respectively; ●——●, intrauterine fetal death.

Table I.   Serum hPL (in micrograms per millilitre) for single and twin pregnancy.

Weeks	Single pregnancy	Both AGA twins	One SGA twin
31–32	6.54 ± 0.97[a]	9.92 ± 2.63	N.S.[b]
33–34	7.26 ± 1.21	11.43 ± 2.65	10.9 ± 1.18
35–36	7.34 ± 1.05	13.19 ± 2.80	12.43 ± 2.44
37–38	8.11 ± 1.32	13.01 ± 0.75	12.57 ± 1.93
39–40	8.31 ± 1.64	12.57 ± 2.30	13.5 ± 3.18

[a]The numbers indicate mean and 1 S.D. values.
[b]Not sufficient for statistical analysis.

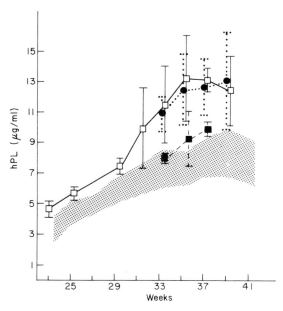

Fig. 2.   hPL values are grouped according to fetal birthweight and related mean and S.D. values are compared with each other for corresponding gestational ages. □, Both AGA twins; ●, one SGA twin; ■, both SGA twins.

E_3 values almost all fell within the normal range for singleton before the 34th week. After this stage the E_3 concentration rose above the normal range in subjects with both fetuses AGA (Fig. 3). As shown in Table II the mean values progressively diverged from the corresponding ones for singleton. In the remaining two groups including one or both SGA twins, the analysis of this parameter was not significant, due to the small numbers of assays. Nevertheless, one relevant finding seemed to be the flattening of E_3 increase in the group with one SGA twin (Fig. 4).

Table II. Serum E_3 (in nanograms per millilitre) for single and twin pregnancy.

Weeks	Single pregnancy	Twin pregnancy[a]
31–32	85.98 ± 28.62[b]	103.44 ± 29.68
33–34	107.73 ± 37.81	124.61 ± 19.21
35–36	132.12 ± 42.36	192.89 ± 39.10
37–38	164.02 ± 54.50	316.52 ± 88.10
39–40	200.36 ± 63.76	363.58 ± 79.05

[a] The values refer to pregnancies with both AGA twins.
[b] The numbers indicate the mean and 1 S.D.values.

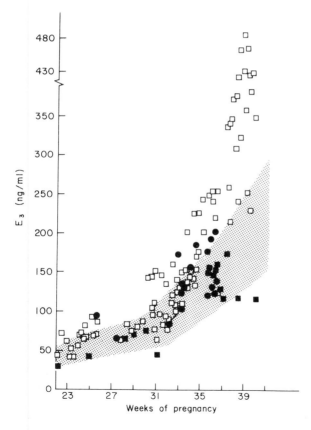

Fig. 3. The distribution of serum E_3 from 20 twin pregnancies is plotted against the normal range (1 S.D.) for singleton pregnancies. □, Both AGA twins; ●, one SGA twin; ■, both SGA twins.

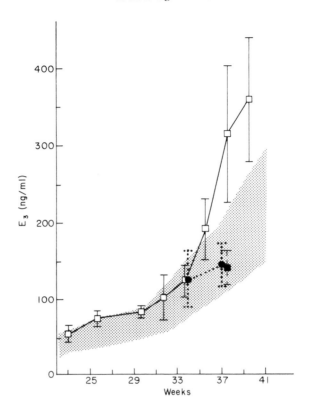

Fig. 4. E₃ values are grouped according to fetal birthweight and related mean and S.D. values are compared with each other for corresponding gestational ages. □, Both AGA twins; ●, one SGA twin; ■, both SGA twins.

Biparietal Diameter Growth

In the group with both AGA twins the individual BPD values were in most cases within the lower part of the normal range and the mean BPD curve ran parallel to that of normal singletons. When both infants were SGA, the mean BPD curve was still parallel, although running at a lower level. The BPD growth rate was similar to that observed in the former group up to 35 weeks of gestation; afterwards a decrease occurred in BPD growth rate. If one member of the pair was SGA, the BPD curves clearly diverged after 35 weeks, due to the flattening of the smaller twin's curve (Fig. 5). These divergent BPD growth rates were in good agreement with the mean birthweights of larger and smaller twins (2.81 kg and 1.87 kg, respectively). Moreover, mean values of BPD measurements of larger twins were consistently higher than those calculated for AGA twins up to 34–35 weeks of gestation.

By means of serial BPD measurements the diagnosis of IUGR was correctly made in 70% of the cases.

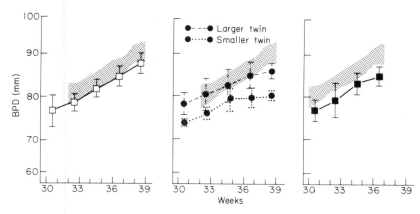

Fig. 5. Behaviour of BPD growth curves (mean and S.D.) in patients with both AGA (□), one SGA (●) and both SGA (■) twins, respectively.

DISCUSSION

The distribution of hPL values in our population of twin pregnancies was clearly above the normal range for singletons and is in good agreement with data obtained by previous investigators (Singer *et al.*, 1970; Spellacy *et al.*, 1971, 1978; Spencer, 1971; Thiery *et al.*, 1977).

The predictive value of this parameter in the diagnosis of IUGR in cases with one SGA infant appeared inconsistent, as in this group hormone levels were not significantly different from those observed in women with both twins AGA.

On the other hand, the clinical usefulness of hPL was evident in cases in which both twins were SGA, as a condition of chronic placental failure might be suggested by the presence of hPL values in the upper zone of the normal range for singletons.

As reported by Duncan *et al.* (1979) for total urinary oestrogens, a significant difference in E_3 serum concentration between singleton and twin pregnancy was not found until 34 weeks and ever after this only the group with both twins AGA showed values above the normal range.

As might be expected, serial estimation of the individual BPD proved to be of clinical importance in the management of twin pregnancy. In the entire group ultrasound BPD evaluation was correct in diagnosing IUGR in 70% of the cases, while it appeared to be 60% correct when the analysis was limited to the group in which both twins were SGA.

With regard to the detection of a twin pregnancy, in the present study the potential usefulness of hormonal parameters was seriously diminished. In fact both hPL and E_3 gave values in the normal range for singletons in the very group of both SGA twins, where an early diagnosis and strict supervision was mandatory.

The integrated use of ultrasound and hormonal parameters seems, therefore, to be an important tool in the diagnosis of IUGR in twin pregnancy. In fact, following ultrasound detection of twins, hPL values were able to demonstrate with a sufficient accuracy an "inadequate" placental function in patients with both SGA twins, while in this group BPD measurements were correct in diagnosing IUGR in only

60% of the cases. Moreover, after 34 weeks' gestation, E_3 levels also showed the possible existence of a condition of chronic fetal distress in women with one SGA twin, although BPD measurements demonstrated a great accuracy (87.5%) in the detection of IUGR of one member of the pair when the other was AGA. In this group fetal malnutrition might be caused by interplacental blood shunts, as the elevated hPL values indicated a normal endocrine function of the placental mass.

In conclusion, a normal growth of both twins may be expected in the presence of elevated hPL and E_3 values and normal BPD curves, while hPL and E_3 concentrations in the normal range for singletons and low BPD curves indicate a condition of poor intrauterine growth of both infants.

The divergence of individual BPD curves, associated with high hPL and apparently normal E_3 values, on the contrary, suggests the fetal malnutrition of one member of the pair, probably due to a twin transfusion syndrome.

REFERENCES

Argelà, R., Pellegrini, A., Elena, G., Bertolini, G., Ciuffi, G., Righi, E., Biso, G., Brugnoli, C. A. and Zacutti, A. (1978). *In* "Medicina Fetale" (F. Destro, ed.), pp. 297–301, Monduzzi, Bologna.

Bessis, R., Brignon, C., Schneider, L. and Coulon, J. (1977). *In* "Symposium international d'echographie obstetricale", pp. 411–413, Glaxo-Evans dietetiques éditions, Paris.

Bleker, O. P., Kloosterman, G. J., Huidekoper, B. L. and Breur, W. (1977). *European Journal of Obstetrics and Gynaecology* **7**, 85.

Dorros, G. (1976). *Obstetrics and Gynecology* **48** suppl. 1, 46s.

Duncan, S. L. B., Ginz, B. and Wahab, H. (1979). *Obstetrics and Gynecology* **53**, 367.

Elena, G., Bertolini, G., Biso, G., Righi, E., Argelà, R., Brugnoli, C. A., Ciuffi, G., Pellegrini, A. and Zacutti, A. (1978). *In* "Medicina Fetale" (F. Destro, ed.), pp. 303–307, Monduzzi, Bologna.

Houlton, M. C. C. (1976). *Obstetrics and Gynecology* **49**, 542.

Klammer, J., Bichler, A. and Brabec, W. (1977). *In* "Poor Intrauterine Fetal Growth" (B. Salvadori and A. Bacchi Modena, eds), pp. 287–289, Centro Minerva Medica, Roma.

Sarramon, M. F., Reme, J. M., Grandjean, H., Favretto, R. and Pontonnier, G. (1977). *In* "Symposium international d'echographie obstetricale", pp. 253–262, Glaxo-Evans dietetiques éditions, Paris.

Scheer, K. (1974). *Journal of Clinical Ultrasound* **2**, 197.

Singer, W., Desiardin, P. and Friesen, H. G. (1970). *Obstetrics and Gynecology* **36**, 222.

Spellacy, W. N., Buhi, W. C., Schram, J. D. and Birk, S. A. (1971). *Obstetrics and Gynecology* **37**, 567.

Spellacy, W. N., Buhi, W. C. and Birk, S. A. (1978). *Obstetrics and Gynecology* **52**, 210.

Spencer, T. S. (1971). *Journal of Obstetrics and Gynaecology of the British Commonwealth* **78**, 232.

Thiery, M., Dhont, M. and Vandekerckhove, D. (1977). *Acta obstetricia et gynecologica scandinavica* **56**, 495.

PHYSIOLOGICAL VARIABILITY OF ENDOCRINE INDICES NORMALLY EMPLOYED IN CLINICAL PRACTICE*

D. Parrini, F. Facchinetti and A. R. Genazzani

Department of Obstetrics and Gynaecology, University of Siena, 53100 Siena, Italy

INTRODUCTION

The assay of plasma concentrations of several hormones in pregnancy has been proposed and extensively utilized to evaluate the well-being of the fetoplacental unit (Klopper, 1976). Although numerous protein and steroid hormones have been proposed as indices, those which have shown general clinical applicability are human placental lactogen (hPL) among the protein hormones and oestriol (E_3) and recently also oestetrol (E_4) among the steroids. hPL has been found to be a valid index of placental function (Genazzani *et al.*, 1972), particularly in view of the close correlation in normal pregnancies between plasma levels of this hormone and the weight of the placenta (Saxena *et al.*, 1969). Since E_3 and particularly E_4 are chiefly of fetal origin (Siiteri and MacDonald, 1963; Zucconi *et al.*, 1967), the measurement of their concentrations may be expected to give a better indication of fetal well-being than hPL (Tulchinsky, 1976). It is important to remember that these steroids circulate in the plasma in both the unconjugated and conjugated forms, notably as sulphates and glucuronates; it has therefore been proposed that, in pregnancy monitoring, both these forms should be measured in the plasma.

Many studies have been carried out regarding the amplitude and period of spontaneous fluctuations of the above hormones. Our previous findings (Genazzani

*Supported by the C.N.R. project "Biology of reproduction".

Serono Symposium No. 35, "The Human Placenta", edited by A. Klopper, A. Genazzani and P. G. Crosignani, 1980. Academic Press, London and New York.

et al., 1977; Facchinetti *et al.*, 1978) are in agreement with those of several authors, e.g. Grumbach *et al.* (1968) and Masson *et al.* (1977), regarding the stability of hPL levels, but disagree with those of Vigneri *et al.* (1975), who found wider fluctuations in this protein. Our findings for the average coefficient of variation of the sub-hourly variation of unconjugated E_3 in the plasma of normal pregnant women at term (Facchinetti *et al.*, 1978; Genazzani *et al.*, 1977) are in complete agreement with those reported by Klopper *et al.* (1977), Allen and Lachelin (1978) and Hull *et al.* (1979) as far as the day-to-day variability is concerned.

Levitz *et al.* (1974) found no particular circadian variation in this index, while Tulchinsky *et al.* (1971), Goebel and Kuss (1974) and Katagiri *et al.* (1976) maintain that the average values are higher in the evening than in the morning. On the other hand, no circadian variations have been reported for unconjugated E_4 (Tulchinsky *et al.*, 1975; Notation and Tagatz, 1977; Parrini *et al.*, 1978).

In the present study we examine the sub-hourly and circadian variations of hPL, progesterone (P) and unconjugated and conjugated oestradiol (E_2), E_3 and E_4.

SUBJECTS AND METHODS

Sub-hourly Variations

Three groups of six normal pregnant women at term (37–40 weeks of gestation) were studied. Twelve heparinized blood samples were taken from each subject every 5, 15 and 30 min for 1, 3 and 6 h respectively. Plasma levels of hPL, P and unconjugated E_2, E_3 and E_4 were measured in each sample.

In a further group of six pregnant women at term, 13 heparinized blood samples were taken every 20 min for 4 h, in order to measure plasma levels of unconjugated and total E_2, E_3 and E_4.

The mean plasma level and relative coefficient of variation (c.v.) of each hormone were determined for each subject. The average c.v. for each sampling period was calculated for each hormone. In addition the percentage difference between the mean plasma hormone level and the 12 or 13 single values which composed it, were calculated for each subject.

The general distribution of these percentage differences (taking into consideration differences of 10% or more) was evaluated for each hormone according to the same sampling interval (5, 15, 20 and 30 min).

Circadian Variations

Two groups of normal pregnant women, nine at 28–34 weeks of gestation, and nine at 36–42 weeks of gestation, were studied. Blood samples were taken at 08.00, 12.00, 16.00, 20.00, 24,00 and 08.00 the following morning. Plasma concentrations of unconjugated and total E_2, E_3 and E_4, hPL and P were measured in each sample. In order to determine the existence of circadian rhythm more accurately, the results were also analysed by calculating the percentage variation of each hormone measurement from the mean of the two 08.00 assays. Statistical analysis of the results was performed using the paired *t*-test.

Methods

All blood samples were immediately centrifuged at 4 °C. The plasma was separated into different tubes and stored at −20 °C until assay. Unconjugated E_2, E_3, E_4 and P were extracted with ethyl ether (1:10) and assayed by radio-immunoassay (RIA). In order to measure the total concentrations (unconjugated and conjugated) of E_2, E_3 and E_4, 50 μl of plasma were incubated at 37 °C for 6 h, with *Helix pomatia* enzyme preparation corresponding to 1000 units of glucuronidase and 10 000 units of sulphatase. At the end of the hydrolysis, the mixture was extracted with ether (1:10) and the various steroids were determined by RIA.

For hPL, free and total E_3 and E_4 assays, CEA-IRE-Sorin kits (Saluggia, Italy) were used with a ^{3}H tracer for E_3 and I^{125}-labelled tracer for E_4 and hPL. Tritiated steroids from NEN (Boston, U.S.A.), specific antisera from Sorin (Saluggia, Italy) and chromatographically pure standard from Vister (Milan, Italy) were used for the measurement of E_2 and P. The RIA was based on an overnight incubation at 4 °C, followed by dextran-coated charcoal separation. The between-assay coefficient of variation of each hormone assay was calculated and is reported in Table I.

RESULTS

The spontaneous fluctuations of the various hormones were evaluated both as c.v. per subject and per sampling period, and as the number of samples for each subject where the hormone concentration varied by 10% or more from the mean value.

Table I. The between assay coefficient of variation of each hormone assay; the average c.v. ± s.d. of each hormone at different sampling intervals and the mean c.v. for all subjects are reported.

Hormone	Method	Spontaneous fluctuations				
		5 min	15 min	20 min	30 min	Mean
hPL	4.3 ± 0.8	8.9 ± 2.0	6.4 ± 1.1		8.3 ± 1.9	7.9 ± 0.6
U-E_2	8.7 ± 1.1	17.8 ± 4.5	16.4 ± 3.1	11.5 ± 1.7	11.7 ± 1.7	14.4 ± 1.5
U-E_3	8.4 ± 0.6	15.7 ± 3.1	19.7 ± 4.2	16.9 ± 2.6	14.7 ± 2.3	16.6 ± 1.4
U-E_4	11.4 ± 1.0	16.2 ± 2.3	13.8 ± 2.0	13.9 ± 2.0	18.4 ± 1.9	15.5 ± 1.1
T-E_2	7.6 ± 1.0			12.3 ± 1.7		12.3 ± 1.7
T-E_3	7.3 ± 0.8			15.6 ± 1.4		15.6 ± 1.4
T-E_4	7.7 ± 1.2			12.9 ± 1.5		12.9 ± 1.5
U-P	9.2 ± 1.3	25.8 ± 4.9	21.7 ± 4.6		12.7 ± 3.9	20.0 ± 2.8

As reported in Table I, the c.v. of hPL plasma ranged from 6.4 to 8.9% of the mean values, and was significantly lower ($p < 0.01$) than those of all other indices. The c.v.s of the total concentrations of the oestrogens were slightly lower than the corresponding unconjugated forms. In this respect, the c.v. of the method was also lower in the assays of the total than of the unconjugated forms. The greatest variability was shown by P values, with a general c.v. of $20.0 \pm 2.8\%$. For each hormone, the c.v.s were similar regardless of the sampling interval.

Table II. General distribution per hormone of single measurements which differ from the mean value (12–13 assays) of each subject by 10%, 10–20% and more than 20%.

Hormone	Time (min)	10%		10–20%		> 20%		Total samples
		n	%	n	%	n	%	
	5	59	81.9	10	13.9	3	4.2	72
hPL	15	64	88.8	8	11.1	–	–	72
	30	57	79.2	11	15.3	4	5.5	72
Total		180	83.3	29	13.4	7	3.2	216
	5	38	54.2	12	17.1	20	28.6	70
U-E_2	15	29	48.3	20	33.3	11	18.3	60
	30	39	68.4	11	19.3	7	12.2	57
	20	45	63.3	21	29.6	5	7.0	71
Total		151	58.5	64	24.8	43	16.7	258
	5	35	48.6	22	30.5	15	20.8	72
U-E_3	15	16	34.7	15	32.6	15	32.6	46
	30	31	50.0	21	33.8	10	16.1	62
	20	33	42.8	28	36.4	16	20.8	77
Total		115	44.7	86	33.5	56	21.8	257
	5	30	44.1	23	33.8	15	22.0	68
U-E_4	15	24	52.1	16	34.8	6	13.0	46
	30	19	42.2	17	37.8	9	20.0	45
	20	45	59.2	21	27.6	10	13.1	76
Total		118	50.2	77	32.8	40	17.0	235
	5	19	31.7	13	21.7	28	46.7	60
U-P	15	24	40.0	16	26.7	20	33.3	60
	30	37	61.0	15	25.0	8	13.3	60
Total		80	44.4	44	24.4	56	31.0	180
T-E_2	20	40	55.5	25	34.7	7	9.7	72
T-E_3	20	39	50.6	28	36.4	10	13.0	77
T-E_4	20	49	63.6	19	24.7	9	11.7	77

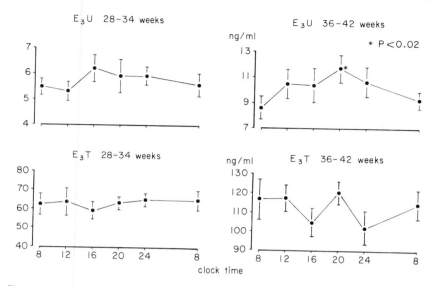

Fig. 1. Circadian variation of plasma concentrations (mean ± S.E.) of unconjugated and total E_2 in two groups of normal pregnant women at 28–34 weeks and 36–42 weeks.

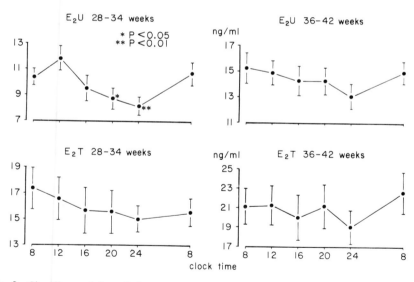

Fig. 2. Circadian variation of plasma concentrations (mean ± S.E.) of unconjugated and total E_3 in two groups of normal pregnant women at 28–34 weeks and 36–42 weeks.

The general evaluation, per hormone, of the number of single measurements which differ from the mean value of each subject by 10%, 10–20% and more than 20% is reported in Table II.

It appears clear that only 3.2% of hPL measurements differ by more than 20% from the mean value, while 83.3% of the readings differ by less than 10%.

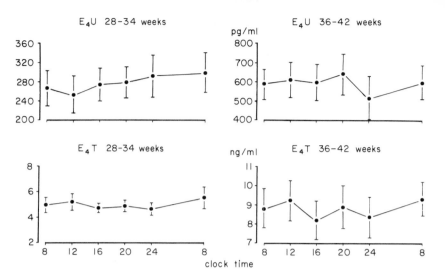

Fig. 3. Circadian variation of plasma concentrations (mean ± S.E.) of unconjugated and total E_4 in two groups of normal pregnant women at 28–34 weeks and 36–42 weeks.

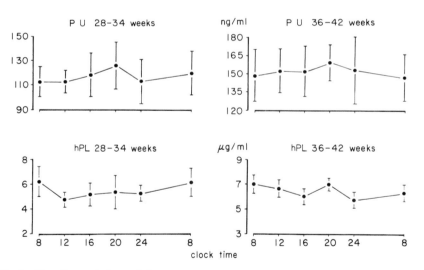

Fig. 4. Circadian variations of plasma concentrations (mean ± S.E.) of unconjugated P and hPL in two groups of normal pregnant women at 28–34 weeks and 36–42 weeks.

A greater number of values exceeding a 10% difference was found in total oestrogens, and even more in the unconjugated forms. Unconjugated E_3 showed 21.8% and unconjugated E_4 17.0% of the readings which differed by more than 20% from the mean value of each subject.

The circadian variability of unconjugated and total E_2, E_3 and E_4 and unconjugated P and hPL is reported in Figures 1–4.

A significant decrease at 20.00 and 24.00 was found in unconjugated E_2 in the 28–34 week group (Fig. 1) and a significant increase in unconjugated E_3 at 20.00 in the 36–42 week group (Fig 2). No significant difference was found in any of the other indices in the two groups. As reported in Table III, the percentage

Table III. Circadian variations of unconjugated and total plasma oestrogens at 28–34 weeks and 38–42 weeks as a percentage difference at various times from the 08.00 mean.

		12.00	16.00	20.00	24.00
A	$U\text{-}E_2$	12.0 ± 7.94	-9.55 ± 6.09	-16.55 ± 5.76^{a}	-22.11 ± 5.80^{b}
	$T\text{-}E_2$	-0.11 ± 4.42	-6.66 ± 5.73	-5.46 ± 7.24	-6.55 ± 7.50
B	$U\text{-}E_2$	-1.33 ± 3.03	-5.88 ± 4.47	-5.55 ± 3.80	-12.00 ± 7.74
	$T\text{-}E_2$	0.85 ± 3.39	-9.94 ± 7.17	0.40 ± 5.50	-11.16 ± 7.40
A	$U\text{-}E_3$	-3.55 ± 6.37	14.88 ± 11.92	6.11 ± 9.04	9.11 ± 6.80
	$T\text{-}E_3$	0.11 ± 7.65	-5.66 ± 7.59	2.44 ± 10.26	6.77 ± 10.86
B	$U\text{-}E_3$	15.66 ± 7.32	15.66 ± 10.31	31.88 ± 9.34	18.55 ± 10.32
	$T\text{-}E_3$	3.75 ± 5.93	-8.55 ± 5.09	8.87 ± 9.74	-11.55 ± 5.65
A	$U\text{-}E_4$	-11.11 ± 2.66	-1.33 ± 7.05	0.20 ± 6.22	2.44 ± 7.04
	$T\text{-}E_4$	2.11 ± 6.32	-5.77 ± 7.97	-0.88 ± 12.21	-6.22 ± 11.23
B	$U\text{-}E_4$	2.43 ± 6.10	0.11 ± 5.09	8.88 ± 9.38	-18.33 ± 9.01
	$T\text{-}E_4$	-3.00 ± 7.01	-14.33 ± 7.34	-8.11 ± 8.73	-13.22 ± 7.42

A = group 28–34 weeks; B = group 36–42 weeks.
[a] $p < 0.05$.
[b] $p < 0.01$.

variations in unconjugated E_2 in the 28–34 week group reached $-16.5 \pm 5.7\%$ at 2000 ($p < 0.05$), and $-22.1 \pm 5.8\%$ at 24.00 ($p < 0.01$). A similar pattern was found in the second group, but was not of significant magnitude (Table III). The unconjugated E_3 increase at 20.00 reached $+31.8 \pm 9.4\%$ in the second group.

DISCUSSION

The sub-hourly variations of the various hormones studied largely corresponded to those reported by previous authors (Table IV). Previously published unconjugated E_2 fluctuations, either on a day-to-day or hourly basis, ranged from 7.2% (Chan and Klopper, 1974) to 16.9% (Hull et al., 1979) as reported in Table IV. Total E_2 variability ($12.3 \pm 1.7\%$) did not differ significantly from unconjugated E_2 ($14.4 \pm 1.5\%$), but very little has been published on this parameter: a c.v. of 7.4% was reported by Chan and Klopper (1974) in the same study in which they reported 7.2% for unconjugated E_2. Authors are generally in agreement on a coefficient of variation of unconjugated E_3 ranging from 13.8 to 19.3% (see Table IV), although in one study Klopper and Shaaban (1974) found a day-to-day variation of 30.9%. Similarly (see Table IV) the total E_3 c.v. ranged from

Table IV. Coefficient of variation of day-to-day and sub-hourly (asterisked) fluctation of oestradiol oestriol, oestetrol and progesterone as reported by various authors.

Reference	Oestradiol		Oestriol		Oestetrol		Progesterone
	Unconjugated (%)	Total (%)	Unconjugated (%)	Total (%)	Unconjugated (%)	Total (%)	Unconjugated (%)
Masson and Wilson, 1972				13.2			
				14.8			
Chan and Klopper, 1974	7.2	7.4					
Klopper and Shaaban, 1974	12.2		30.9				21.9
Klopper et al., 1975							18.9
Klopper et al., 1977			16.5	15.0			
Masson et al., 1977	16.5		16.5	13.9			
Allen et al., 1978	12.7		14.1	15.8			14.2
Buster et al., 1978	15.6*		19.3*				13.4
	14.6*		18.8*				16.5
	16.9		15.6				
Hull et al., 1979	16.1*		13.8*				
Present data	14.4	12.3	16.6	15.6	15.5	12.9	20.0

13.2% (Masson and Wilson, 1972) to 15.8% (Allen and Lachelin, 1978). These results confirm that the sub-hourly variations of unconjugated and total E_2 and E_3 plasma levels are very similar and that in clinical practice differences of more than 20% may be accounted for by changes in the fetoplacental output of these steroids.

The present measurements of unconjugated (15.5 ± 1.1%) and total (12.9 ± 1.5%) E_4 variability did not differ from those of the steroid discussed above.

As reported in Table IV, plasma P showed a slightly greater variability and its c.v. ranged from 13.4% (Hull *et al.*, 1979) to 21.9% (Klopper and Shaaban, 1974). The c.v. found in the present study (20.0 ± 2.8%) was the highest of all the steroids examined.

The relative stability of hPL was confirmed (Grumbach *et al.*, 1968; Genazzani *et al.*, 1977; Masson *et al.*, 1977). Only 3.2% of measurements differed by 20% from the average hormone concentrations per subject, which strongly supports the validity of single hPL assays in clinical practice.

As regards unconjugated oestrogens, 24.8% of the E_2 and 33.5% of the E_3 measurements differed by more than 10% and less than 20%, and 16.7% of the E_2 and 21.8% of the E_3 measurements differed by more than 20% from the mean concentrations. Total oestrogens gave more or less similar results.

These findings suggest that even if the c.v.s seem to indicate the relative stability of these indices, there is still a frequent occurrence of measurements differing significantly from the average plasma concentrations.

The similarity of results obtained by sampling at different time intervals from 5 to 30 min for 1–6 consecutive hours, suggests that an unconjugated or total oestrogen plasma assay is best done on a pool of two or more samples collected even at short time intervals. This may reduce spontaneous fluctuations and make the results more useful in clinical practice, as suggested also by Buster *et al.* (1978). However, the findings of Klopper *et al.* (1975) indicate that sub-hourly variation is different and greater in pre-eclamptic subjects than in normal pregnancy. It may therefore be interesting to investigate the degree of variability of each index proposed in fetoplacental monitoring in all the different pathological conditions of pregnancy, so as to be able to use the best sampling schedule for each index.

The study of the circadian variation of the different hormones showed the existence of significant changes in unconjugated E_2 in 28–34 week subjects, with minimum values at 24.00 h. A similar pattern was also observed in unconjugated E_2 in 38–42 week subjects, but although the range of the variations differed from subject to subject, the trend was not significant.

The only other hormone showing circadian variations was unconjugated E_3 in the groups of advanced pregnancies where minimum values were found at 08.00 and maximum values at 20.00. In the group of 28–34 week subjects this was not so evident. The difference in absolute E_3 levels in these two groups and the relatively greater distribution volume of unconjugated E_3 in the earlier group may explain these discrepancies. The unconjugated E_2 circadian variation is similar to that reported by Munson *et al.* (1972) and Townsley *et al.* (1973) while Tulchinsky *et al.* (1971), Allen and Lachelin (1978) and Patrick *et al.* (1979) found only minor and insignificant circadian variation in this hormone.

Controversial findings are reported on both unconjugated and total E_3 circadian variations. Our results on unconjugated E_3 correspond to those reported by

Tulchinsky *et al.* (1971) and Goebel and Kuss (1974), who demonstrated the same 31% change in unconjugated E_3 values at 20.00. More recently, Patrick *et al.* (1979) also reported a similar or even more marked pattern in unconjugated E_3. Total E_3 which failed to show any significant circadian variations in the studies of Macourt *et al.* (1971), Levitz *et al.* (1974) and in the present study, showed a significant increase from 10.00 to 12.00 in Townsley *et al.* (1973) and an afternoon and evening decrease in Katagiri *et al.* (1976). A late morning decrease in total E_3 was also reported by Allen and Lachelin (1978) in pre-eclampsia. The inverse pattern of unconjugated E_2 and E_3 may be related to their different origin: the former being the placental metabolite of dehydro-epiandrosterone sulphate (DHAS) which is 50% of maternal origin (Gurpide *et al.*, 1966) while 90% of E_3 is derived from fetal DHAS (Siiteri and MacDonald, 1963, 1966). The circadian variability of the maternal adrenal gland clearly demonstrated by plasma cortisol changes (Genazzani *et al.*, 1978) may induce, by the transplacental passage of this steroid (Simmer *et al.*, 1974), a contrary circadian variation in the fetal hypothalamus–pituitary–adrenal axis. The lack of circadian variations in both unconjugated and total E_4 seems to indicate that the supposed circadian rhythm of the hypothalamus–pituitary–adrenal axis of the fetus and the circadian variation of maternal E_4 do not influence the total 15α-hydroxylation capacity of the fetal liver. The stability of unconjugated E_4 was also reported by Tulchinsky *et al.* (1975).

Lowest levels of P were reported at 08.00 by Runnebaum *et al.* (1972) and Allen and Lachelin (1978), while Craft *et al.* (1969), Teoh *et al.* (1973), Lindberg *et al.* (1974) and the present findings do not support any consistent circadian trend in this steroid.

In conclusion, the present findings (i) indicate that plasma hPL levels are more stable than unconjugated or total oestrogens; (ii) confirm the amplitude of sub-hourly variations of these steroids as reported previously; (iii) suggest that a pool of two or three samples collected from the same subject even at brief intervals may give more reliable information on the average plasma concentrations of unconjugated or total oestrogens; and (iv) support the existence of inverse circadian variations in unconjugated E_2 and E_3 related to the different maternal and fetal origin of their precursors.

REFERENCES

Allen, E. I. and Lachelin, G. C. L. (1978). *British Journal of Obstetrics and Gynaecology* **85**, 278–292.

Buster, J. E., Meis, P. J., Hobel, C. J. and Marshall, J. R. (1978). *Journal of Clinical Endocrinology and Metabolism* **46**, 907–910.

Chan, T. and Klopper, A. (1974). *Journal of Obstetrics and Gynaecology of the British Commonwealth* **80**, 357–360.

Craft, I., Wyman, H. and Sommerville, I. F. (1969). *Journal of Obstetrics and Gynaecology of the British Commonwealth* **76**, 1080–1086.

Facchinetti, F., Nasi, A., Parrini, D., Danero, S., Franchi, F., De Leo, V. and Genazzani, A. R. (1978). *Atti della Società Italiana di Ostetricia e Ginecologia* **59**, 858–863.

Genazzani, A. R., Cocola, F., Neri, P. and Fioretti, P. (1972). *Acta endocrinologia, Copenhagen* **71**, Suppl. 167, 5–39.

Genazzani, A. R., Parrini, D., Centini, G., Facchinetti, F., Massafra, C. and De Leo V. (1978). *Atti della Società Italiana di Ostetricia e Ginecologia* **59**, 864–871.

Genazzani, A. R., Nasi, A., Medda, F., Facchinetti, F., Demurtas, M., Parrini, D., D'Antona, N. and Fioretti, P. (1977). *In* "Poor Intrauterine Fetal Growth" (B. Salvadori and A. Bacchi, eds), pp. 377–380, Minerva Medica, Parma.

Goebel, R. and Kuss, E. (1974). *Journal of Clinical Endocrinology and Metabolism* **39**, 969–972.

Grumbach, M. M., Kaplan, S. L., Sciarra, J. J. and Burr, I. M. (1968). *Annals of the New York Academy of Science* **148**, 501–531.

Gurpide, E. E., Schwers, J., Welch, M. T., Vande Wiele, R. L. and Leberman, S. (1966). *Journal of Clinical Endocrinology and Metabolism* **26**, 1355–1365.

Hull, M. G. R., Monro, P. P., Morgan, R. J. M. and Murray, M. A. F. (1979). *Clinical Endocrinology* **11**, 179–185.

Katagiri, A., Distler, W., Freeman, R. K. and Goebelsmann, U. (1976). *American Journal of Obstetrics and Gynecology* **124**, 272–280.

Klopper, A. (ed.) (1976). "Plasma Hormone Assays in Evaluation of Fetal Well-being", Churchill Livingstone, Edinburgh.

Klopper, A. and Shaaban, M. M. (1974). *Obstetrics and Gynecology* **44**, 187–193.

Klopper, A., Jandial, V. and Wilson, G. (1975). *Journal of Steroid Biochemistry* **6**, 651–656.

Klopper, A., Wilson, G. R. and Masson, G. M. (1977). *Obstetrics and Gynecology* **49**, 459–461.

Levitz, M., Slyper, A. J. and Selinger, M. (1974). *Journal of Clinical Endocrinology* **38**, 698–700.

Lindberg, B. S., Johansson, E. D. B. and Nilsson, B. A. (1974). *Acta obstetrica et gynecologia, scandinavica* **33**, Suppl., 21–36.

Macourt, D., Corker, C. S. and Naftolin, F. (1971). *Journal of Obstetrics and Gynaecology of the British Commonwealth* **78**, 335–340.

Masson, G. M. and Wilson, G. R. (1972). *Journal of Endocrinology* **54**, 245–250.

Masson, G. M., Klopper, A. and Wilson, G. R. (1977). *Obstetrics and Gynecology* **50**, 435–438.

Munson, A. K., Yannone, M. E. and Mueller, R. (1972). *Acta endocrinologia, Copenhagen* **69**, 410–412.

Notation, A. D. and Tagatz, G. E. (1977). *American Journal of Obstetrics and Gynecology* **128**, 747–756.

Parrini, D., Centini, G., Inaudi, P., De Leo, V., Pecciarini-Snickars, L. and Genazzani, A. R. (1978). *Atti della Società Italiana di Ostetricia e Ginecologia* **59**, 872–877.

Patrick, J., Challis, J., Natale, R. and Richardson, B. (1979). *American Journal of Obstetrics and Gynecology* **135**, 791–798.

Runnebaum, B., Rieben, W., Bierwirth, V., Münstermann, A. M. and Zander, J. (1972). *Acta endocrinologia, Copenhagen* **69**, 731–738.

Saxena, B. N., Emerson, K. and Selenkow, H. A. (1969). *New England Journal of Medicine* **281**, 225–231.

Siiteri, P. K. and MacDonald, P. C. (1963). *Steroids* **2**, 713–720.

Siiteri, P. K. and MacDonald, P. C. (1966). *Journal of Clinical Endocrinology and Metabolism* **26**, 751–761.

Simmer, H. H., Tulchinsky, D., Gold, E. M., Frankland, M., Greipel, M. and Golda A. S. (1974). *American Journal of Obstetrics and Gynecology* **119**, 283–290.

Teoh, E. S., Dawood, M. Y., Ratnam, S. S., Ambrose, A. and Das, N. P. (1973).

Australian and New Zealand Journal of Obstetrics and Gynaecology **13**, 198–202.

Townsley, J. D., Dubin, N. H., Frannis, G. F., Gartman, L. J. and Crystle, C. D. (1973). *Journal of Clinical Endocrinology and Metabolism* **36**, 289–295.

Tulchinsky, D. (1976). *In* "Plasma Hormone Assays in Evaluation of Fetal Well-being" (A. Klopper, ed.), p. 75, Churchill Livingstone, Edinburgh.

Tulchinsky, D., Hobel, C. J. and Korenman, S. G. (1971). *American Journal of Obstetrics and Gynecology* **111**, 311–318.

Tulchinsky, D., Frigoletto, F. D., Kenneth, J. R. and Fishman, J. (1975). *Journal of Clinical Endocrinology and Metabolism* **40**, 560–567.

Vigneri, R., Aquatrito, S., Spezzino, V., Cinquervi, E., Proto, S. and Montoneri, C. (1975). *Journal of Clinical Endocrinology and Metabolism* **40**, 506–510.

Zucconi, G., Lisboa, B. P., Simonitsch, E., Roth, L., Hagen, A. A. and Diczfaluzy, E. (1967). *Acta endocrinologia, Copenhagen* **56**, 413–422.

Section Four

PROTEIN SYNTHESIS IN THE PLACENTA

PROTEIN SYNTHESIS AND RELEASE BY THE HUMAN PLACENTA IN ORGAN CULTURE

J. Hustin, U. Gaspard, A. Reuter, J. C. Hendrick and P. Franchimont

Departments of Gynaecology and Radioimmunology, University of Liège, Liège, Belgium

INTRODUCTION

Since 1969, we have been involved in the study of protein hormone production by the human placenta in normal and pathological pregnancies. In order to elucidate further the capacity of the trophoblast to withstand adverse conditions, we have developed a tissue culture model. Preliminary reports have been published (Gaspard and Franchimont, 1972; Franchimont *et al.*, 1972), describing a progressive decrease in chorionic gonadotrophin (hCG) and placental lactogen (hPL) production while the α-subunit of hCG increased steadily. We have also shown (Hustin and Gaspard, 1977) that the syncytiotrophoblast of human placental villi placed in organ culture conditions in a chemically defined medium was soon altered, while cytotrophoblastic cells did not seem to be affected.

In order to relate these findings to the alterations in hCG and hPL production, we performed organ cultures of first trimester placentae using the same method as in previous studies. We have tried to define the requirements of human placenta for protein synthesis and have measured at various intervals different placental and embryonic markers in the tissue and in the culture medium.

Serono Symposium No. 35, "The Human Placenta", edited by A. Klopper, A. Genazzani and P. G. Crosignani, 1980. Academic Press, London and New York.

MATERIAL AND METHODS

Tissue Culture of Placentae

Eight placentae were obtained from therapeutic abortions. Four cases were of less than 10 weeks gestational age, three cases were between 10 and 13 weeks, and one was 17 weeks. All specimens were collected under strict aseptic conditions. Preparation of the explants was performed immediately according to previously described techniques (Gaspard and Franchimont, 1972; Hustin and Gaspard, 1977).

The medium was TS 199 (Difco) (2.5 ml per 35 mm petri dish) to which penicillin was added at a concentration of 400 IU/ml. Incubation was carried out at 37 °C. For each case nine petri dishes containing one to three explants were prepared. At various intervals (days 1, 3 and 5) media and the corresponding explants were separately collected and stored at −20 °C for subsequent assay. Some explants were routinely fixed in Bouin's fluid and processes for light microscopic examination in order to assess the viability of the cultures.

Radioimmunoassay Procedures

Human chorionic gonadotrophin in its undissociated form (u-hCG) as well as its α- and β-subunits (α-hCG and β-hCG), human placental lactogen (hPL), alpha-fetoprotein (AFP), carcinoembryonic antigen (CEA) and kappa casein (K-cas) were simultaneously assayed in the media according to procedures already described (Reuter *et al.*, 1976; Gaspard *et al.*, 1973; Franchimont *et al.*, 1973, 1975; Hendrick *et al.*, 1976). The explants were disrupted by sonication after defreezing and the same RIA procedures were applied to the homogenates. It should be noted that only three experiments were assayed for hPL.

RESULTS

Undissociated hCG and its Subunits

Before the initiation of the culture, the tissue content of u-hCG and its subunits was, of course, much elevated. Within the limits of the experiment, there seemed to be some decrease in the placental content of u-hCG and β-hCG in samples of more than 10 weeks gestational age (Fig. 1).

Table I.   u-hCG and subunits in placental tissue during organ culture (mean ± 2 S.D., in nanograms per milligram of protein).

	Preculture	Day 1	Day 3	Day 5
u-hCT	1445 ± 1260	533 ± 505	638 ± 613	593 ± 585
α-hCG	607 ± 460	978 ± 272	163 ± 21[a]	1060 ± 530
β-hCG	590 ± 540	539 ± 275	423 ± 410	664 ± 595

[a]This value differs significantly (*p* < 0.05) from preculture and day 1 and day 5 values.

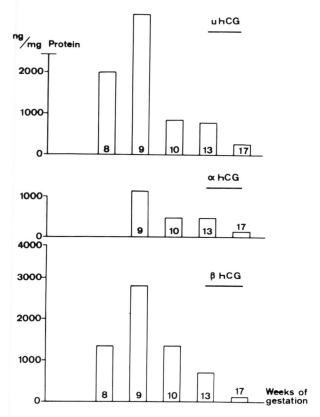

Fig. 1. Tissue concentration of u-hCG and its subunits prior to the cultures. Note that the highest values correspond to very early placentae.

The tissue content of the explants did not show any variation of the β-subunit throughout the week of observation. On the other hand, there was a sharp decrease in u-hCG content after 1 day to about 40% preculture values; u-hCG remained constant in the tissue thereafter. As regards αhCG, a temporary decrease was evident at day 3, but at the end of the observation period preculture values had been resumed (Table I).

Table II.   u-hCG and subunits in the culture medium (mean ± 2 s.ɛ. in nanograms per millilitre).

	Day 1	Day 3	Day 5
u-hCG	952 ± 916	1009 ± 996	980 ± 953
β-hCG	94 ± 75	108 ± 82	196 ± 159
α-hCG	257 ± 107	850 ± 440[a]	1042 ± 880[a]

[a]These values differ significantly ($p < 0.01$) from day 1 values.

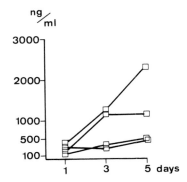

Fig. 2. Evolution of α-hCG concentration in the medium (four cultures). There is a marked increase in concentration.

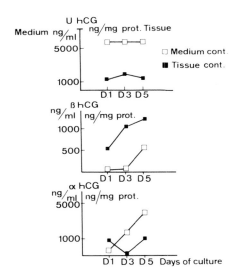

Fig. 3. Comparative evolution of tissue and medium concentrations in u-hCG and its sub-units in a given culture (No. 139). In this instance, u-hCG remained constant in the medium and the tissue while *both* subunits increased in the medium and the tissue (9 week placenta).

In the medium (Table II), u-hCG and β-hCG remained constant throughout the observation period. On the other hand, the α-subunit was present in much increased amounts (300% and 400% increase at days 3 and 5 respectively) (Fig. 2). It should be noted, however, that some specimens displayed a somewhat different behaviour. In the particular case depicted in Fig. 3, it is noteworthy that u-hCG content remained stable in the medium throughout 1 week while β-hCG and α-hCG increased in similar fashion in the medium and the tissue.

hPL

Three cultures were observed in different gaseous conditions: In an atmosphere of 95% O_2 –5% CO_2, no change in hPL production was evident in one case, while in the two other specimens a noticeable increase in hPL concentration could be noted at day 3. However, in cultures gassed with air this increase in peptide liberation was not apparent (Fig. 4).

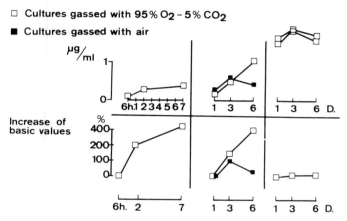

Fig. 4. hPL liberation in the medium. Three cultures (from left to right, respectively 8 week, 10 week and 13 week placentae). There is an increase in hPL liberation only in the cultures of early placentae.

It is noteworthy that the most important increment was observed with two cultures of 8 weeks and 10 weeks placental age where hPL production was modest, while in the third case (13 weeks) overall production was higher but it remained constant in the medium.

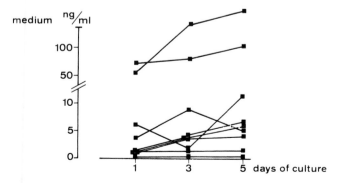

Fig. 5. CEA release in organ culture. There are only two instances of elevated values which correspond to 8 and 9 week placentae.

Embryonic Markers

CEA production in the medium was usually lower than 10 ng/ml. However, there were two experiments dealing with very early pregnancies (8 and 9 weeks) where elevated values were obtained, with a regular increase throughout the culture period. These high values in the medium corresponded to elevated tissue values (Fig. 5).

AFP values were often high from the beginning in the medium, but only in cultures gassed with 95% O_2-5% CO_2. When the gassing medium was air no AFP production could be noted (Fig. 6). In the tissues, AFP was most often under the lower limit of sensitivity of the assay method.

Finally, K-cas was present in the media and the tissues in very low values, which did not change during the culture period.

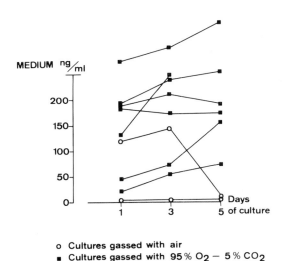

o Cultures gassed with air
■ Cultures gassed with 95 % O_2 — 5 % CO_2

Fig. 6. AFP release in organ culture. High values are present in cultures gassed with 95% O_2-5% CO_2.

DISCUSSION

From the data presented here, it is clear that the human placenta placed *in vitro* in a medium completely lacking in any protein supplementation is still capable of some peptide synthesis. Embryonic markers are usually not represented in the placental tissue. However, there was a progressive and cumulative increase of AFP in the medium. This marker might be progressively liberated from fetal blood vessels. This does not seem to be the case for CEA, which was present in the placental tissue of two early pregnancies. This may point to the persistence of primary trophoblast with all its potentiality.

Placental lactogen increased in the medium of two cultures and remained stable in a third experiment. This is somewhat at variance with earlier findings of

Gaspard and Franchimont (1972) and Franchimont *et al.* (1972). Golander *et al.* (1978) dealt with term placentae and showed a rapid decrease of hPL within 2 days. Hall *et al.* (1977), using midterm (13 weeks) and term placentae, demonstrated the same decrease of production. So also did Belleville *et al.* (1978) for two first trimester placentae. The sole explanation for this discrepancy resides in the very young age of the placentae we used. In both specimens, hPL from the beginning was present in very low values and the increase, though significant, was moderate.

The fact that with a 13 week old placenta, no increased production was found, points to a decreased capacity of ageing trophoblast to synthesize hPL. Interestingly enough, the older the placenta, the more elevated hPL values at the initiation of cultures. This corroborates the increasing plasma and tissue levels observed with advancing pregnancy (Gaspard *et al.*, 1973).

In contrast, u-hCG and its subunits presented consistent and interesting variations. In the tissue, u-hCG and the β-subunit remained more or less constant. In the medium there was a tendency towards a moderate and steady increase of β-hCG while u-hCG remained constant. The α-subunit was liberated in the medium in increasing amounts while its tissue values decreased at day 3 but resumed elevated values thereafter; this points to a true synthesis. Franchimont *et al.* (1972) and Gaspard and Franchimont (1972) described this evolution for second and third trimester placentae. It thus seems that preferential synthesis of α-hCG occurs *in vitro*, whatever the gestational age. Other papers dealing with hCG production by the human placenta *in vitro* have not mentioned this fact. Indeed, Hall *et al.* (1977) claimed that midterm placentae produced increasing amounts of hCG (β-hCG). Golander *et al.* (1978) demonstrated the same finding for term placentae, while Belleville *et al.* (1978) showed high sustained hCG production in first trimester placentae compared to very low values in term placentae. It must be kept in mind that all those papers dealt with cultures supplemented with protein. This might easily explain the higher production rates which were observed.

In our experiments, cultures of younger placentae produced much more hCG and β-hCG than cultures of placentae 10 weeks or more old. This finding must be related to the presence of CEA and hPL in such very young placentae. It is tempting to say that early placenta retain more capabilities *in vitro* than older ones. However, incubation in air instead of 95% O_2 produced, in all cases, a marked reduction in the liberation of peptides. This is another interesting point. In this study, α-hCG levels increased markedly in the medium; β-hCG seemed to increase moderately, but there was no simultaneous increase of the levels of u-hCG. It may be that synthesis of both subunits occurs when sufficiently viable trophoblast remains, but in our culture conditions no recombination to form the undissociated molecule was apparent. This inability to recombine may be related to progressive trophoblastic alterations. MacLennan *et al.* (1972) produced ultrastructural evidence that in organ culture conditions the integrity of the trophoblast was maintained up to 96 h. We have shown (Hustin and Gaspard, 1977) that the syncytiotrophoblast was damaged from the third day on *in vitro*, while cytotrophoblastic cells began to thrive.

Further work from this laboratory (U. Gaspard and J. Hustin, to be published) is in progress which concerns the site of protein hormones within placental explants maintained in organ culture conditions. After several days, only viable areas of syncytiotrophoblast retain their immunocytochemical reaction for u-hCG and β-hCG while a marked positive reaction for the α-subunit can be demonstrated in the cytotrophoblastic cells. Cytotrophoblastic cells are generally considered as reserve cells capable of proliferation under hypoxic conditions in order to replace the damaged syncytium (Fox, 1970).

Derepression, at the cytotrophoblastic level, of the ancestral gene controlling the synthesis of the α-subunit may also be induced by the same trigger. Increased synthesis would ensue and explain the autonomous high levels of α-hCG released in the medium.

REFERENCES

Belleville, F., Lasbennes, A., Nabet, P. and Paysant, P. (1978). *Acta endocrinologica, Copenhagen* **88**, 169.

Fox, H. (1970). *American Journal of Obstetrics and Gynecology* **107**, 1058.

Franchimont, P., Debruche, M. L., Zangerle, P. F. and Proyard, J. (1973). *Annales d'immunologie* **124**, 619.

Franchimont, P., Gaspard, U., Reuter, A. M. and Heynen, G. (1972). *Clinical Endocrinology* **1**, 315.

Franchimont, P., Zangerle, P. F., Debruche, M. L., Proyard, J., Simon, M. and Gaspard, U. (1975). *Annales de biologie clinique* **33**, 139.

Gaspard, U. and Franchimont, P. (1972). *Comptes rendus hebdomadaires des séances de l'Académie des sciences* **275**, 1661.

Gaspard, U., Hendrick, J. C., Reuter, A. M. and Franchimont, P. (1973). *Annales de biologie clinique* **31**, 447.

Golander, A., Barrett, J. R., Tyrey, L., Fletcher, W. H. and Handwerger, S. (1978). *Endocrinology* **102**, 597.

Hall, C. S. G., James, T. E., Goodyer, C., Branchaud, C., Guyda, H. and Giroud, C. J. P. (1977). *Steroids* **30**, 569.

Hendrick, J. C., Thirion, A. and Franchimont, P. (1976). *In* "Cancer Related Antigens" (P. Franchimont, ed.), pp. 51–57, North-Holland Publishing Co., Amsterdam.

Hustin, J. and Gaspard, U. (1977). *British Journal of Obstetrics and Gynaecology* **84**, 210.

MacLennan, A. H., Sharp, F. and Shaw-Dunn, J. (1972). *Journal of Obstetrics and Gynaecology of the British Commonwealth* **79**, 113.

Reuter, A. M., Schoonbroodt, J. and Franchimont, P. (1976). *In* "Cancer Related Antigens" (P. Franchimont, ed.), pp. 237–249, North-Holland Publishing Co., Amsterdam.

BIOSYNTHETIC PATHWAY OF CORTICOTROPHIN AND RELATED PEPTIDES OF THE HUMAN PLACENTA: *IN VITRO* DEMONSTRATION

A. S. Liotta and D. T. Krieger

Neuroendocrinology Laboratory, Division of Endocrinology, Department of Medicine, Mount Sinai School of Medicine, New York, New York 10029, U.S.A.

INTRODUCTION

The synthesis of substances similar to pituitary hormones by the human placenta has been established. Some of these substances include chorionic gonadotrophin, chorionic somatomammotrophin and chorionic thyrotrophin. Immunoassayable and bioassayable corticotrophin (ACTH) (Genazzani *et al.*, 1974, 1975; Liotta *et al.*, 1977; Rees *et al.*, 1975), immunoassayable α-melanotrophin (α-MSH), β-lipotrophin (β-LPH) and β-endorphin (Nakai *et al.*, 1978) have been demonstrated in extracts of human placenta. Table I illustrates typical immunoassayable values obtained in our laboratory for these activities.

Utilizing *in vitro* tissue incubation techniques, Liotta *et al.* (1977) and Genazzani *et al.* (1974) have presented evidence consistent with, but not definitive proof of, human placental synthesis of ACTH-like material. In two previous studies employing radioimmunoassay and molecular sieve chromatography, high molecular weight (HMW) forms of placental immunoreactive ACTH (Liotta *et al.*, 1977) and β-endorphin (Nakai *et al.*, 1978) have been detected. The last finding is of interest because ACTH, β-lipotrophin and β-endorphin have been demonstrated to be contained within, and are post-translationally derived from the same HMW glycoprotein precursor molecule which is present in the anterior and intermediate lobes

Serono Symposium No. 35, "The Human Placenta", edited by A. Klopper, A. Genazzani and P. G. Crosignani, 1980. Academic Press, London and New York.

Table I. ACTH-related immunoreactivity; term human placenta.

	Immunoreactivity (pmol/g placenta)			
ACTH (NH$_2$-terminal)	0.54	0.65	2.9	0.97
ACTH (mid-portion)	0.21	0.39	0.93	0.52
β-Lipotropin	0.32	0.43	0.86	0.39
β-Endorphin	0.26	0.31	0.69	0.26
α-MSH	0.15	0.29	0.40	0.17

Freshly obtained term human placentas were trimmed of cord and membranes, washed extensively with isotonic saline at 10°C and homogenized in 0.2 M HCl containing 0.1% bovine serum albumin. The extracts were purified by methods previously reported from our laboratory and subjected to radioimmunoassay. The NH$_2$-terminal ACTH antiserum reacts with mouse precursor ACTH/β-endorphin, while the mid-portion antiserum reacts poorly with precursor-like material (approximately 5–10%, in a non-parallel manner) and not at all with α-MSH. It reacts with ACTH(11–24), ACTH(1–24) and ACTH(1–39) on a near equimolar basis. The β-LPH antiserum is NH$_2$-terminal directed and reacts with β- and γ-LPH equally, but not at all with β-endorphin. The β-endorphin antiserum is COOH-terminal directed, reacting with β-LPH and β-endorphin on an equimolar basis. The β-endorphin values listed were obtained after β-LPH immunoreactivity was first removed from the extract by affinity chromatography. The α-MSH antiserum is highly specific for α-MSH, ACTH(1–13) and ACTH(1–39), exhibiting less than 0.2% cross-reactivity on a molar basis. Each column represents values obtained for one placenta ($n = 4$).

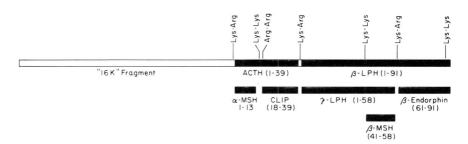

Fig. 1. Peptide backbone of the murine and bovine pituitary common precursor of ACTH and related peptides. Note the location of the paired basic amino acids which can be proteolytically cleaved to yield the component peptides.

of the normal murine and bovine pituitary, and in a mouse pituitary tumor cell line (Mains *et al.*, 1977; Roberts *et al.*, 1978; Nakanishi *et al.*, 1979). Figure 1 depicts the peptide backbone of the murine and bovine pituitary precursor of ACTH and related peptides. Note the location of the paired basic amino acids which can be cleaved proteolytically to yield the component peptides.

The present study unequivocally demonstrates human placental synthesis of immunoreactive ACTH, α-MSH, β-LPH and β-endorphin-like material and establishes that these peptides are derived from an HMW precursor. The placental biosynthetic pathway is thus similar to that described for pituitary.

SUMMARY OF METHODOLOGICAL APPROACH

Briefly, the trophoblastic shell with any adhering decidual tissue was dissected from fresh term human placenta. It was then mechanically and enzymatically dispersed to obtain a cell suspension (Liotta and Krieger, 1977; Liotta *et al.*, 1979). The cells were maintained in culture for 4 days prior to use and then incubated for 30 min or 6 h in the presence of $[^{35}S]$methionine and $[^3H]$lysine. Cell extracts were put on affinity columns of immobilized ACTH and β-endorphin antisera in order to detect and purify specifically labelled material. These immobilized antisera preparations will subsequently be referred to as immunoadsorbents. Radiolabelled material eluted from these immunoadsorbents was subjected to the following procedures: (a) sodium dodecyl sulfate (SDS)–polyacrylamide gel electrophoresis; (b) sequential binding to both the ACTH and β-endorphin immunoadsorbents, in order to determine if any immunoreactive material contained the dual antigenic determinants of ACTH and β-endorphin; (c) Sephadex gel filtration; (d) ability to bind to concanavalin-A, as an indication of the presence or absence of carbohydrate; (e) isoelectric focusing; and (f) partial tryptic mapping and identification of two of the fragments generated.

RESULTS

SDS–Polyacrylamide Gel Electrophoresis (SDS–PAGE)

Figure 2 illustrates the SDS-PAGE Profiles obtained for the 30 min incubation cell extracts. Radiolabelled material specifically retained and eluted from the ACTH immunoadsorbent (Fig. 2A) and the β-endorphin immunoadsorbent (Fig. 2B) display nearly identical profiles. This material was resolved into at least two size classes, with apparent molecular weights (M_r) of 35 000 ± 1700 and 47 000 ± 1100 daltons. These values represent the average and s.d. from six gel runs.

Sequential Use of Immunoadsorbents

To ascertain whether the nearly identical SDS-PAGE profiles obtained for immunoreactive ACTH and β-endorphin represented HMW material containing both immunoreactive ACTH and β-endorphin determinants or two (or more) separate species, each containing a single determinant, the immunoadsorbents were used sequentially. An aliquot of cell extract derived from the 30 min incubation was reacted with the ACTH immunoadsorbent and, after washing, specifically retained material was eluted with excess synthetic hACTH(1–39) solution. The eluted radiolabelled material was then reacted with the β-endorphin immunoadsorbent, washed and specifically retained activity was eluted with excess synthetic β_h-endorphin solution. This manipulation demonstrated that > 83% of the HMW material present in the SDS-PAGE profiles represented molecules which contained the dual antigenic determinants of ACTH and β-endorphin.

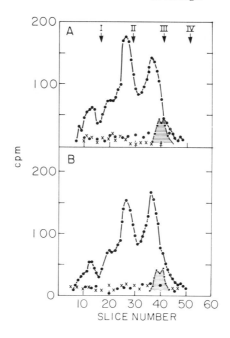

Fig. 2. SDS gel electrophoresis of cell extracts after the 30 min incubation. Specification retained immunoreactive material eluted from the ACTH (A) and β-endorphin (B) immuno-adsorbents was denatured in 2.5% SDS and 5% dithiothreitol at 90 °C for 10 min and applied to 2.5% stacking/10% separation tube gels. The solid circles and crosses represent the profiles obtained when immunoadsorption was performed in the presence of two different concentrations of excess synthetic ligand ((A) ACTH(1–39) for (B) $β_h$-endorphin). The shaded area represents the immunoreactive profile of mouse pituitary precursor ACTH/β-endorphin. The > 67 000 dalton peak has subsequently been shown to be dissociable into M_r = 35 000 and 47 000 dalton material following more rigorous conditions of reduction and denaturation. The arrows indicate the peak elution positions of the calibration proteins: (I) M_r = 67 000; (II) 43 000; (III) 30 000; and (IV) 20 100 daltons.

Concanavalin-A Binding

HMW ACTH/β-endorphin obtained by immunoadsorption was applied to concanavalin-A–Sepharose microcolumns in the presence of Mn^{2+} and Ca^{2+}. An average of 77.6% (n = 6) of the applied material was retained on the column. Parallel columns were eluted with either D-mannose buffer or buffer containing synthetic hACTH(1–39) plus $β_h$-endorphin. When D-mannose was used, an average of 82% of the retained material was eluted, while < 6% of the activity was eluted with the peptide solution.

Isoelectric Focusing of HMW ACTH/β-Endorphin

HMW ACTH/β-endorphin was subjected to polyacrylamide gel flat-bed iso-electric focusing. This material was focused into multiple peaks between pH 8.5 and pH 9 at the cathode strip. For comparison, highly purified natural hACTH (1–39) was focused into three components in the pH range 6.7–8.0.

Sephadex Gel Filtration of HMW ACTH/β-Endorphin

Since molecular weights of glycoproteins and basic proteins by SDS-PAGE tend to be overestimated due to the anomalous behaviour of these classes of proteins (Weber and Osborn, 1975, HMW material eluted from the ACTH immuno-

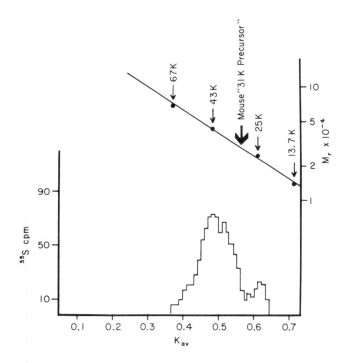

Fig. 3. Sephadex G-200 gel filtration of immunoreactive HMW material eluted from the ACTH immunoadsorbent. Cell extract obtained from the 30 min incubation was reacted with the ACTH immunoadsorbent, specifically retained activity eluted and incubated in a minimum volume of 6 M urea containing 5% dithiothreitol before being applied to a 0.9 cm × 60 cm Sephadex G-200 column. Elution was performed with 6 M urea containing 0.05% human serum albumin. The material eluting with apparent $M_r \cong 19\,000$ daltons was shown to contain only the ACTH antigenic determinant. The calibration proteins are indicated.

adsorbent was subjected to Sephadex G-200 gel filtration under denaturing conditions (Fig. 3). The molecular weight estimates for the two poorly resolved HMW species are $M_r = 42\,500$ and $33\,000$ daltons.

Partial Tryptic Analysis of HMW ACTH/β-Endorphin

[³⁵S]Methionine- and [³H]lysine-labelled HMW ACTH/β-endorphin was subjected to carboxymethyl–Sepharose cation exchange chromatography (Fig. 4). At least five peaks are evident in the profile, presumably indicating the presence of at least five methionine residues in this HMW material.

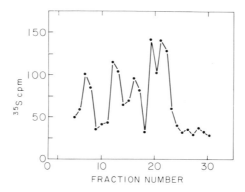

Fig. 4. Carboxymethyl–Sepharose cation exchange chromatography of HMW ACTH/β-endorphin tryptic digest. After overnight trypsinization, the products were applied to the cation exchange column and elution was performed with sodium acetate–acetic acid buffer. Since the HMW material was labelled with [^{35}S] methionine, each peak presumably represents a separate methionine-containing fragment.

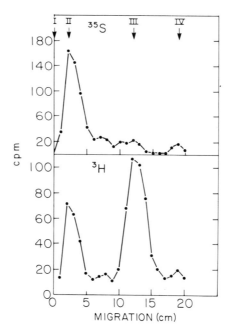

Fig. 5. Identification of two tryptic fragments of placental HMW ACTH/β-endorphin. High voltage paper electrophoresis of antisera-purified tryptic digest of HMW material. Cells were incubated in the presence of [^{35}S]methionine and [^{3}H]lysine. After electrophoresis the paper was cut, eluted and counted in a dual channel β-liquid scintillation counter. Arrows indicate (I) origin; (II) synthetic β-endorphin(1–9); (III) synthetic ACTH(9–15); and (IV) lysine.

Further characterization of the tryptic digests by immunoprecipitation with affinity-purified ACTH and methionine encephalin antisera followed by high voltage paper electrophoresis of the precipitated material revealed the presence of two radiolabelled fragments physicochemically identical to the ACTH(9–15) and β-endorphin(1–9) sequences (Fig. 5). It can be seen that the ACTH(9–15)-like fragment contains only ^{3}H activity while the β-endorphin(1–9)-like fragment possesses both ^{3}H and ^{35}S activity. This result is consistent with the primary sequences of the corresponding synthetic marker peptides, since ACTH(9–15), contains lysine, but not methionine, while β-endorphin (1–9) contains one methionine and one lysine residue.

Six Hour Incubation of Placental Cells with Radiolabelled Amino Acids

Following a 6 h incubation of placental cells with the radiolabelled amino acids, the cell extracts were purified on immunoadsorbents and the specifically retained material was eluted and chromatographed on Sephadex G-75 superfine columns (Fig. 6). Immunoreactive ACTH consisted of at least four components.

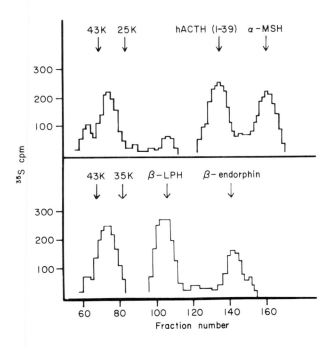

Fig. 6. Sephadex G-75 profile of 6 h incubation cellular extracts. Immunoreactive ACTH (upper panel) eluted in positions corresponding to HMW ACTH/β-endorphin, hACTH(1–39) and α-MSH. Immunoreactive (lower panel) β-endorphin eluted in positions corresponding to HMW ACTH/β-endorphin, $β_h$-LPH and $β_h$-endorphin. (Note that $β_h$-LPH contains two methionine residues, while $β_h$-endorphin contains only one.) The arrows indicate the elution positions of the calibration proteins and peptides.

This material co-eluted with hACTH(1–39) and α-MSH markers in approximately equimolar quantities, as well as eluting in the HMW region (Fig. 6, lower panel). Immunoreactive β-endorphin co-eluted with β_h-LPH and β_h-endorphin markers, in near equimolar quantities, as well as eluting in the HMW region (Fig. 6, lower panel).

Pulse–Chase Experiment

Cells were pulse-labelled in the presence of $[^{35}S]$ methionine for 30 min and the fate of the label incorporated into immunoreactive HMW material was followed by utilizing chase periods of 30, 45, 60, 120 and 240 min. Label disappeared progressively from the HMW material and appeared in smaller molecules containing either the ACTH or β-endorphin antigenic determinant according to the following scheme:

(a) immunoreactive ACTH: HMW ACTH/β-endorphin → 22–17K ACTH → 4.5K ACTH → α-MSH;

(b) immunoreactive β-endorphin: HMW ACTH/β-endorphin → β-LPH → β-endorphin.

The disappearance of HMW material and the corresponding appearance of label in progressively smaller molecular species is consistent with a precursor–product relationship for this material.

CONCLUSIONS

In summary, we conclude that the human placenta synthesizes glycoprotein(s) containing the dual antigenic determinants of ACTH and β-endorphin; that such material exhibits apparent size heterogeneity and is larger than the reported mouse pituitary forms. Partial tryptic mapping of this precursor-like material reveals fragments which are physiochemically similar to fragments generated by trypsinization of hACTH(1–39) and of β_h-endorphin. Two of these fragments have been identified. Finally, this precursor-like material is processed into smaller molecular species physiochemically similar to hACTH(1–39), α-MSH, β-LPH and β_h-endorphin. The physiological roles of these placental peptides remain to be elucidated.

REFERENCES

Genazzani, A. R., Hurliman, J., Fioretti, P. and Felber, J. P. (1974). *Experientia* **30**, 430.

Genazzani, A. R., Fraioli, F., Hurliman, J., Fioretti, P. and Felber, J. P. (1975). *Clinical Endocrinology* **4**, 1.

Liotta, A. S., Osathanondth, R., Ryan, K. J. and Krieger, D. T. (1977). *Endocrinology* **101**, 1552.

Liotta, A. S. and Krieger, D. T. (1977). *Endocrine Research Communications* **4**, 159.

Liotta, A. S., Gildersleeve, D., Brownstein, M. J. and Krieger, D. T. (1979). *Proceedings of the National Academy of Sciences of the U.S.A.* **76**, 1448.

Mains, R. E., Eipper, B. A. and Ling, N. (1977). *Proceedings of the National Academy of Sciences of the U.S.A.* **74**, 3014.

Nakai, Y., Nakao, K., Oki, S. and Imura, H. (1978). *Life Sciences* **23**, 2013.

Nakanishi, S., Inoue, A., Kita, T., Nakamura, M., Chang, A. C. Y., Cohen, S. N. and Numa, S. (1979). *Nature, London* **278**, 423.

Rees, L. H., Burke, C. W., Chard, T., Evans, S. W. and Letchworth, A. T. (1975). *Nature, London* **254**, 620.

Roberts, J. L., Phillips, M., Rose, P. A. and Herbert, E. (1978). *Biochemistry* **17**, 3609.

Weber, K. and Osborn, M. (1975). *In* "The Proteins' (H. Neurath and R. L. Hill, eds), Vol. 1, pp. 179–223, Academic Press, London and New York.

SOMATOSTATIN-LIKE ACTIVITY IN PLACENTA, AMNIOTIC FLUID AND UMBILICAL CORD PLASMA

H. Etzrodt, K. Musch, K. E. Schröder, and E. F. Pfeiffer

Departments of Internal Medicine and Gynaecology, University of Ulm, Ulm/Donau, German Federal Republic

INTRODUCTION

The polypeptide somatostatin (SRIF) was originally discovered in extracts of the hypothalamus. It received its name because of its inhibiting effect on the secretion of growth hormone. Later, SRIF was also found in other tissues, especially in the gastrointestinal tract and the pancreas, where it inhibited the secretion of endocrine and exocrine systems. It was also proved that many other exocrine and endocrine systems were dependent on, or could be inhibited by, SRIF. Because of the multiplicity of the action of SRIF, a paracrine function on the surrounding cells was assumed.

Among all endocrine glands the placenta holds a unique position both with regard to the number of hormones it produces (steroid as well as polypeptide hormones) and that these different hormone systems are found in close proximity to each other. Because of the supposed paracrine function of SRIF, it seemed interesting to investigate the presence of SRIF in placenta.

METHODS

Radioimmunoassay of Somatostatin

For the radioimmunoassay of SRIF (Etzrodt *et al.*, 1979) Tyr-1-SRIF, kindly provided by Serono-Freiburg, was labelled with ^{125}I by the chloramine-T method

Serono Symposium No. 35, "The Human Placenta", edited by A. Klopper,
A. Genazzani and P. G. Crosignani, 1980. Academic Press, London and New York.

(Hunter and Greenwood, 1962). The iodinated Tyr-1-SRIF was purified by ion exchange carboxymethyl cellulose (Whatman no. 52) in a discontinuous ammonium acetate buffer (pH 4.6) according to Arimura *et al.* (1975). Antiserum was raised in goats by injection of SRIF coupled to human albumin by glutaraldehyde. The radioimmunoassay buffer consisted of 0.01 M phosphate (pH 6.8), 0.15 M NaCl, 0.001 M ethylenedichlorotetraacetic acid (EDTA) and 0.1% Tween 20 (v/v). Tracer (0.1 ml containing 10 000 c.p.m.) and 0.1 ml of sample or standard were added to 0.1 ml antiserum at a final dilution of 1:600. After incubation for 18 h at 4 °C the free and antiserum-bound tracer were separated by addition of 0.1 ml human serum and 1.5 ml of 20% (w/v) polyethylene glycol 6000 in 0.005 M phosphate buffer. The sensitivity of the radioimmunoassay was 3 pg/ml. At the top end of the range, 50 pg/ml SRIF displaced 50% of the tracer from the antiserum. Hormones other than SRIF were not able to compete with the tracer.

Placental Extraction

Full term human placentae, obtained directly after normal or surgical delivery, were extensively washed with ice-cold saline solution to remove all traces of blood. Several small pieces were cut off and homogenized either in hypotonic buffer (0.001 M $NaHCO_3$, 0.5 mM $CaCl_2$, pH 7.4) or in 0.25 M sucrose; 1 g tissue to 5 ml solution. These homogenates were subjected to one of the following treatments:

(a) Homogenate (1 ml) was adjusted with concentrated acetic acid to a concentration of 1 N acetic acid and heated for 5 min in a waterbath. After centrifugation the supernatant was lyophilized.

(b) Homogenate (1 ml) was added to 8 ml of the organic phase of a *n*-butanol–2 N acetic acid mixture (4:5 v/v). After thorough mixing, the samples were centrifuged and the upper phase dried and used for the radioimmunoassay.

(c) The homogenate was centrifuged at 100 000 g, the supernatant (cytosol) was treated either with acetic acid and heating (treatment (a)) or the upper phase of butanol–acetic acid (treatment (b)).

Gel Chromatography of Placental Extract

Two millilitres of the 100 000 g supernatant were subjected to gel chromatography on Sephadex G-25m (25 cm × 1.5 cm) in 0.1 M ammonium acetate, pH 4.6. Fractions of 2.5 ml were collected, lyophilized and their SRIF-like immunoreactivity (SLI) was determined by the radioimmunoassay. The butanol-extracted cytosol was also subjected to the same chromatographic procedure and checked for SLI.

Comparison between SLI in Placenta and SRIF Standard Curve

Several dilutions were made from the butanol-extracted cytosol and were compared with serial dilutions of cold SRIF (standard curve) in the radioimmunoassay.

Determination of SLI in Amniotic Fluid and Umbilical Cord Plasma

SLI in amniotic fluid and umbilical cord plasma was determined as described earlier (Etzrodt *et al.*, 1979). Eight millilitres of the upper phase of *n*-butanol-2 N acetic acid (4:5, v/v) were added to 1 ml umbilical cord plasma or amniotic fluid. The preparation was mixed, centrifuged and the supernatant dried after addition of 10 μl of a 10% (v/v) solution of Tween 20 in water. For the radio-immunoassay the dried residue was reconstituted with the radioimmunoassay buffer.

RESULTS

In the radioimmunoassay for FLI (SRIF-like immunoreactivity), extracts from human placental tissue displace the tracer from its binding to the antiserum.

Gel Chromatography of the 100 000 g Supernatant from the Placental Homogenate on Sephadex G-25m

The eluted fractions were tested for SLI in the radioimmunoassay. As shown in Fig. 1, one peak of activity was found corresponding to a molecular weight of 1600 daltons. When iodinated SRIF was chromatographed in the same way, the peak of radioactivity was detected in similar fractions. Chromatography of the butanol-extracted cytosol showed results similar to the chromatography of native cytosol.

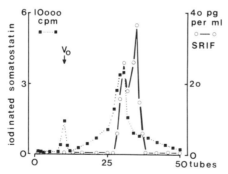

Fig. 1. Gel chromatography of the 100 000 g supernatant of placental homogenate and of the iodinated Tyr-1-SRIF on Sephadex G-25m in 0.1 M ammonium acetate, pH 4.6. Fractions of 2.5 ml were collected, dried and tested for somatostatin-like immunoreactivity by radio-immunoassay.

Serial Dilutions of Butanol-extracted Cytosol

In the radioimmunoassay, the displacement of the tracer by different concentrations of cytosol extracts was found to be parallel with that of the standard curve (Fig. 2).

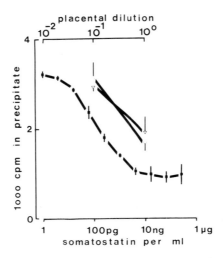

Fig. 2. Radioimmunoassay of SRIF and dilutions of the butanol–acetic acid extract from two different placentae. Standard deviations of three different pieces from each placenta are indicated.

Table I. Somatostatin-like immunoreactivity in placental extracts. The placentae had been homogenized in 1 mM $NaHCO_3$, 0.5 mM $CaCl_2$ [a] or in 0.25 M sucrose solution. [b] The concentrations are given in nanograms of SLI per gram of tissue (wet weight).

Extraction with	Homogenate	Cytosol
Acetic acid and heating	2.7 (± 1.3)[a]	2.8 (± 0.9)[a]
	1.6 (± 0.5)[b]	1.3 (± 0.5)[b]
Butanol–acetic acid	2.9 (± 1.0)[a]	3.2 (± 1.3)[a]
	1.5 (± 0.6)[b]	1.3 (± 0.5)[b]

[a] Homogenization in 1 mM $NaHCO_3$, 0.5 $CaCl_2$.
[b] Homogenization in 0.25 M sucrose.

Extraction Procedures

Native homogenate and native 100 000 g supernatant could not be used for determination of SLI because of non-parallelism with the SRIF standard curve. Extraction of SLI by heating in 1 N acetic acid and extraction with the organic phase of *n*-butanol-2 *N* acetic acid yielded reproducible SLI values. Serial dilutions showed parallelism with the SRIF standard curve in buffer. Addition of exogenous SRIF to extracts of placenta exhibited the same parallelism to the curve.

When the tissue was homogenized in 1 mM $NaHCO_3$, SLI of 2.9 (± 1.1) ng/g wet tissue or 120 (± 50) pg/ml supernatant protein was found for both extraction methods (Table I). After homogenization in 0.25 M sucrose solution, 1.4 (± 0.6) ng/g wet tissue or 50 (± 20) pg/mg supernatant protein was found.

SLI in Amniotic Fluid and Umbilical Cord Plasma

The concentration of SLI in amniotic fluid from three full-term patients was 35 (± 25) pg/ml. In umbilical cord plasma the SLI values were 50 (± 40) pg/ml.

DISCUSSION

Our results demonstrate the presence of a substance in placental tissue which behaves similarly to the synthetic SRIF in the radioimmunoassay for SRIF. This substance has a molecular weight of the same order of magnitude as that of the iodinated SRIF tracer. Extraction procedures that determine the SLI of other tissues can be used successfully. In serial dilutions the substance behaves similarly to the SRIF standard curve. We therefore assume the substance we are measuring in placental tissue to be somatostatin.

We found that SLI could only be demonstrated when the tissue had been extracted either with acetic acid and heating or with the upper phase of butanol–acetic acid. For our purposes the latter technique was the method of choice. Higher SLI values were obtained by homogenization of the tissue in 1 mM $NaHCO_3$ than in 0.25 M sucrose solution. This may be due to the more thorough cell lysis in hypotonic medium. Extraction of the homogenate and of the 100 000 g supernatant yielded the same SLI values. As the 100 000 g supernatant does not contain organelles, one might assume that SLI is cytoplasmic. Because of low SLI values found in both amniotic fluid and umbilical cord plasma, the possibility of contamination of the placental homogenate by these substances can be eliminated.

Japanese researchers have described somatostatin-like immunoreactivity in placenta by radioimmunoassay and immunofluorescence techniques (Nishihira and Yagihashi, 1978; Kumasaka *et al.*, 1978). In early pregnancy, cells containing SLI can be detected in the cytotrophoblastic layer. Kumasaka *et al.* (1978) indicated a concentration of 300 pg/g dry weight.

In comparison to the levels of SLI in other tissues, the placenta appears to contain low amounts of SLI. In the central nervous system the levels of SLI are about 100 times higher than in the placenta (Brownstein *et al.*, 1974). In the gastrointestinal tract, values of 33 ng/g tissue for pancreas and 50 ng/g tissue for the antrum of stomach were found (McIntosh *et al.*, 1978). The concentration of the hormone should not be correlated to its significance for the gland because of its paracrine action. In the surroundings of the SRIF secreting cell, much higher concentrations than are indicated by the overall concentration in the placenta may be assumed.

ACKNOWLEDGEMENTS

We thank Ms A. Held and Ms M. A. Zang for their valuable technical assistance. The investigation was supported by Deutsche Forschungsgemeinschaft, SFB 87, Ulm.

REFERENCES

Arimura, A., Sato, H., Coy, D. H. and Schally, A. V. (1975). *Proceedings of the Society for Experimental Biology and Medicine* **148**, 784.

Brownstein, M., Arimura, A., Sato, H., Schally, A. and Kizer, J. S. (1974). *Endocrinology* **96**, 1456.

Etzrodt, H., Schröder, K. E., Rosenthal, J. and Pfeiffer, E. F. (1979). *Acta endocrinologica, Copenhagen*, Suppl. 225, 224.

Hunter, W. M. and Greenwood, F. C. (1962). *Nature, London* **194**, 495.

Kumasaka, T., Nishi, N., Yaoi, Y., Suzuki, A., Saito, M., Okayasu, I., Hatakeyama, S., Sawano, S. and Kokubu, T. (1978). *Nippon Naibunpi Gakkai Zasshi* **54**, 779.

McIntosh, C., Arnold, R., Bothe, E., Becker, H., Köbberling, J. and Creutzfeldt, W. (1978). *Gut* **19**, 655.

Nishihira, M. and Yagihashi, S. (1978). *Tohoku Journal of Experimental Medicine* **126**, 397.

HUMAN PLACENTAL AMINOPEPTIDASES

S. Lampelo and T. Vanha-Perttula

*Department of Anatomy, University of Kuopio, P.O. Box 138,
70101 Kuopio 10, Finland*

INTRODUCTION

Homogenates of human placenta inactivate oxytocin enzymatically (Ryden, 1966). Besides the natural substrates, this enzyme also hydrolyses several synthetic substrates, e.g. L-cystinedi-β-naphthylamide (CysNA) and L-leucine-β-naphthylamide (LeuNA) (Tuppy and Nesvadba, 1957). Oxytocinase and cystine aminopeptidase are considered to be the same enzyme (Tuppy and Nesvadba, 1957). The enzyme is present in high concentration in human placental tissue (Lampelo and Vanha-Perttula, 1979).

Placental tissue is also known to contain arylamidase activity. The most generally used substrate for determining its activity is LeuNA (James, 1966; Warwas *et al.*, 1972). Arylamidase has been shown to split leucine peptides, but its biological substrate is not known (Patterson *et al.*, 1963).

Cystine aminopeptidase levels show a progressive rise throughout normal pregnancy, reaching a maximum in the last trimester (Gazarek *et al.*, 1976). The enzyme level in the maternal serum is supposed to reflect the activity of the placental tissue (Ryden, 1972).

Normal serum contains aminopeptidase (Yman, 1970*b*). The activity of an arylamidase hydrolysing LeuNA has been known to increase during pregnancy and has been considered to be mainly due to cystine aminopeptidase (oxytocinase) (Hiwada *et al.*, 1978), which shows a broad substrate specificity (Yman, 1970*b*).

Serono Symposium No. 35, "The Human Placenta", edited by A. Klopper,
A. Genazzini and P. G. Crosignani, 1980. Academic Press, London and New York.

This report is concerned with the fractionation by gel filtration of amino-peptidases in human placentae as well as in sera from pregnant and non-pregnant women. The biochemical properties of the separate enzyme activities were then characterized after pooling the activity peaks.

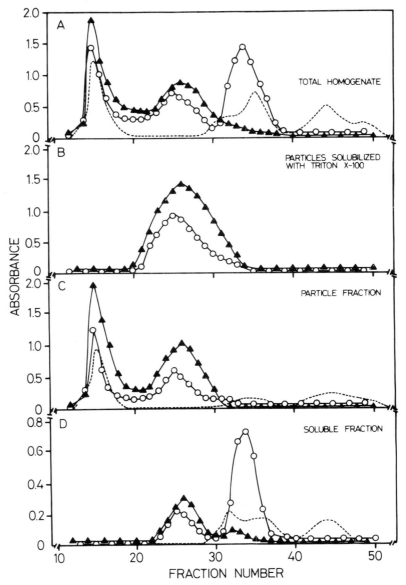

Fig. 1. Elution patterns of the enzymes hydrolysing LeuNA (▲) and CysNA (○) after Sepharose 6B filtration of human placentae. (A) Total homogenate; (B) particles solubi-lized with Triton X-100; (C) unsolubilized particle fraction; and (D) soluble fraction. The pro-tein content of the 10 ml fractions is given as the absorbance at 280 nm (- - -). (Reproduced from Lampelo and Vanha-Perttula (1979), with permission.)

PLACENTAL TISSUE PREPARATIONS

Gel filtration of the total placental homogenate on Sepharose 6B revealed three peaks of cystine aminopeptidase and two of arylamidase with CysNA and LeuNA as substrates, respectively (Fig. 1(A)). Elution of the placental particle fraction (obtained after centrifugation of homogenate prepared in 0.25 M sucrose at 105 000g for 1 h) resulted in peaks which were coincident with the two first activities of the total homogenate with both substrates (Fig. 1(C)). When the particle fraction was treated with Triton X-100 (0.3%) prior to elution, the first peak disappeared, whereas the second peak became stronger (Fig. 1(B)). Further studies showed that enzymes in these two peaks have identical biochemical characteristics. It is therefore concluded that these peaks represent the placental particle-bound enzyme(s), which can be released by the detergent.

The supernatant of the placental tissue after centrifugation resulted in two peaks with CysNA and in one peak with LeuNA as substrate (Fig. 1(D)). The first peak with both substrates was coincident with that of the solubilized enzyme peak of the particle fraction. This was called cystine aminopeptidase I and arylamidase I, respectively. CysNA gave, in addition, a separate smaller peak (cystine amino-peptidase II) in later fractions devoid of any arylamidase activity.

SERUM SAMPLES

Total cystine aminopeptidase (CysNA) and arylamidase (LeuNA) activities were significantly higher in maternal serum than in control serum ($p < 0.001$)

Table I. Hydrolysis of various amino acid naphthylamides by control and maternal sera.

Substrate	Control serum (C)	Maternal serum (M)	M:C
CysNA	0.02 ± 0.001 (7)	0.25 ± 0.01 (8)	12.5
LeuNA	0.46 ± 0.06 (7)	3.82 ± 0.25 (8)	8.3
AlaNA	1.44 ± 0.17 (3)	2.40 ± 0.23 (3)	1.6
ArgNA	0.39 ± 0.03 (3)	1.68 ± 0.11 (4)	4.3
GlyNA	0.07 ± 0.003 (3)	0.16 ± 0.01 (4)	2.3
HisNA	0.04 ± 0.002 (3)	0.14 ± 0.01 (4)	3.5
IleNA	0.03 ± 0.003 (3)	0.11 ± 0.01 (4)	3.7
LysNA	0.20 ± 0.02 (3)	1.60 ± 0.11 (3)	8.0
MetNA	0.93 ± 0.02 (3)	3.05 ± 0.13 (3)	3.3
ThrNA	0.03 ± 0.0 (3)	0.17 ± 0.1 (4)	5.7

Values are mean ± S.E.M. for the number of experiments indicated in parentheses, and are given as micromoles of β-naphthylamine liberated per minute per milligram of protein.

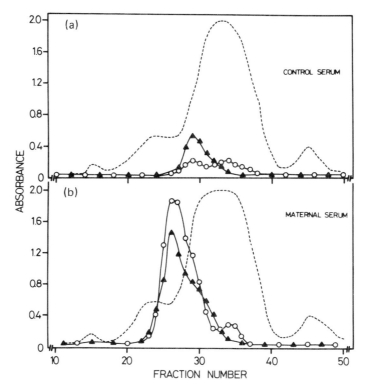

Fig. 2. Elution patterns of enzymes hydrolysing CysNA (○) and LeuNA (▲) after Sepharose 6B gel filtration of (a) control serum and (b) maternal serum of women. The protein content of the 10 ml fractions is given as the absorbance at 280 nm (- - -).

(Table I). In both sera CysNA was hydrolysed more slowly than LeuNA. However, during pregnancy CysNAhydrolysis increased about 12.5-fold and LeuNAhydrolysis about 8.3 times compared to the activities in the control sera. Using other amino acids naphthylamidases as substrates the increase of hydrolysis was even smaller than with LeuNA (Table I).

Elution of the control serum on Sepharose 6B (Fig. 2(a)) resulted in one peak with LeuNA as substrate arylamidase I_c), while CysNA gave additionally a second peak in later fractions (cystine aminopeptidase II). Fractionation of the maternal serum (Fig. 2(b)) showed a new enzyme activity. It eluted before arylamidase I_c and was able to hydrolyse both CysNA (cystine aminopeptidase I_m) and LeuNA (arylamidase I_m). This peak partially overlapped arylamidase I_c. A separate cystine aminopeptidase II in later fractions hydrolysed only CysNA.

pH OPTIMA AND MOLECULAR WEIGHTS

Pooled preparations of enzymes were obtained from gel filtration of placental homogenate (cystine aminopeptidase I and II, arylamidase I) as well as of control serum (arylamidase I_c) and maternal serum (cystine aminopeptidase I_m and II,

Table II. The pH optima and molecular weights of the human placental and serum aminopeptidases.

	Placental enzymes		
	Cystine aminopeptidase I	Aryl amidase I	Cystine aminopeptidase II
pH	6.5	7.5	6.0
Molecular weight (daltons)	309 000	309 000	76 000

	Serum enzymes			
	Cystine aminopeptidase I_m	Aryl amidase I_m	Cystine aminopeptidase II	Aryl amidase I_c
pH	6.5	7.5	6.0	7.0 with LeuNA 5.25–5.5 with CysNA
Molecular weight (daltons)	309 000	309 000	76 000	130 000

arylamidase I_m). Table II summarizes the pH optima and molecular weights of these activities. The placental enzyme(s) I, cystine aminopeptidase I_m and arylamidase I_m had pH optima at 6.5 with CysNA and pH 7.5 with LeuNA. These enzymes had a molecular weight of 309 000 daltons. Arylamidase I_c hydrolysed LeuNA optimally at pH 7.0 and CysNA at pH 5.25–5.5. Its molecular weight was 130 000 daltons. Cystine aminopeptidase II obtained from the maternal and control sera as well as from the placenta hydrolysed CysNA optimally pH 6.0 and had a molecular weight of 76 000 daltons.

MODIFIERS

Both maternal (Fig. 3a) and control serum enzymes I (I_m and I_c) were highly sensitive even to as low a concentration of ethylenediaminotetraacetic acid (EDTA) as 0.001 mM. The placental enzyme(s) I had a similar response to EDTA. On the other hand, neither placental nor serum cystine aminopeptidase II (Fig. 3) was inhibited. Other chelating agents (2,2'-dipyridyl, Fig. 3b; ethylene glycol tetraacetic acid, 1,10-phenanthroline) had no similar differential inhibition on these enzymes.

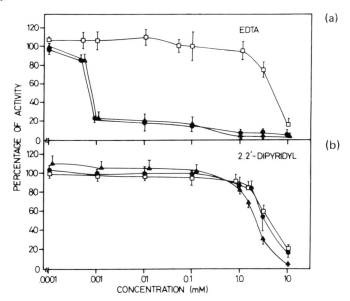

Fig. 3. Effect of various EDTA and 2,2'-dipyridyl concentrations on the hydrolysis of CysNA and LeuNA by the maternal serum enzyme preparations, cystine aminopeptidase I_m (○); cystine aminopeptidase II (●) and arylamidase I_m (▲). The results of five duplicate experiments are given as percentages (± S.E.M.) of the appropriate duplicate controls (100%).

After EDTA pretreatment (Fig. 4) Co^{2+} and Zn^{2+} re-activated cystine aminopeptidase I_m, arylamidase I_m, and arylamidase I_c. At the highest concentrations Zn^{2+} was inhibitory. Cystine aminopeptidase I_m, arylamidase I_m (Fig. 4) and arylamidase I_c were also re-activated by Ni^{2+}, but only when CysNA was used as substrate. Mn^{2+} caused only a partial (40%) re-activation.

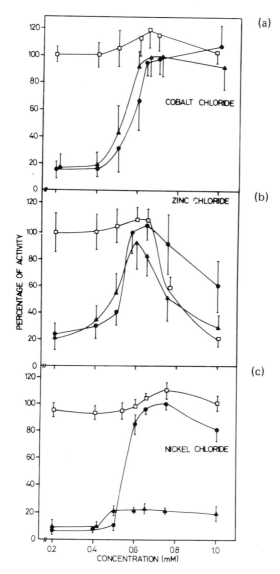

Fig. 4. Effect of various concentrations of (a) Co^{2+}, (b) Zn^{2+} and (c) Ni^{2+} after a 90 min pretreatment with 0.75 mM EDTA on the hydrolysis of CysNA and LeuNA by the maternal serum enzyme preparations, cystine aminopeptidase I_m (●), cystine aminopeptidase II (□) and arylamidase I_m (▲). The results of five or six duplicate experiments are given as percentages (± S.E.M.) of the appropriate duplicate controls (100%).

Cystine aminopeptidase II did not respond to Co^{2+}, Mn^{2+} and Ni^{2+} after EDTA treatment, but Zn^{2+} caused a marked inhibition at the high (above 0.6 mM) concentrations. When the effect of the metal ions was tested alone it was found that Ni^{2+} inhibited the maternal and control serum enzymes I (I_m and I_c) more effectively than cystine aminopeptidase II ($p < 0.01$ at 0.2 mM, $p < 0.001$ above 0.6 mM Ni^{2+}). Zn^{2+} was clearly inhibitory to all of the enzymes already at 0.2 mM.

The enzymes also had differences in their response to L-methionine. Serum (Fig. 5(a)) and placental cystine aminopeptidase II was not inhibited, but the placental and serum enzymes I showed a gradual inhibition with increasing levels

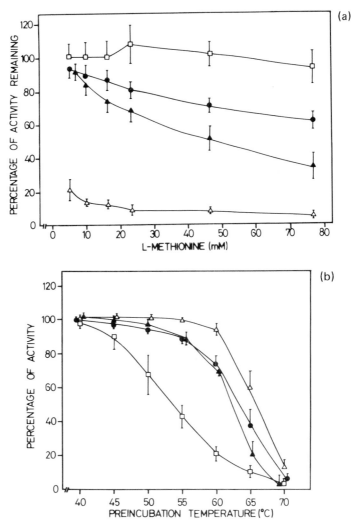

Fig. 5. Effect of (a) various L-methionine concentrations and (b) temperature on the hydrolysis of CysNA and LeuNA by the pooled serum enzyme preparations, cystine aminopeptidase I_m (●); cystine aminopeptidase II (□); arylamidase I_m (▲); arylamidase I_c with LeuNA and CysNA as substrate (△). The results are given as percentages (± S.E.M.) of the appropriate duplicate controls (100%) for five duplicate experiments in (a) and of the uninhibited duplicate control values for four duplicate experiments in (b).

of L-methionine. On the other hand, arylamidase I_c was highly sensitive even at the lowest (5 mM) concentration tested.

Arylamidase I_c was the most resistant and serum cystine aminopeptidase II the most sensitive to thermal treatment (Fig. 5(b)). The placental enzymes I and II behaved in a similar way as the maternal enzymes I and II, respectively.

DISCUSSION

Our results showed that the human placenta contains both particle-bound and soluble enzymes hydrolysing the synthetic substrate, CysNA, used for estimation of oxytocinase. The particle-bound enzyme(s) could easily be solubilized by detergent. Previously Oya *et al.* (1976) have suggested that one cystine amino-peptidase activity in placenta is a lysosomal enzyme. Since the new enzyme(s) appearing in the serum during pregnancy (cystine aminopeptidase I_m, arylamidase I_m) were similar to the enzyme which could be extracted from placentae, it is apparent that secretory granules may also be involved.

The soluble placental cystine aminopeptidase II had the same biochemical characteristics as the maternal in both normal and maternal serum. It had the lowest molecular weight (76 000 daltons) and hydrolysed only CysNA. No similar activity has previously been reported. It does not seem, however, to be involved in the placental secretory activity, since the relative size of the enzyme peak in the fractionation of normal and maternal serum did not change.

The secretory placental enzyme had the highest molecular weights (309 000 daltons). Previously, the molecular weights of human cystine aminopeptidases from placenta (Mäkinen and Raekallio, 1974) and retroplacental serum (Yman and Sjöholm, 1967) were found to be 320 000 and 325 000 daltons by gel filtration on Sephadex G-200, respectively. More recently, slightly higher values (340 000 daltons) for serum and placental activities have been reported by Hiwada *et al.* (1978) using Sepharose 4B. It is possible that this enzyme is a glycoprotein (Yman, 1970a), like some other secretory products (e.g. hCG, hCT) of the placenta.

The release of the secretory placental enzyme into the maternal blood caused a marked increase in the hydrolysis rates of all substrates tested. The relative increase, however, was variable, which suggests a difference in the substrate specificity of the enzyme(s) in the control serum and the new activity(ies) appearing during pregnancy. From the small selection of substrates utilized it can be concluded that AlaNA is preferred by enzyme(s) in normal serum, whereas CysNA and LeuNA are more readily split by the placental secretory activity(ies).

The sensitivity to EDTA of the particle-bound secretory placental enzyme(s) and the arylamidase of the normal serum indicated that they are dependent on metal ions. The re-activation of these enzymes after EDTA pretreatment by Co^{2+}, Ni^{2+} and Zn^{2+}, and partially by Mn^{2+}, confirmed this hypothesis. In contrast, cystine aminopeptidase II did not respond to EDTA and does not seem to have any metal ion in the active centre. Previously, Werle and Semm (1956) have shown that the tissue oxytocinase activity of human erythrocytes, as well as of pancreas and ovaries from swine, is not inhibited by EDTA, whereas oxytocinase in pregnant serum is suppressed by this agent.

The differences of the placental and serum enzymes in pH, substrate specificity, response to EDTA, metal ions, L-methionine, thermal treatment, etc., can be utilized as criteria to establish methods for their differential quantitation. On the basis of the present findings it appears probable that a highly specific enzymatic assay for the secretory placental cystine aminopeptidase is possible. However, a more sensitive method would be radioimmunoassay with a highly purified enzyme preparation as tracer and used as antigen for antibody production.

REFERENCES

Gazarek, F., Pohanka, J., Talas, M., Fingerova, H., Janouskova, M., Krikal, Z. and Hamal, Z. (1976). *Endocrinologia experimentalis* **10**, 283.

Hiwada, K., Saeki-Yamaguchi, C., Inaoka, Y. and Kokubu, T. (1978). *Biochemical Medicine* **20**, 296.

James, N. T. (1966). *Nature, London* **210**, 1276.

Lampelo, S. and Vanha-Perttula, T. (1979). *Journal of Reproduction and Fertility* **56**, 285.

Mäkinen, P. -L. and Raekallio, J. (1974). *Biochemical Medicine* **11**, 210.

Oya, M., Wakabayashi, T., Yoshino, M. and Mizutani, S. (1976). *Physiological Chemistry and Physics* **8**, 327.

Patterson, E. K., Hsiao, S. -H. and Keppel, A. (1963). *Journal of Biological Chemistry* **238**, 3611.

Ryden, G. (1966). *Acta obstetricia et gynecologica scandinavica* **45**, Suppl. 3, 1.

Ryden, G. (1972). *Acta obstetricia et gynecologica scandinavica* **51**, 329.

Tuppy, H. and Nesvadba, H. (1957). *Monatshefte für Chemie,* **88**, 977.

Warwas, M., Dobryszycka, W. and Sward, J. (1972). *Enzyme* **14**, 340.

Werle, E. and Semm, K. (1956). *Archiv für Gynäkologie,* **187**, 449.

Yman, L. (1970a). *Acta pharmaceutica suecica* **7**, 29.

Yman, L. (1970b). *Acta pharmaceutica suecica* **7**, 75.

Yman, L. and Sjöholm, I., (1967). *Acta pharmaceutica suecica* **4**, 13.

BINDING OF ANDROGENS AND PROGESTERONE TO EXTRACTS OF HUMAN PLACENTAL NUCLEI

K. Musch, A. S. Wolf and Ch. Lauritzen

Department of Gynaecology and Obstetrics, University of Ulm, D-7900 Ulm/Donau, German Federal Republic

INTRODUCTION

The steroid hormone dehydroepiandrosterone (DHA) has an important role in the fetoplacental unit. This steroid is termed an oestrogen precursor. since it is metabolized by the placental aromatase system to oestrogens. It is synthesized in the fetal adrenals—the zona reticularis—at the very high rate of 75 mg/day at the end of pregnancy. This corresponds well to the upper levels of oestrogen excretion, with a maximum rate of 70 mg/day. DHA is used for functional tests of the fetoplacental unit; after injection of this steroid into pregnant women the placental function is evaluated by determination of the increase of oestrogens in the peripheral blood of the mother.

From these findings, the question arose whether DHA is acting at a molecular level. This concept stimulated investigation of steroid binding by cytoplasmatic and nuclear compounds.

MATERIALS AND METHODS

Preparation of Human Placental Nuclei

Human term placentae were used immediately after normal or surgical delivery. Small pieces of placental tissue were washed several times in ice-cold saline and then homogenized with a Polytron homogenizer, either in a hypotonic medium (1 mM

Serono Symposium No. 35, "The Human Placenta", edited by A. Klopper, A. Genazzani and P. G. Crosignani, 1980. Academic Press, London and New York.

$NaHCO_3$, 0.5 mM $CaCl_2$, pH 7.4), or buffered 0.25 M sucrose. After filtration through four layers of cheesecloth, a crude nuclear fraction was obtained by centrifugation of the filtered homogenate for 15 min at 1500g. The sediments were then used for the preparation of placental nuclei either by the method of Hogeboom and Schneider (1952) or by the two-phase polymer method by Brunette *et al.* (1968). The nuclei were suspended in 0.05 M Tris buffer, pH 7.4 and stored frozen.

Demonstration of Steroid Binding to
Extracts of Human Placental Nuclei

Placental nuclear suspensions were incubated with 50 000 c.p.m. of ^{3}H-labelled steroids for 60 min at 0 °C in a glass–Teflon homogenizer with agitation every 5 min. The nuclei were then extracted with solutions of increasing ionic strength: 0.4 M KCl, 1 M NaCl, 3 M NaCl or 1 N HCl, and 2 N NaOH. The extracts were centrifuged at 10 000g for 10 min and the macromolecular content of the supernatants separated by gel filtration on Sephadex G-75 using a Tris–HCl buffer, pH 7.4. Fractions of 2 ml (80 drops) were collected and investigated for radioactivity.

The question of possible multiple forms of steroid binding macromolecules was investigated by gel chromatography with Sephadex G-150.

The activity of the nuclear marker enzyme, ATP: NMN-adenylylphosphotransferase (EC 2.7.7.1), was determined according to the method of Kornberg (1955). DNA (Schneider, 1957) and RNA (Lusena, 1957) were assayed by colorimetric methods.

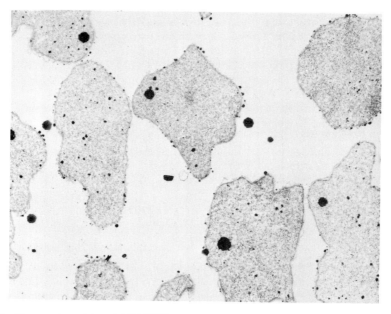

Fig. 1. Human placental nuclei (× 6200).

RESULTS

Quality of Isolated Placental Nuclei

The nuclei obtained from placental tissue indicated very little cytoplasmatic contamination (Fig. 1), as shown by electron microscopy.

Other criteria for the purity of isolated nuclei were concerned with the ATP:NMN-adenylyphosphotransferase, (NAD-pyrophosphorylase, EC 2.7.7.1) and the determination of the RNA:DNA ratio. These results are shown in Table I. The

Table I. Specific activity (in micromoles of NAD per milligram of protein per hour) of the nuclear marker enzyme ATP:NMN-adenylyltransferase (NAD-pyrophosphorylase, EC 2.7.7.1) in human placental homogenate ($n = 4$) and purified nuclei ($n = 4$) and RNA:DNA ratio of the purified nuclei.

	Homogenate	Nuclei
Specific activity	0.18 ± 0.02	1.66 ± 0.34
Purification		$9.2 \times$
RNA:DNA ratio		0.22 ± 0.07

activity of the marker enzyme in the purified nuclei is increased about 10-fold when compared to the homogenate. This is comparable to data published by others. Corresponding to this, we found a sufficiently low RNA:DNA ratio of 0.22 ± 0.07, which is also in the range of published data.

Demonstration of ^{3}H-Labelled Steroid Bound to Macromolecules

As shown in Fig. 2 (top), it is possible to extract a binding molecule for ^{3}H-labelled dehydroepiandrosterone (DHA) from placental nuclei, using gel chromatography for separation of bound and free steroids. This binding activity is found only in the 0.4 M KCl extract. Extracts with higher ionic strength do not contain ^{3}H-labelled DHA associated to macromolecules. This complex obviously undergoes denaturation by storage (Fig. 2 (middle)). When different androgenic steroids are investigated for formation of the complex in the extract, it is found that only DHA and Δ_4-androstene-3, 17-dione are bound, and not testosterone (T) or DHA sulphate (DHA-S) (Fig. 2 (bottom)).

From the asymmetric distribution of radioactivity in the fractions collected by gel chromatography on Sephadex G-150, one may conclude that several DHA-binding forms exist (Fig. 3).

Placental nuclei obviously contain an additional binding compound for progesterone. Since this macromolecule is extractable only by 1 N HCl, it may consist of basic proteins, e.g. histones (Fig. 4).

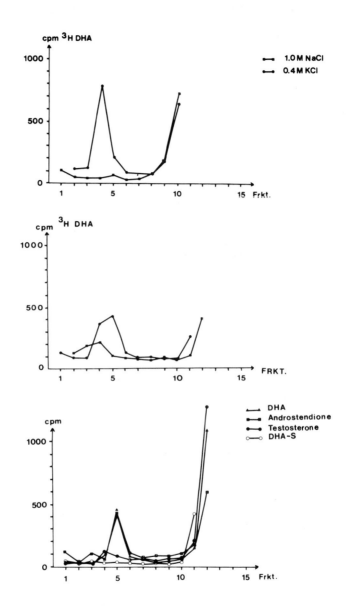

Fig. 2. (*Top*) Extraction of placental nuclei with 0.4 M KCl and 1 M NaCl after incubation of nuclei with ³H-labelled DHA and separation of free and bound steroids by gel chromatography (on Sephadex G-75) (□). (*Middle*) Denaturation of the DHA-binding macromolecule by storage of the complex for 48 h (■—■) compared to the control experiment without storage (●—●). (*Bottom*) Incubation of different steroids with placental nuclei, extraction of nuclei by 0.4 M KCl and separation by gel chromatography.

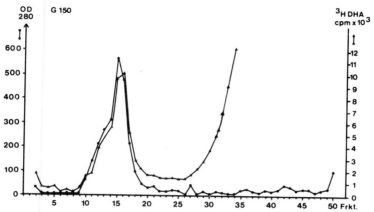

Fig. 3. Separation of the ³H-DHA-labelled nuclear extract by gel chromatography on Sephadex G-150 (1.5 cm × 90 cm, 0.05 M Tris–HCl, pH 7.4).

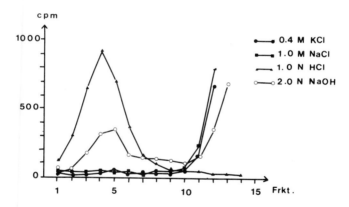

Fig. 4. Incubation of placental nuclei with ³H-labelled progesterone and extraction of the nuclei by solutions of different ionic strength, HCl and NaOH. Separation of free and bound steroid by gel chromatography (Sephadex G-75).

DISCUSSION

Although human placenta is a readily available tissue, no investigations have been published to our knowledge with regard to steroid binding of cytoplasmatic or nuclear origin. Only experiments with rodents have been performed for the investigation of corticosterone receptors (Wong and Burton, 1973).

Human placental nuclei obviously contain a compound which binds DHA and A. There are several requirements for the binding of steroids to this nuclear compound. As shown by the binding of DHA and A, the 17-keto group is essential. In addition, the configuration of the A ring of the steroid is important, since DHA-S and oestrone are not bound. Furthermore, this binding specificity distinguishes plasma steroid-binding globulins from the nuclear macromolecule. Plasma proteins bind DHA and DHA-S; the nuclear compound binds only the DHA.

Probably several forms of this binder exist, as may be concluded from gel chromatography on Sephadex G-150. The investigation of this question, however, requires a different methodological approach.

In addition to the androgen-binding compound, the placental nuclei contains a macromolecule which binds progesterone. Since it is extractable only by use of 1 N HCl, this compound might be a basic protein, or associated with these kinds of proteins (e.g. histones).

From these results, it is concluded that there must be another role for DHA in the fetoplacental unit other than being a precursor for oestrogen biosynthesis. With regard to the placental progesterone receptor, similar mechanisms for hormone action may exist, as have been shown for the chick oviduct progesterone receptor.

REFERENCES

Brunette, D. M., McCulloch, E. A. and Till, J. E. (1968). *Cell and Tissue Kinetics* **1**, 319–329.

Hogeboom, G. H. and Schneider, W. T. (1952). *Journal of Biological Chemistry* **197**, 611–620.

Kornberg, A. (1955). *Methods in Enzymology* **2**, 670–672.

Lusena, C. V. (1957). *In* "Medizinische Chemie" (K. Hinsberg and K. Lang, eds), p.718, Urban and Schwarzenberg, München.

Schneider, W. C. (1957). *Methods in Enzymology* **3**, 680–684.

Wong, M. D. and Burton, A. F. (1973). *Biochemical and Biophysical Research Communications* **50**, 71–79.

ANDROGEN-BINDING MACROMOLECULE IN
HUMAN PLACENTA

G. Barile[1], S. Giani, P. Scirpa, D. Mango, P. Fiorillo[1], A. Montemurro
and A. Bompiani

*Istituto di Ostetricia e Ginecologia, Università Cattolica del Sacro Cuore,
Largo A. Gemelli 8, Rome, Italy, and
[1]Laboratorio Tecnologie Biomediche, Consiglio Nazionale dell Ricerche,
Via G. B. Morgagni 30/E, Rome, Italy*

INTRODUCTION

It is well established that the human placenta utilizes mainly C_{19} steroidal compounds of fetal origin for the synthesis of oestrogens (Diczfalusy and Mancuso, 1969). Although the main metabolic pathways are well known (Makin, 1975; Ferreiros *et al.*, 1975), the biological significance and the mechanism of action of the steroids produced by the fetoplacental unit are not yet clear.

Protein receptors for glucocorticoids and oestrogens have been found in the placenta of the rat and the mouse (McCormack and Glasser, 1976; Wong and Burton, 1974). Recently, in human placental cytosol, a specific macromolecule binding testosterone was found. It had some physicochemical characteristics of steroid receptors (Barile *et al.*, 1978, 1979).

In this work we report further studies on the specific macromolecule binding labelled testosterone in human placental cytosol and on the analysis of the nuclear uptake after *in vitro* incubation at 37 °C of placental tissue with labelled steroids.

Serono Symposium No. 35, "The Human Placenta", edited by A. Klopper,
A. Genazzani and P. G. Crosignani, 1980. Academic Press, London and New York.

MATERIALS AND METHODS

Chemicals

[1, 2, 6, 7-^{3}h] Testosterone (specific activity 88.5 Ci/mmol), [2, 4, 6, 7-^{3}H] oestradiol (specific activity 104 Ci/mmol) and [1, 2, 6, 7-^{3}H] androstenedione (specific activity 99 Ci/mmol) were purchased from Radiochemical Centre (Amersham, U.K.); [7-^{3}H] dehydroepiandrosterone (specific activity 20 Ci/ mmol) was purchased from NEN (Frankfurt, German Federal Republic). Radio-ligands were purified before use by thin layer chromatography (TLC). Unlabelled steroids were purchased from Sigma (St. Louis, U.S.A.) and from Makor Chemicals Ltd (Jerusalem, Israel). Lumagel was purchased from Lumac System (Basel, Switzerland). General reagents and sheets of aluminium oxide F_{254} neutral were purchased from Merck (Darmstadt, German Federal Republic).

General Procedure

Full term placentas obtained from normal vaginal deliveries were used. Tissue and cytosol preparations, competitor studies and sucrose gradient analysis were performed as previously described (Barile *et al.*, 1979).

Column Chromatography on Sephadex G-100

For the gel filtration experiments a column (1.5 cm × 140 cm) of Sephadex G-100 Superfine was equilibrated in 10 mM Tris, 1.5 mM ethylenediaminotetracetic acid (EDTA), 0.15 M NaCl, 1 mM mercaptoethanol, 10% glycerol, 0.02% NaN$_3$ with or without 5 mM MgCl$_2$. The column was calibrated with Dextran blue 2000, bovine serum albumin ovalbumin and ^{3}H-labelled testosterone. The samples were applied in a final volume of 2 ml. The column was eluted at a flow rate of 2 ml/h and 3.5 ml fractions were collected.

Incubation of Tissue and Preparation of Purified Nuclei

Fragments of human placenta were incubated at 37 °C for 1 h with 4.3 × 10^{-8} M ^{3}H-labelled testosterone or 3.9 × 10^{-8} M ^{3}H-labelled oestradiol or 4.0 × 10^{-8} M ^{3}H-labelled androstenedione or 4.2 × 10^{-8} M ^{3}H-labelled dehydroepiandrosterone. The incubation medium was doubly distilled water containing 5 mM MgCl$_2$, pH 7.4. Some incubations were carried out with ^{3}H-labelled testosterone in the presence or absence of 5 × 10^{-7} or 5 × 10^{-6} M cold testosterone. At the end of incubation the fragments were washed with cold 10 mM Tris containing 1.5 mM EDTA, 1 mM mercaptoethanol, 5 mM MgCl$_2$, 10% glycerol, pH 7.4 (buffer A) and then homo-genized in the same buffer (1 : 4 w/v) with an Ultra-Turrax at 4 °C. The 800 g pellet was washed three times and each was followed by centrifugation at 800g for 10 min at 4 °C. The resuspended pellet was filtered through a double layer of gauze and recentrifuged. The crude nuclei were resuspended in 2 ml of buffer A and centrifuged at 45 000g for 60 min at 2 °C through 7 ml of buffer A containing 2.25 M sucrose. The purified nuclei were resuspended in 5 ml and the pellet extracted for 30 min with 1 ml 10 mM Tris containing 1.5 mM EDTA, 0.5 M KCl, pH 7.4. One extraction with 1 ml of absolute ethanol followed for 30 min. In some experiments the purified nuclei were directly extracted with absolute ethanol.

Thin Layer Chromatography

TLC was performed by drying the nuclear or cytoplasmatic extract with ethanol or diethyl ether respectively, on an aluminium sheet. The run was carried out at room temperature in the systems benzene–ethanol (95:5) and benzene–diethylether (4:5). Testosterone, oestrone, oestradiol, dehydroepiandrosterone, 5α-dihydrotestosterone and androstenedione were used as standards. At the end of the run the area on the sheet, where the sample was dried, was cut into 30 cm × 0.5 cm sections and each one placed in vials containing 10 ml of Lumagel, while the standards area was stained with iodine bisublimate and then treated with H_2SO_4 plus $K_2Cr_2O_7$ to bring out all the standards.

Protein and DNA Assay

Protein was determined using the method of Lowry *et al.* (1951), with bovine serum albumin as standard. The DNA content of placental nuclei was determined using the diphenylamine method of Burton (1956).

Measurement of Radioactivity

The radioactivity was counted in a Nuclear Chicago Mark II liquid scintillation spectrometer with 45% counting efficiency for tritium.

RESULTS

Cytoplasmatic Binding

Cytosol from human placenta contains a specific macromolecule binding testosterone. Figure 1 shows the ^{3}H-labelled testosterone binding at 4 °C and 30 °C. At these two temperatures, in a cell-free system, no conversion of labelled testosterone occurs. Indeed the radioactivity bound to the cytoplasmatic macromolecule, extracted with diethyl ether and analysed on TLC, gives a radioactivity peak which can be ascribed to testosterone (Fig. 2). Specific binding shows saturation at a ^{3}H-labelled testosterone concentration of 2×10^{-8}–3×10^{-8} M. The apparent dissociation constant has a wide range and the mean of six experiments yielded a K_d of 11×10^{-9} M ± 2.6 (S.D.) at 4 °C.

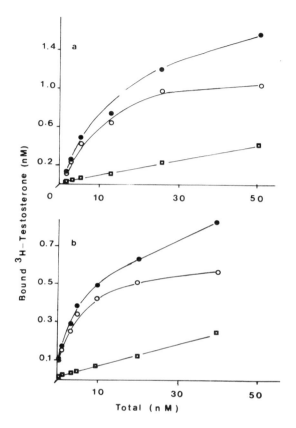

Fig. 1. Increasing amounts of labelled testosterone (5×10^{-10} –5×10^{-8} M) or (1×10^{-10} – 5×10^{-8} M) were added to cytosol in the presence or absence of cold testosterone (5×10^{-5} M). Total (●—●), specific (○—○), and unspecific (□—□) binding sites were measured. (a) Cytosol incubated at 4 °C for 3 h; (b) cytosol made up to 0.5 M KCl and then incubated at 4 °C for 3 h followed by an incubation at 30 °C for 1 h.

Column Chromatography on Sephadex G-100

At near physiological ionic strength, 0.15 M NaCl, the macromolecule binding labelled testosterone elutes from a Sephadex G-100 column as a peak after the void volume (Fig. 3). Aggregates before the elution of Dextran blue 2000 are also observed. Cytosol containing 5 mM $MgCl_2$, incubated with labelled testosterone and then eluted on the same column with buffer containing 5 mM $MgCl_2$, results in a more pronounced radioactivity peak in the same area.

Competitor Studies

The cytoplasmatic binding stereospecificity for labelled testosterone was studied at 4 °C using various cold steroids as cold competitors. Table I shows that

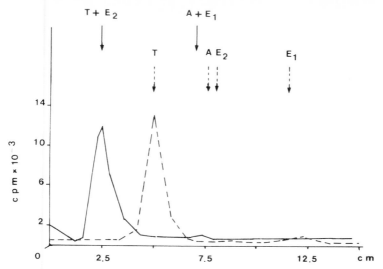

Fig. 2. Cytosol was incubated with 5×10^{-8} M ^{3}H-labelled testosterone at 4 °C for 3 h and then at 30 °C for 1 h. After cooling at 4 °C for 10 min the cytosol was treated with dextran-coated charcoal at 4 °C for 15 min and the radioactivity bound extracted with diethyl ether. TLC was performed in benzene–ethanol (95:5) (——) and in benzene/diethyl ether (4:5) (- - - - -). The arrows represent the run of the main standards used.

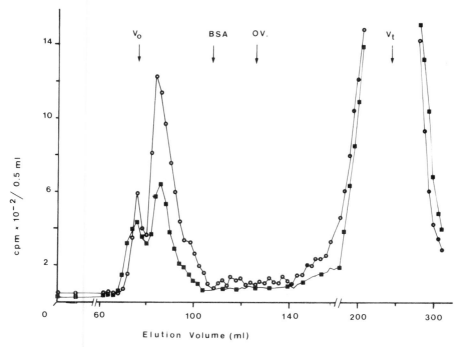

Fig. 3. Cytosol was incubated with 5×10^{-8} M ^{3}H-labelled testosterone at 4 °C for 6 h and then applied to a column of Sephadex G-100. Elution pattern of cytosol in absence of 5 mM $MgCl_2$ (■—■) and elution pattern of cytosol obtained from tissue homogenized in presence of 5 mM $MgCl_2$ (○—○). Dextran blue 2000, bovine serum albumin, ovalbumin and ^{3}H-labelled testosterone were used as external standards.

Table I. Percentage of labelled testosterone bound in the presence of cold steroids.[a]

Cold steroids	Competitor concentration		
	3×10^{-7} M	3×10^{-6} M	3×10^{-5} M
5-Dihydrotestosterone	28.0 ± 5.7	9.5 ± 2.6	5.6 ± 0.4
Testosterone	31.0 ± 4.3	10.0 ± 1.3	5.0 ± 0.4
Androstenedione	44.0 ± 8.3	17.5 ± 4.0	10.0 ± 3.8
Dehydroepiandrosterone	61.5 ± 9.6	35.0 ± 10.6	22.0 ± 7.3
Oestradiol	73.8 ± 4.6	41.0 ± 11.3	36.5 ± 12.7
Cyproterone	92.5 ± 0.5	84.0 ± 1.2	56.5 ± 4.3
17-Hydroxyprogesterone[b]	—	—	63.0
Progesterone	—	—	84.5
Pregnenolone	—	—	93.0
17-Hydroxypregnenolone	—	—	89.0
Oestriol	—	—	98.0
Cortisol	—	—	99.0
Androstenediol	50.0	48.5	46.0
Methyltestosterone	56.0	43.0	34.0

[a] The results are expressed as percentage of labelled testosterone bound in the presence of cold steroids, relative to the control (no steroid added). The binding capacity of control incubation (assigned as 100% of binding) was 25 610 ± 1603 c.p.m./mg protein (mean of four experiments ± S.D.).
[b] The binding capacity of control was 27 000 c.p.m./mg protein.

cold testosterone and 5α-dihydrotestosterone compete for ³H-labelled testosterone binding sites. Methyltestosterone, androstenediol and cyproterone acetate at high concentrations also compete, but less intensely. The inhibitory capacity of dehydro-epiandrosterone, androstenedione and oestradiol varied in the different placentas. Very little or no effect was observed for progesterone, 17-hydroxyprogesterone, pregnenolone, 17-hydroxypregnenolone, oestriol and cortisol.

Sucrose Gradient Analysis

The macromolecule binding labelled testosterone sediments with bovine serum albumin marker under low and high salt condition (Fig. 4). Labelled oestradiol binds the 4.6 s component to a slight extent, while cold cortisol does not decrease the ³H-labelled testosterone binding significantly (Fig. 4).

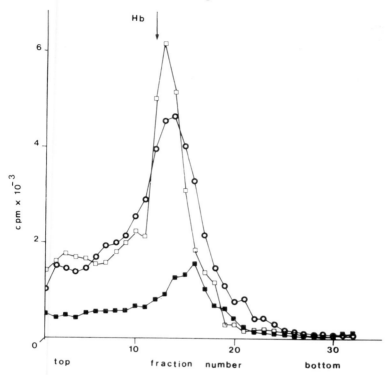

Fig. 4. Sucrose density gradient analysis was performed by layering 0.3 ml of cytosol, pre-incubated with labelled steroids and treated with dextran-coated charcoal, over 5–20% sucrose density gradient made in buffer A containing 0.5 M KCl. Cytosol incubated with 3×10^{-8} M ^{3}H-labelled testosterone alone (□—□), in the presence of 5×10^{-8} M cold cortisol (○—○), and with 3×10^{-8} M ^{3}H-labelled oestradiol (■—■). The gradient was centrifuged at 48 000 r.p.m. in a SW50 rotor (Beckman centrifuge L5 65) at 2°C for 16–17 h. Haemoglobin (Hb) was used as external standard. Fractions of five drops were collected from the top of the tube.

Nuclear Uptake

Fragments of whole tissue were incubated with labelled testosterone at 37 °C in the presence or absence of 10- or 100-fold excess of cold testosterone. Figure 5 shows the pattern of nuclear radioactivity extracted with 0.5 M KCl and then with absolute ethanol. The nuclear radioactivity extracted with ethanol and analysed by TLC gives a radioactivity peak which does not correspond to testosterone marker. The labelled metabolite migrates as oestrone marker (Fig. 5, inset). In Table II, the R_f values of standards used both in the benzene–ethanol (95:5) system and the benzene-diethyl ether (4:5) system are reported. On the other hand after incubation at 4 °C, under the same experimental conditions, no radioactivity is detectable from purified nuclei. When labelled oestradiol or androstenedione or dehydroepiandrosterone or testosterone were incubated at 37 °C with tissue fragments, a nuclear radioactivity was extracted with ethanol, as reported in Fig. 6.

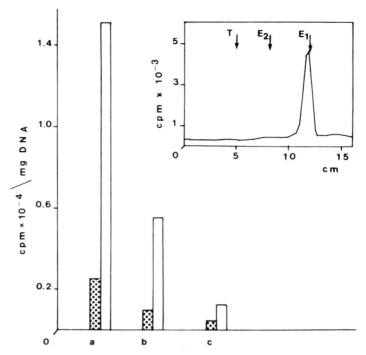

Fig. 5. Pattern of radioactivity extracted from purified nuclei with 0.5 M KCL ▨▨ and that with ethanol □. (a) Nuclear radioactivity from tissue incubated with 5×10^{-8} M ^{3}H-labelled testosterone alone or (b) in the presence of 5×10^{-7} M cold testosterone or (c) in the presence of 5×10^{-6} M cold testosterone. In the inset the pattern of nuclear radioactivity from experiment (a) is shown after TLC on benzene–diethyl ether (4:5). The arrows represent the run of the main standard used.

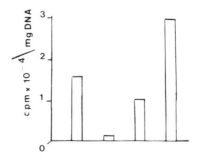

Fig. 6. Pattern of radioactivity extracted from purified nuclei with ethanol. From left to right, nuclear radioactivity extracted from tissue incubated at 37 °C with ^{3}H-labelled oestradiol, ^{3}H-labelled androstenedione, and ^{3}H-labelled testosterone.

Table II. R_f value of steroid standards and of the labelled metabolite extract from purified nuclei. TLC was performed in the benzene–ethanol (95:5) (A) and benzene–diethyl ether (4:5) (B) systems.

	A	B
Testosterone	0.16	0.33
Oestradiol	0.18	0.53
Dehydroepiandrosterone	0.20	0.42
5α-Dihydrotestosterone	0.20	0.45
Androstenedione	0.44	0.50
Oestrone	0.44	0.78
Labelled metabolite[a]	0.42	0.77

[a]The labelled metabolite was extracted from purified nuclei after tissue incubation at 37 °C for 1 h with labelled testosterone.

DISCUSSION

The results presented clearly demonstrate the presence of a macromolecule binding testosterone in human placental cytosol. The binding occurs at 4 °C. At 30 °C it begins to dissociate and this can be avoided by making up the cytosol to 0.5 M KCl. Both at 4 °C and at 30 °C, in a cell-free system, no conversion of labelled testosterone occurs. On Sephadex G-100 the macromolecule is eluted after the void volume, showing a molecular weight not far from 100 000 daltons. A more accurate measurement of molecular weight is under investigation.

As reported elsewhere (Barile *et al.*, 1979) the ^{3}H-labelled testosterone cytoplasmatic binding is stable during the incubation time. However, it is destroyed by heat at 45 °C.

In competition studies, cold testosterone, 5α-dihydrotestosterone, androstenedione and dehydroepiandrosterone are the most active competitiors, despite their structural differences. Cyproterone acetate, dehydroepiandrosterone and androstenedione compete to some degree for the ^{3}H-labelled testosterone binding, and this indicates that the macromolecule studied is not SHBG.

The macromolecule sediments on sucrose gradient analysis at 4.6 s under low and high salt conditions, and this is in agreement with the results of McCormack and Glasser (1976), who found a sedimentation value (4 s) for oestrogen-binding protein in rat placental trophoblast.

After *in vitro* incubation at 37 °C with labelled testosterone we find a nuclear radioactivity extractable with ethanol which can be ascribed to oestrone. At 4 °C no nuclear radioactivity is detectable due to the lack of metabolization of labelled testosterone. Indeed it is well known that androgens are metabolized at 37 °C into oestrogens by *in vitro* incubation of placental tissue (Makin, 1975). On the other hand, labelled steroids such as androstenedione, dehydroepiandrosterone and oestradiol did not have a nuclear uptake like that found for labelled testosterone. Hence, in an *in vitro* system, without the presence of oestrogen cofactors, the highest amount of extractable nuclear radioactivity comes from the metabolization of labelled testosterone to oestrone.

Even though we do not know the role of the macromolecule binding testosterone in human placental cytosol, or its relation to the nuclear uptake, we think that androgens, and in particular testosterone, could have an endocrine function during or after the transformation into oestrogens in the human placenta.

REFERENCES

Barile, G., Montemurro, A., Scirpa, P. and Mango, D. (1978). *Journal of Steroid Biochemistry* **9**, 828.

Barile, G., Giani, S., Montemurro, A., Scirpa, P. and Mango, D. (1979). *Journal of Biochemistry* in press.

Burton, K. (1956). *Biochemical Journal* **62**, 315.

Diczfalusy, E. and Mancuso, S. (1969). *In* "Foetus and Placenta" (A. Klopper and E. Diczfalusy, eds), p. 191, Blackwell Scientific Publications, Oxford.

Ferreiros, H. P., Vega Ramos, P., Montemurro, A., Mango, D., Scirpa, P. and Menini, E. (1975). *Annali Ostetricia e Ginecologia Medicale Perinatale* **1**, 19.

Lowry, O. H., Rosebrough, W. J., Farr, A. L. and Randall, R. J. (1951). *Journal of Biological Chemistry* **193**, 265.

McCormack, S. A. and Glasser, S. R. (1976). *Endocrinology*, **99**, 701.

Makin, H. L. J. (1975). *In* "Biochemistry of Steroid Hormones" (H. L. J. Makin, ed.) p. 105, Blackwell Scientific Publications, Oxford.

Wong, M. D. and Burton, A. F. (1974). *Canadian Journal of Biochemistry* **52**, 190.

hPL RECEPTORS IN PLACENTAL MEMBRANES

O. Genbačev, B. Čemerikić and B. Marinković

Department of Physiology and Radiobiology, INEP, Zemun, Yugoslavia

INTRODUCTION

Possible target sites for hormone action may be identified by the detection of specific hormone binding. The type of specificity displayed may provide some clues to the physiological role these hormones play.

In order to search for possible target tissues of placental lactogen, various tissues obtained from pregnant animals and from fetuses have been examined for specific binding sites (Chan *et al.*, 1978; Sakai and Kohmoto, 1976; Sheth *et al.*, 1974).

The binding of human placental lactogen (hPL) to placental membrane preparations was tested by Haour and Bertrand 1974. They did not succeed in demonstrating the presence of hPL receptors in placentae at term. However, displacement of prolactin from placental and lung preparations by hPL was demonstrated by Josimovich 1977.

The purpose of this study was to investigate the binding of hPL to membranes of placentae of different gestational age and to examine the factors that regulate hPL receptors in placentae.

MATERIALS AND METHODS

Clinical Material

Fresh human placentae were obtained from legal abortions (8–10 week pregnancies) and in two cases from hysterotomies on patients with mental

Serono Symposium No. 35, "The Human Placenta", edited by A. Klopper,
A. Genazzani and P. G. Crosignani, 1980. Academic Press, London and New York.

O. Genbačev et al.

retardation who were 24–26 weeks pregnant. Full-term placentae were obtained from women with uncomplicated pregnancies who delivered spontaneously at the Clinic for Gynaecology and Obstetrics, Faculty of Medicine, Belgrade.

Methods

Isolation of Cell Membranes

Fresh human placental tissue was homogenized in 10 volumes of Tris–sucrose (10 mM Tris-HCl, pH 7.0, containing 250 mM sucrose, 1 mM $CaCl_2$, 1 mM dithriothreitol, 0.1% NaN_3 and 0.1% bovine serum albumin). After centrifugation for 10 min at 1000g, the supernatant fraction was again centrifuged for 45 min at 10 000g. The 10 000g pellet was resuspended in 10 volumes of Tris–sucrose for use in binding studies (Wright et al., 1979).

Isolation of Microsomal Pellet

Placental tissue was minced in ice-cold 0.3 M sucrose, homogenized in five volumes of sucrose solution and the homogenate filtered through two layers of cheesecloth. The filtrate was centrifuged at 1500g for 20 min at 4 °C. The supernatant was centrifuged at 15 000g for 20 min and the pellet was discarded. The supernatant was centrifuged at 100 000g for 90 min to obtain the total microsomal pellet. The microsomal pellet was resuspended in 0.025 Tris–HCl buffer, pH 7.6, containing 10 mM $CaCl_2$ (Shiu et al., 1974).

Binding Studies

The assay procedure which was employed was essentially the same as described by Shiu et al. (1974) for prolactin binding assay.

Non-specific binding was determined using 10 μg of hPL per assay tube.

Incubation of Placental Tissue Fragments

The incubation studies were performed as previously described (Genbačev et al., 1977).

RESULTS

Characteristics of hPL Binding to Placental Cell Membranes

Human placental lactogen binds specifically to cell membranes and to the 100 000g fractions of human placentae of different gestational age.

In placental membrane preparations specific binding of ^{125}I-labelled hPL ranged from 5 to 8% and binding to 100 000 g pellets from 7 to 11%. Non-specific binding was 1–3%. Using different concentrations of membrane preparations, expressed as milligrams of protein per tube, the difference in specific binding was achieved. Maximal binding was obtained at a protein concentration of 1 mg protein per tube (Fig. 1). The binding of ^{125}I-labelled hPL was inhibited

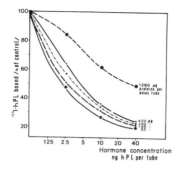

Fig. 1. Radioreceptor assay for hPL using different concentrations of placental membrane preparation. The amount of radioactivity bound in the absence of hPL was taken to be equal to 100%. The specific binding of ^{125}I-labelled hPL was 5–8%.

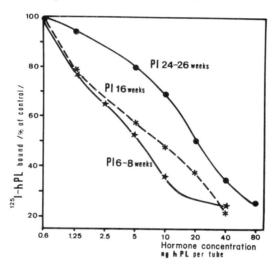

Fig. 2. Radioreceptor assay for hPL using membrane fractions from placentas of different gestational age. 1000 μg protein was used per assay tube and percentage of specific binding was 6% for 6–8 and 16 week placentae, and 8% for 24–26 week placentae.

by unlabelled hPL in a dose-dependent manner (Fig. 2). Competitive inhibition of hPL binding to placental membranes preparation was obtained by unlabelled prolactin (Fig. 3).

Scatchard analysis of the binding of hPL to 100 000g fraction of 6–8 week placentae and placentae at term revealed the presence of high affinity saturable binding sites (Fig. 4). The binding activity was determined as 0.85 ng/mg protein for 6–8 week placentae and 2.5 ng/mg protein for term placentae. The non-linear plot for the first trimester placentae indicates two binding sites, a high affinity, low capacity site, usually associated with specific receptors, and a low affinity, high capacity or non-specific site.

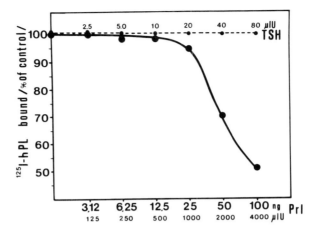

Fig. 3. The inhibition of ^{125}I-labelled hPL binding by prolactin. The amount of radioactivity bound in the absence of prolactin was taken to be equal to 100%. There was no
inhibition of the binding of ^{125}I-labelled hPL by luteinizing hormone (hLH), thyroid
stimulating hormone (hTSH), or hCG.

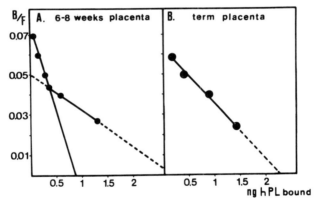

Fig. 4. Scatchard analysis of hPL binding to 105 000 g pellet of term and 6–8 week old
human placentae. The ordinate represents the ratio of bound: free hormone and the abscissa
the amount of hPL bound. The intercept on the x-axis is the total amount of hPL bound to
1 mg protein of 105 000 g pellet.

Control of hPL Binding Sites

The experiments were performed to examine the *in vitro* effect of prostaglandin
$F_{2\alpha}$ ($PGF_{2\alpha}$) and chorionic gonadotrophin (hCG) on hPL binding to human
placental membranes. The first task was to see if placental membranes retain their
ability to bind hPL under the *in vitro* conditions. Our results proved that short
incubations do not alter the specific binding of hPL. In order to study the possible
role of prostaglandin and hCG in the regulation of hPL receptors the incubation
of placental tissue fragments was carried out for 60 min in the presence of different concentrations of $PGF_{2\alpha}$ and hCG. After the end of incubation placental

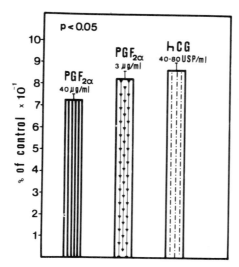

Fig. 5. PGF$_{2\alpha}$ and hCG *in vitro* effect on ^{125}I-labelled hPL binding to membrane fractions of 6–8 week palcentae. A significant decrease in specific binding was obtained with high doses of PGF$_{2\alpha}$

tissue was used for membrane preparation and testing of binding activity.

The results are summarized in Fig. 5. It can be seen that prostaglandin treatment *in vitro* depresses the hPL binding to the membrane fraction by about 25%. Lower doses of PGF$_{2\alpha}$ and hCG than those in Fig. 5 did not alter the hPL binding significantly.

DISCUSSION

Evidence of specific, high affinity and low capacity binding of hPL to membrane preparations and 100 000g pellets of human placentae of different gestational age has been presented. The binding of ^{125}I-labelled hPL is a saturable process that is dependent on time, pH, temperature and protein concentration in assay. The ^{125}I-labelled hPL was displaced by cold hPL in all placentae studied. Although the sites which bind hPL exhibit a high degree of specificity for this hormone, the competitive displacement studies demonstrate that these sites can also bind human prolactin. Relative activities of hPL and prolactin for competitive displacement of ^{125}I-labelled hPL indicate that these binding sites exhibit the greatest affinity for hPL.

Scatchard analysis of hPL binding to the placental membrane fraction and the microsomal pellet revealed two classes of binding sites in placentae from the first and second trimester; the high affinity, low capacity, specific binding sites, and low affinity, high capacity, non-specific sites. The physiological significance of this binding remains to be investigated.

The distribution of binding between membrane fraction and microsomal pellet indicates that about 60% of total hPL binding is present in the microsomal pellet.

No significant difference was obtained in specific binding of hPL to placental membranes of different gestational age expressed per milligram of protein. However, total organ binding by placenta increases with age of gestation in proportion to increase in weight.

The *in vitro* experiment with placental tissue fragments incubated in the presence of $PGF_{2\alpha}$ and hCG offers the possibility of using this approach in the study of regulation of hPL receptors. After 1 h of incubation, placental membranes retain the ability to bind ^{125}I-labelled hPL. The addition of high doses of $PGF_{2\alpha}$ to the incubation medium decreases the ^{125}I-labelled hPL binding to membrane preparation. This effect was obtained with the first and second trimester placentae and was not demonstrated in full-term placentae.

It was reported previously (Genbačev *et al.*, 1975) that *in vitro* $PGF_{2\alpha}$ treatment results in the inhibition of hPL synthesis by the tissue slices of mid-gestational placentae, and the hypothesis that this effect is initiated by the decrease of hPL binding to placental membranes seems very attractive but needs further confirmation.

ACKNOWLEDGEMENT

Special thanks are due to Dr V. Šulović, Medical School, University of Belgrade, for collaboration and supplying placentae which were used in the binding studies. We thank Mrs Kostić Gordana for preparing figures and Mrs Mirjana Momčilović for secretarial help.

Prostaglandin $PGF_{2\alpha}$ used in incubation experiments was a generous gift from Dr John E. Pike, The Upjohn Co.

This research was supported by the Republic Fund for Scientific Work of SR Serbia.

REFERENCES

Chan, J. S. D., Robertson, H. A. and Friesen, H. G. (1978). *Endocrinology* **102**, 632.

Genbačev, O., Kraincanić, M. and Šulović, V. (1975). In "Physical and Chemical Bases of Biological Information Transfer" (J. G. Vassileva-Popova, ed.), pp. 147–155, Plenum Press, New York.

Genbačev, O., Ratković, M., Kraincanić, M. and Šulović, V. (1977). *Prostaglandins* **13**, 723.

Haour, F. and Bertrand, J. (1974). *Journal of Clinical Endocrinology and Metabolism* **38**, 334.

Josimovich, J. B. (1977). In "Prolactin and Human Reproduction" (P. G. Crosignani and C. Robyn, eds), Serono Symposium No. 11, pp. 27–36, Academic Press, London and New York.

Sakai, S. and Kohmoto, K. (1976). *Endocrinologia Japonica* **23**, 499.

Sheth, N. A., Ranadive, K. J. and Sheth, A. R. (1974). *European Journal of Cancer* **10**, 653.

Shiu, R. P. C. and Friesen, H. G. (1974). *Biochemical Journal* **140**, 301.

Wright, K., Luborsky-Moore, J. L. and Behrman, H. R. (1979). *Molecular and Cellular Endocrinology* **3**, 25.

VARIOUS HUMAN CHORIONIC GONADOTROPHIN-LIKE ENTITIES IN BIOLOGICAL FLUIDS AND IN PITUITARY GLANDS OF NON-PREGNANT SUBJECTS*

A. Pala, G. Marinelli, R. Di Gregorio, M. Moro and L. Carenza

II Clinica Ostetrica e Ginecologica, Università di Roma, Rome, Italy

INTRODUCTION

The presence of immunoreactive chorionic gonadotrophin-like (hCG-like) materials in a pituitary extract and in plasma from a woman submitted to intravenous administration of luteinizing hormone releasing hormone (LHRH), and in fluid from an ovarian cyst is reported.

It is known that hCG is present in the blood and in the urine of normal pregnant women. The detection of measurable levels of the hormone in peripheral blood indicates the differentiation of the trophoblast from the remainder of the blastocyst.

Following the development of highly sensitive and specific methods for measuring the hormone, the possible use of hCG measurement has been proposed for the early diagnosis of non-trophoblastic cancers as well as for studying the clinical course of the disease in response to therapy (Braunstein *et al.*, 1973; Golde *et al.*, 1974, Rosen *et al.*, 1975; Samann *et al.*, 1976; Stone *et al.*, 1977; Rutanen and Seppälä, 1978).

As regards production of the hormone in non-malignant conditions, the presence of an antigenically active fraction similar to hCG has been recently

*Supported by C.N.R. project "Biology of reproduction".

Serono Symposium No. 35, "The Human Placenta", edited by A. Klopper, A. Genazzani and P. G. Crosignani, 1980. Academic Press, London and New York.

demonstrated in normal human testis (Braunstein *et al.*, 1975), pituitary gland (Chen *et al.*, 1976), liver and colon (Yoshimoto *et al.*, 1977) and in kidney, lung, ovary, pancreas and spleen (Braunstein *et al.*, 1978).

The purpose of this study was to investigate further the hCG-like materials present in extracts from the pituitary of normal subjects, as well as in ovarian cystic fluids from patients with benign ovarian tumours.

MATERIALS AND METHODS

Ovarian cystic fluid samples were obtained from 15 patients with benign tumours. Serum samples were collected from one normally ovulating woman at $-15, 0$, 15, 30, 60, 90 and 120 min after intravenous administration of a bolus of 200 μg of synthetic LHRH. The regular function of the hypothalamic–pituitary–ovarian axis was previously ascertained by determining the circulating hormone profile over the course of a month. The biological fluids were frozen until assayed for hCG. The serum sample and the ovarian cystic fluid with the highest hCG concentration were ultrafiltrated on Amicon Diaflo PM-30 membrane followed by gel chromatography carried out at 4 °C on a 2.6 cm × 85 cm Sephadex G-150 column.

A pool of 30 human pituitaries obtained at autopsy from non-pregnant subjects without apparent neoplasia was studied. The glands were minced and washed in acetone, homogenized in 0.05 M Tris–HCl buffer solution, pH 7.5, 0.1 M KCl, centrifuged at 25 000 g for 1 h at 4 °C and concentrated by ultrafiltration on a Diaflo PM-30 membrane before gel chromatography on a Sephadex G-100 Superfine column.

Gel Chromatography

Columns (2.6 cm × 100 cm) were packed with Sephadex G-100 Superfine or Sephadex G-150 equilibrated with 0.05 M Tris–HCl buffer, pH 7.5, containing 0.1 M KCl. After determination of the void volume (V_0) with dextran blue 2000, the elution volumes (V_e) of highly purified hCG, β-hCG, α-hCG and pituitary luteinizing hormone (LH), labelled with ^{125}I, were determined.

Radioimmunoassay

All radioimmunoassays (RIA) were performed using the double antibody technique described by Midgley (1966). Immunochemicals used for RIA were described previously (Pala *et al.*, 1979).

An antiserum raised against the β-hCG peptide sequence 111–145 provided by Dr V. C. Stevens, Columbus, Ohio, U.S.A., was also used for assaying the pituitary extract.

Concanavalin-A (Con-A) Affinity Chromatography

Sepharose 6B was coupled to Con-A through the divinylsulphonyl bridge, as described by Sairam and Porath (1976). Fifty milligrams of Con-A were coupled to each millilitre of settled Sepharose.

Aliquots of the gel chromatographic eluate were applied to the column in 0.01 M acetate buffer, pH 6.0, containing 10^{-3} M Mg^{2+}, Ca^{2+} and Mn^{2+}. This was then washed with the same solution and by the elution with a linear gradient of methyl-α-D-glucopyranoside (MEG) from 0 to 1.0 M.

In vitro Bioassay

The radioligand assay of Hour and Saxena (1974) was used for measuring LH and hCG activity.

RESULTS AND DISCUSSION

Partially purified LH (LER 907) gave a 0.17% cross-reaction with the hCG antiserum. The same LH preparation showed no cross-reactivity to the anti-β-hCG (111–145) peptide serum over a range of 0–50 000 mIU/ml. The β-hCG immunogens found in the biological fluids or in the chromatographic eluates were therefore not likely to be due to cross-reactivity of the antiserum to hLH.

Using anti-β-hCG serum, values as high as 48 mIU/ml were found in the serum sample at 45 min after the LHRH injection and became undetectable at 90 min. Evidence that hCG-like materials are secreted in such conditions can be deduced from parallelism of inhibition curves of the hCG standard and the serum samples in the β-hCG RIA.

The serum sample was subjected to ultrafiltration on a Diaflo PM-30 membrane before gel chromatography of the higher molecular weight fraction on a Sephadex G-150 column.

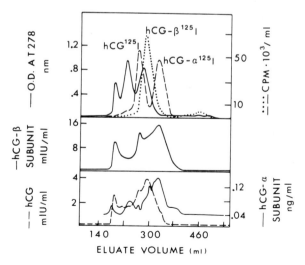

Fig. 1. The Sephadex G-150 gel chromatographic pattern of a serum sample from one patient after LHRH i.e. Upper panel: protein pattern and elution volumes of different tracers used for column calibration. Other panels: immunoreactivity patterns as determined by β-hCG, hCG and α-hCG RIA systems.

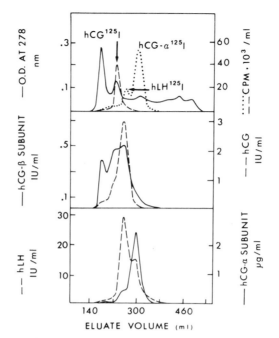

Fig. 2. The Sephadex G-150 gel chromatographic pattern of an ovarian cyst fluid. Upper panel: protein pattern and elution volumes of different tracers used for column calibration. Other panels: immunoreactivity patterns as determined by β-hCG, hCG, α-hCG and LH RIA systems.

The profiles of β-hCG, hCG and α-hCG immunoactivities are shown in Fig. 1. The first anti-β-hCG immunoreactive peak was eluted in the V_0, whereas the second and the third were eluted in the hCG zone and in that of α-hCG respectively.

β-hCG concentrations in four of the 15 ovarian cyst fluids were between 8 and 60 mIU/ml. The fluid with the highest concentration of β-hCG was concentrated by ultrafiltration on Diaflo PM-30 membrane and then chromatographed on a Sephadex G-150 column. The immunological pattern of the eluate is shown in Fig. 2. An anti-β-hCG immunoactive material is shown in the V_0 of the column, whereas a second peak with a V_e/V_0 ratio similar to that of hCG was found in the other fractions.

Material with β-hCG immunoactivity, but a higher molecular weight, was also present in the pituitary extract. Sephadex G-100 Superfine gel chromatography (Fig. 3) revealed three peaks with β-hCG immunoactivity; the first in the V_0, the second in the hCG zone and a third in that of LH. The latter was probably due to the high levels of LH in the eluate and presented a hCG/LH ratio 50 times lower than the V_0 peak.

The material eluted in the V_0 was further purified by affinity chromatography on Sepharose–Con-A. Three major peaks were observed when a linear gradient of MEG from 0 to 1.0 M was used as eluent. The LH and β-hCG radioimmunological profiles are shown in Fig. 4.

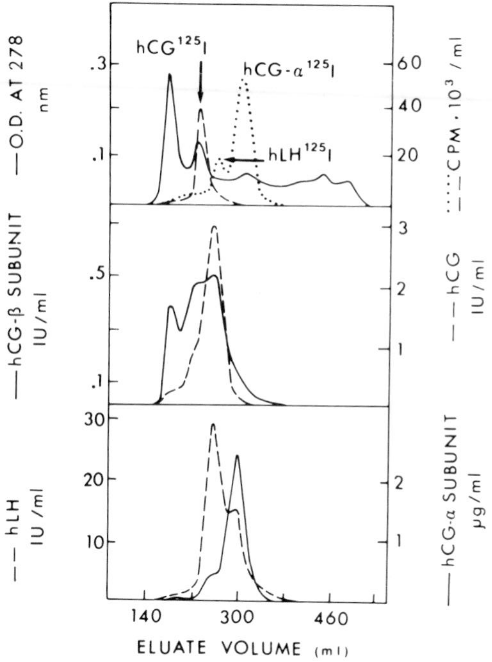

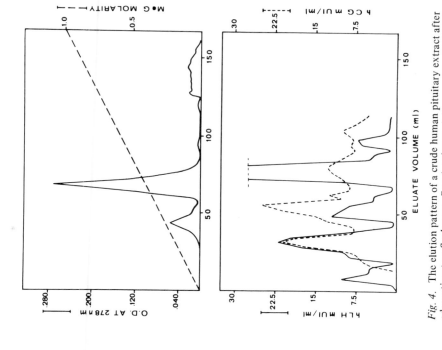

Fig. 4. The elution pattern of a crude human pituitary extract after adsorption to a Sepharose–Con-A column. A linear gradient of methyl-α-D-glucopyranoside has been used for desorption.

Fig. 3. The Sephadex G-100 Superfine gel chromatographic pattern of a crude pituitary extract. Upper panel: protein pattern and elution volumes of different tracers used for column calibration. Other panels: immunoreactivity patterns as determined by β-hCG, hCG, α-hCG and LH RIA systems.

When the three peaks were assayed in the radioligand assay using receptors prepared from bovine corpora lutea, hCG activity was detected in all three peaks.

Although a trypsin-like protease present in tissues has been found to interfere in the assay systems used to measure hCG (Segal *et al.*, 1979), the data presently available suggest that more than one hCG-like substance is present in pituitary glands as well as in peripheral blood after hypophysiotropic stimulation.

Data presented elsewhere (see Pala and Carenza, this volume) show that hCG-like materials are present in all normal sera and that they may be assayed under adequate unblocking conditions. Therefore the ectopic production of hCG no longer appears likely since this production would have to be considered as unblocked hormone circulation.

REFERENCES

Braunstein, G. D., Vaitukaitis, J. L., Carbone, P. P. and Ross, G. T. (1973). *Annals of Internal Medicine* **78**, 39.

Braunstein, G. D., Rasor, J. and Wade, M. E. (1975). *New England Journal of Medicine* **293**, 1339.

Braunstein, G. D., Kamdar, V., Rasor, J., Swaminathan, N. and Wade, M. E. (1978). Paper presented at the 60th Annual Meeting of the Endocrine Society (abstract no. 44).

Chen, H. C., Hodgen, H. C., Matsuura, S. *et al.* (1976). *Proceedings of the National Academy of Sciences of the U.S.A.* **73**, 2885.

Golde, D. W., Schambelan, M., Weintraub, B. D. and Rosen, S. W. (1974). *Cancer* **33**, 1048.

Hour, F. and Saxena, B. B. (1974). *Journal of Biological Chemistry* **249**, 2195.

Midgley, A. R., Jr (1966). *Endocrinology* **79**, 10.

Pala, A., Donini, P. and Carenza, L. (1979). *In* "Recent Advances in Reproduction and Regulation of Fertility" (Talwar G. P. ed.) pp. 439–451, Elsevier/North Holland Biomedical Press, Amsterdam.

Rosen, S. W., Weintraub, B. D., Vaitukaitis, J. L. *et al.* (1975). *Annals of Internal Medicine* **82**, 71.

Rutanen, E. M. and Seppälä, M. (1978). *Cancer* **41**, 692.

Sairam, M. R. and Porath, J. (1976). *Biochemical and Biophysical Research Communications* **69**, 190.

Samann, N. A., Smith, J. P., Rutledge, F. N. and Schultz, P. N. (1976). *American Journal of Obstetrics and Gynecology* **126**, 186.

Segal, S. J., Maruo, T., Adejuwon, C. and Koide, S. (1979). *In* "Recent Advances in Reproduction and Regulation of Fertility" (Talwar G. P. ed.) pp. 399–413, Elsevier/North Holland Biomedical Press, Amsterdam.

Stone, M., Bagshawe, K. D., Kardana, A. and Searle, F. (1977). *British Journal of Obstetrics and Gynaecology* **84**, 375.

Yoshimoto, Y., Wolfsen, A. R. and Odell, W. D. (1977). *Science, New York* **197**, 575.

Section Five

PLACENTAL MORPHOLOGY

PLACENTAL PRODUCTS AND QUANTITATIVE MORPHOLOGY

R. C. W. Vermeulen, P. H. J. Kurver, H. van Kessel and L. A. M. Stolte

*Department of Obstetrics and Gynaecology, Free University,
Amsterdam, The Netherlands*

INTRODUCTION

To establish the relation of the placental production rate of proteins and hormones to fetal growth has been the aim of numerous studies in the last decades. This placental activity is said to be reflected by the concentration of the products in the blood or by the quantity excreted in the urine. In the evaluation of each newly discovered placental product as a reflection of placental function, the actual relation to fetal growth plays an important role.

In fetal monitoring, less attention has been given to microscopy of the placental tissue, probably because of the fact that the results can only be obtained after delivery and because of the mainly qualitative aspect of this type of investigation. The introduction, however, of quantitative morphology in microscopy of the placenta might enable us to reach a better understanding of the processes of production and nutritive transport.

Quantitative microscopic data of the placenta seem to be clearly related to results of oxytocin challenge tests (Sanchez-Ramos *et al.*, 1976) and to birthweight (Aherne and Dunnill, 1966). The technique used in processing the placenta greatly influences the morphological picture. In particular, the time of the clamping of the cord proved to be of the utmost importance (Bouw *et al.*, 1976).

Serono Symposium No. 35, "The Human Placenta", edited by A. Klopper,
A. Genazzani and P. G. Crosignani, 1980. Academic Press, London and New York.

In our study we aim to investigate the relation between the quantitative morphological characteristics of the placenta and some biochemical placental parameters.

PATIENTS AND METHODS

The subjects were randomly selected from patients attending the antenatal clinic of the Department of Obstetrics of the Academic Hospital of the Free University of Amsterdam. After informed consent, blood was taken and urine collected at T_1 (244-261 days of amenorrhoea) and T_2 (261-280 days).

The completeness of the urine collection was checked by the assay of the urinary creatinine. The total urinary oestrogens were assayed by means of an automated Ittrich procedure (Van Kessel *et al.*, 1969). The pregnanediol was measured by means of gas-liquid chromatography of the tetrachloromethane extracts of acid hydrolysed urines (courtesy of Dr A. C. Akkerman-Faber, Laboratory of Endocrinology, Free University, Amsterdam). The oxytocinase was measured kinetically in a Zeiss PM4 spectrophotometer at 30 °C using S-benzyl-L-cysteine-*p*-nitroanilide as substrate (Van Oudheusden, 1971).

At delivery (256-294 days of amenorrhoea) the cord was clamped within 10 s of the appearance of the feet. The placenta was suspended from its membranes at room temperature in a 4% formalin, pH 7.0, phosphate buffer of 0.7 mol/l for at least 2 weeks. The net placental volume was assessed by measuring the fluid displacement when the fixed placenta, free from membranes and cord, was submerged in saline. Six pieces of tissue (3 mm × 20 mm × 30 mm) were randomly selected for microscopy, and 7 μm thick sections prepared. Periodic acid Schiff (PAS) staining was used.

For the assessment of the volume percentage of the trophoblast in the placental tissue the microscopic picture (× 750) was projected on a screen provided with a grid of 20 points and the number of points coinciding with the trophoblast were counted (Bouw *et al.* 1978). Forty projections were counted per slide. The percentage arrived at in this way has a 95% confidence limit of ± 10%.

For the surface density, i.e. the amount of surface per unit of volume, the microscopic picture (× 456) was projected on a screen provided with a line of given length and the intersections with the villi were counted (Bouw *et al.*, 1978). Sixty projections were counted per slide. The surface density arrived at in this way has a 95% confidence limit of ± 5%. The volume percentage and the surface density were multiplied by the net placental volume to obtain the volume and the surface of the trophoblast.

The percentile of the birthweight was derived from the data of Kloosterman (1977).

The probabilities of no correlation were computed using the Spearman test.

RESULTS

The findings obtained in this study are summarized in Table I. As is shown in this table, the volume of the trophoblast was determined in 26 placentae only.

Table I. Numbers, minima, medians and maxima of amenorrhoea, pregnanediol and oxytocinase at T_1 = 244–261 and T_2 = 261–280 days of amenorrhoea and birth weight, percentile, net placental volume and the surface and volume of the trophoblast at birth.

		n	Minimum	Median	Maximum
Amenorrhoea (days)	T_1	48	244	252	260
	T_2	42	261	266	279
	Delivery	53	256	281	294
Oestrogens (μmol/day)	T_1	46	62	126	384
	T_2	42	56	151	315
Pregnanediol (μmol/day)	T_1	36	71	119	161
	T_2	36	66	114	193
Oxytocinase (IU/l)	T_1	44	49	103	239
	T_2	40	56	120	276
Birthweight (g)		53	1970	3260	4080
Percentile		53	0.4	30.8	89.0
Net placental volume (ml)		45	320	520	785
Surface area of trophoblast (m^2)		42	6.7	12.2	22.3
Volume of trophoblast (ml)		26	42.0	53.5	91.0

Table II. The correlation between the surface and the volume of the trophoblast, the net placental volume and the birthweight and percentile of the child. The values shown are probabilities of no correlation computed with the Spearman test.

	Net placental volume	Surface area of trophoblast	Volume of trophoblast
Surface area of trophoblast	< 0.01		
Volume of trophoblast		< 0.01	
Net placental volume			< 0.01
Birthweight	< 0.01	< 0.01	0.06
Percentile	< 0.01	< 0.01	0.05

This low number was due to technical difficulties. This group of 26 patients is not a representative sample of the whole population since the mean of the amenorrhoea is significantly lower (275 days) than in the remaining group (285 days).

The statistical analysis shows that the surface and the volume of the trophoblast correlate strongly with the net placental volume, and also between themselves. These three placental parameters are correlated with the fetal weight at birth and accordingly with the percentile of the birthweight (Table II).

Table III. The correlation between the oestrogens, pregnanediol and oxytocinase at T_1 = 244–261 and T_2 = 261–280 days of amenorrhoea and their correlation with the surface and volume of the trophoblast, the birthweight and the percentile. The values shown are probabilities of no correlation computed with the Spearman test.

	Oestrogens		Pregnanediol		Oxytocinase	
	T_1	T_2	T_1	T_2	T_1	T_2
Surface area of trophoblast	0.15	0.02	0.36	0.01	0.05	< 0.01
Volume of trophoblast	0.51	0.18	0.72	0.25	0.01	0.02
Net placental volume	0.27	0.08	0.45	0.02	0.08	0.01
Birthweight	0.08	0.03	0.03	0.03	0.81	0.13
Percentile	0.06	0.03	0.04	0.01	0.24	0.09
Oxytocinase	0.16	0.01				
Oestrogens			0.11	0.01		
Pregnanediol					0.41	< 0.01

The oxytocinase at T_1 and T_2 is significantly correlated with the surface of the trophoblast and with the net placental volume. The urinary steroids do not show a correlation with the surface of the trophoblast and the net volume of the placenta at T_1, but they do show a correlation at T_2. In the group of 26 patients in which both surface and volume were determined, the oxytocinase correlated with the surface and the volume of the trophoblast, but did not correlate with the birthweight and the percentile. The oestrogens in this group did not correlate with any of the morphological parameters, nor with the birthweight or percentile (Table III).

The steroid values, particularly at T_2, show a fair correlation with birthweight and percentile. The oxytocinase levels at T_1 clearly show an absence of relation with birthweight and percentile. The levels obtained at T_2 also fail to show a significant correlation.

DISCUSSION

The obvious relationship of the trophoblastic surface with the fetal growth, expressed by the weight at birth, or even better by the percentile, is in harmony with the concept that the trophoblast surface determines the transport of nutrients. The equally obvious relationship of the trophoblast surface with the net volume of the placenta indicates that the development of the surface is accompanied by an increase of placental volume. Consequently, we observed a fair correlation of the net placental volume with birthweight and percentile.

The values obtained for the steroids and for the oxytocinase at T_2, close to the time of spontaneous delivery, are clearly correlated with the trophoblast surface. The values obtained for the steroids 2 weeks earlier do not show this pattern. It is not clear whether this is caused by a change in the steroid production or by a change in the surface of the trophoblast. The fact that the early (T_1) oxytocinase values also correlated with the placental surface area points to the first possibility.

The discrepancy in the group of 26 patients between the correlation of the oxytocinase and the placental parameters on the one hand and the birthweight on the other, and the absence of a correlation with the oestrogens, will be the subject of a further study.

REFERENCES

Aherne, W. and Dunnill, M. S. (1966). *Journal of Pathology and Bacteriology* **91**, 133.

Bouw, G. M., Stolte, L. A. M., Baak, J. P. A. and Oort, J. (1976). *European Journal of Obstetrics and Gynaecology and Reproductive Biology* **6**, 325.

Bouw, G. M., Stolte, L. A. M., Baak, J. P. A. and Oort, J. (1978). *European Journal of Obstetrics and Gynaecology and Reproductive Biology* **8**, 31.

Kloosterman, G. J. (1977). *In* "De voortplanting van de mens" (G. J. Kloosterman *et al.*, eds), pp. 82–83, Center Press, Bussum.

Sanchez-Ramos, J. E., Fabre, E., Sandoval, C. and Botella-Llusia, J. (1976). *Journal de gynécologie, obstétrique et biologie de la reproduction* **5**, 761.

Van Kessel, H., Seitzinger, R., Schreurs, J. and Versteeg, M. (1969). *Nederlandsch Tijdschrift voor Verloskunde en Gynaecologie* **69**, 81.

Van Oudheusden, A. P. M. (1971). *Clinica chimica acta* **32**, 140.

THE RELATION OF PLACENTAL MORPHOLOGY TO HORMONAL STATUS IN PRE-ECLAMPSIA AND IN WOMEN WHO SMOKE

F.-J. Kaltenbach

Universitätsfrauenklinik, Albert-Ludwigs-Universität, Freiburg, German Federal Republic

INTRODUCTION

Cigarette smoking results in a significant reduction of the fetal birthweight (Simpson, 1957). No clear information is known about the placental function and morphological size in smokers. Stereological measurements were therefore undertaken to investigate different quantitative placental parameters in relation to hormonal status, as measured by plasma placental lactogen (hCS) and urinary oestriol excretion. The results were compared with placental and hormonal data of pregnancies complicated by pre-eclampsia.

MATERIAL AND METHODS

Placentae from 10 women without complications, 10 with mild pre-eclampsia and 10 with severe pre-eclampsia were studied. Placentae from non-smokers ($n = 11$) and pregnant women who smoked six ($n = 10$), 7-15 ($n = 12$) and 15-20 ($n = 11$) cigarettes per day were also analysed.

Two other groups of patients were eliminated and analysed separately. One group ($n = 6$) stopped smoking during pregnancy, the other group ($n = 5$) were patients who smoked and showed signs of pre-eclampsia.

Serono Symposium No. 35, "The Human Placenta", edited by A. Klopper,
A. Genazzani and P. G. Crosignani, 1980. Academic Press, London and New York.

Placental lactogen was determined using a commercial radioimmunoassay kit (Phadebas).

The oestrogens in the 24 h urine were measured by the modified fluorescence method described by Ittrich (1958).

Macroscopic Preparation Procedure

After macroscopic examination placentae were fixed in formalin, having removed membranes and umbilical cord. The placental volume was determined by the water displacement method. The fixed placentae were then cut into sections of 1 cm. Infarcted areas of more than 0.5 cm in diameter were examined planimetrically and their volumes calculated. The functioning placental volume was estimated by subtracting the infarct volume from the placental volume.

Histological Preparation Procedure

Tissue samples were taken of each placenta, embedded in paraffin wax and stained with haematoxylin and eosin and Goldner's stain.

Stereological Method

The stereological data were obtained by the method of Hennig (1956, 1958). The following parameters were determined: total placental villous area (S_T), placental villous volume (V), relative villous surface area ($S_R = S_T/V_T$), capillary volume of the villi (C_T), capillary density (C_V), surface density (S_V), placental capacity, degree of villous ramification, degree of villous vascularization. To estimate the morphological alterations we used a modified semiquantitative placental morphological index taking into account syncytial knots, intervillous fibrin deposits, fibrinoid necrosis of villi, fibrosis of villi, placental maturity, state of placental vessels, microinfarction of villi, dilatation of intervillous space, and congestion of villous capillaries.

Statistics

The data were examined by statistical methods, especially by determining the distribution of t and the sample correlation coefficient, r.

RESULTS

Pre-eclampsia

The clinical and stereological data are summarized in Table I. It is evident that the cases with severe gestosis are different from the normal ones and from cases with mild gestosis. The increase of the placental morphological index (PMI) is striking. In severe gestosis the mean birthweight decreased, and increases in both systolic and diastolic blood pressure were highly significant. (The degree of oedema and albuminuria expressed by the Goecke index (Goecke, 1970) was compared with the χ-squared test and showed no significant relationship.)

Table I. Placental morphometry in relation to pre-eclampsia.

Parameter	I Normal cases $n = 10$	II Mild gestosis $n = 10$	III Severe gestosis $n = 10$	p (I:III)[a]
Fetal birth weight (g)	3434	3102	2430	< 0.001
Systolic blood pressure (mmHg)	125.0	138.5	151.5	< 0.001
Diastolic blood pressure (mmHg)	82.5	94.5	104.6	< 0.001
Oestrogens (mg/24 h urine)	42.6	36.8	20.8	< 0.05
hPL (10^{-6} g/ml)	5.4	6.5	4.02	< 0.05 (II:III)
Placental weight (g)	563.5	574.0	404.0	< 0.05
Placental volume (cm^3)	473.0	464.0	332.0	< 0.05
Placental morphologic index (PMI)	12.7	20.0	21.7	< 0.001
Villous volume (cm^3)	308.0	310.0	242.0	< 0.05
Total villous surface area (m^2)	12.87	11.89	7.16	< 0.001
Relative villous surface area (cm^2)	3.2	3.2	2.8	< 0.01
Degree of ramification	419.9	385.0	305.9	< 0.001
Degree of vascularization	33.6	29.2	28.8	N.S.[b]

[a]p = probability.   [b]N.S., not significant.

The hPL concentration and the excretion of oestrogens in the 24 h urine are significantly diminished in group III.

Severe gestosis also influences the placental volume and weight. There is a significant reduction of the mean values.

The mean total villous surface area was found to be 12.8 m² (Adelstein and Frerrick, 1978). The exchange area is significantly different between groups I and III and II and III. In the last group the villous surface area is reduced by half to 7.16 m² (Fig. 1).

In contrast to normal pregnancy the relative villous surface area was significantly decreased.

All parameters were correlated and the correlation coefficient was calculated. The most frequent correlations were found for the systolic blood pressure. The oestrogens in the 24 h urine were correlated only with the placental morphologic index. But hPL correlated with placental weight, placental volume, placental villous surface area and placental villous volume.

Placental villous volume and placental volume and hPL values were closely

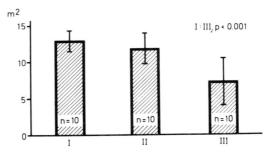

Fig. 1. Total villous surface area (in square metres) and severity of pre-eclampsia. I, normal cases; II, mild pre-eclampsia; III, severe pre-eclampsia.

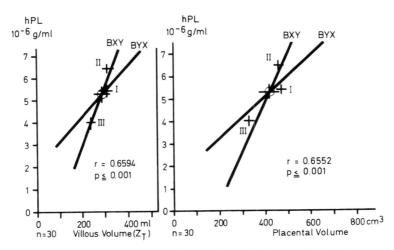

Fig. 2. Pre-eclampsia. Placental villous volume, placental volume and hPL values are closely correlated.

Table II. Placental morphometry in relation to cigarette smoking

Parameter	I Normal cases n = 11	II Smokers n = 10 (1–6 cigarettes/day)	III Smokers n = 12 (7–15 cigarettes/day)	IV Smokers n = 11 (15–20 cigarettes/day)	p (I:IV)[a]
Fetal birth weight (g)	3447	3420	3287	3345	N.S.[b]
Oestrogens (mg/24 h urine)	50.3	35.5	36.3	51.4	N.S.[b]
hPL (10^{-6} g/ml)	5.5	7.8	9.2	8.9	< 0.05
Placental weight (g)	558.18	550.00	625.00	700.91	< 0.001
Placental volume (cm^3)	463.64	471.00	530.00	619.09	< 0.001
Placental morphologic index (PMI)	9.09	10.4	11.0	11.5	< 0.01
Villous volume (cm^3)	322.09	357.56	398.90	457.25	< 0.001
Total villous surface area (m^2)	12.8	13.7	16.0	18.9	< 0.001
Relative villous surface area (cm^2)	31.95	36.24	41.37	46.76	< 0.001
Degree of ramification	40.09	38.2	40.4	41.3	N.S.[b]
Degree of vascularization	0.26	0.23	0.25	0.28	N.S.[b]
Capillary volume (cm^3)	85.01	80.93	101.94	127.50	N.S.[b]
Capillary density (cm^2/cm^3)	0.18	0.17	0.19	0.21	N.S.[b]
Surface density (cm^3/cm^3)	276.7	289.4	302.5	304.9	< 0.05
Placental capacity	3.37	3.08	4.10	5.2	< 0.05

[a] p = probability.   [b] N.S., not significant.

correlated (Fig. 2). Severe gestosis with high blood pressure was associated with the most striking reduction in plasma hPL concentration, placental surface area and placental volume.

The quantitative morphological findings in cases with severe gestosis are marked by the close correlation between plasma hPL concentration, total villous surface area and fetal birthweight.

All babies with a birthweight under 1600 g, plasma hPL concentration under 3 μg/ml and an exchange area under 6 m^2 died.

Cigarette Smoking

The quantitative macroscopic and microscopic results are shown in Table II. It is evident that smoking habits have a particular influence on the parameters under investigation.

The fetal birthweight was not significantly reduced in the smokers' group. The placental data were influenced macroscopically and microscopically. Placental volume (V) and weight increased in the heavy smokers. Increasing cigarette consumption also influenced the size of the total and relative placental villous surface area (Fig. 3). There is a highly significant increase in the mean values.

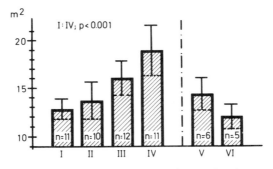

Fig. 3. Total villous surface area (in square metres) and increasing cigarette consumption. I, non-smokers; II–IV, mild–strong smokers; V, stopped smoking during pregnancy; VI, smokers and pre-eclampsia combined.

The total villous surface area (S_T) in non-smokers was found to be 12.8 m^2; in the group of heavy smokers (IV) it was 18.9 m^2. The surface density (S_V), representing the villous surface area contained in 1 cm^3 of the placenta, was significantly higher in the group of heavy smokers (IV).

Placental villous volume (Z_T) and placental capacity (villous surface area × degree of vascularization) were found to be significantly higher in the group of heavy smokers (IV). The degree of vascularization and ramification of villi, the capillary density (C_V) and capillary volume (in cubic centimetres) were not influenced.

The increase in the placental morphological index was striking. The most important parameter was the excessive formation of syncytial knots.

The hPL levels were significantly elevated in women who smoke. In contrast to these results the oestrogen excretion was not altered (Fig. 4).

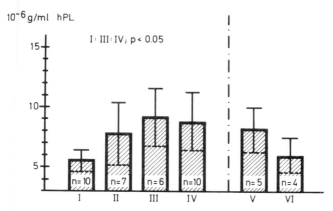

Fig. 4. hPL levels and increasing cigarette consumption. I, non-smokers; II–IV, mild–strong smokers; V, stopped smoking during pregnancy; VI, smokers and pre-eclampsia combined.

Close correlations were found between placental surface area (S_T) and placental weight $(r = 0.73; p < 0.001)$ and between placental surface area (S_T) and villous surface density (S_V) $(r = 0.6; p < 0.001)$. A positive correlation existed between relative surface area (S_R) and surface area $(r = 0.64; p < 0.001)$ and between relative surface area (S_R) and surface density (S_V). We also found a close correlation between placental villous volume (Z_T) and placental weight $(r = 0.69; p < 0.001)$. There was a negative correlation between the degree of ramification and villous volume $(r = 0.57; p < 0.001)$ and between the degree of vascularization and the placental morphological index $(r = 0.41; p < 0.01)$.

DISCUSSION

Pre-eclampsia

Our findings confirm that placental and fetal birthweight decrease in correlation with severity of gestosis and blood pressure (Hölzl, 1973; Kaltenbach *et al.*, 1977; Kraus *et al.*, 1968).

The plasma hPL levels and the excretion of oestrogens in 24 h urine are significantly diminished in cases with severe gestosis.

The comparison of hPL values with placental volume and weight and fetal birthweight showed close correlation between hPL and placental weight and volume. But there was no correlation between hPL levels and fetal weight. Most authors confirm our results (Josimovich, 1970; Saxena, 1969; Singer, 1970; Spellacy, 1966).

The total villous surface area is an important parameter for characterizing placental damage and infarction in gestosis. In cases with severe gestosis the total villous surface area was only half the size of that in normal pregnancies.

The relative villous surface area (the ratio between the total surface of a placenta available for exchange and the tissue volume) (Baur, 1973) decreased significantly in severe gestosis.

The closest correlations existed between hPL and fetal birthweight, placental weight, placental volume, placental villous surface area and blood pressure. The correlation of oestrogen excretion with blood pressure and placental morphological index was negative. These results demonstrate the close relationship of hPL to the placental structure including stroma and trophoblast cells (Klopper *et al.*, 1977; Sciarra, 1968).

As hPL is synthesized by the syncytiotrophoblast, which is part of the placental surface, the decrease of hPL level could be the result of diminishing villous surface (Sciarra *et al.*, 1963).

Cigarette Smoking

In cases of heavy smokers our results demonstrate an evident increase in most of the parameters studied.

With smokers there was a reduction of the mean fetal birthweight of about 104 g. The mean birthweight with smokers combined with gestosis was 329 g less, and therefore evidently lower (Adelstein and Frerrick, 1978; Russel *et al.*, 1968). In contrast to these findings, the placental volume and weight were higher with heavy smokers.

Targett *et al.* (1973) and Asmussen (1977) have described lower placental weights in smokers, but Spellacy *et al.* (1977) and Wingerd *et al.* (1976) found higher placental weight in heavy smokers.

The increase of the total and relative placental villous surface area and of the placental surface density was a striking result. The surface density, which is a measure of the enlargement of the exchange surface area caused by the placental villi, increased more than 15% in heavy smokers.

The placental villous volume also increased, but placental capillary volume and degree of vascularization did not change. The placental capacity (villous surface area × degree of vascularization) was significantly higher with heavy smokers. This suggests that the placentae of smokers are able to adapt their filtration capacity better by enlarging the surface area or degree of vascularization (Bender, 1974).

To clarify the histology of the placenta we calculated the placental morphological index (PMI). The PMI increased with the number of cigarettes. The most evident findings were the excessive proliferation of syncytial knots. This is a well-known state under hypoxic conditions (Fox, 1970, 1978; Kaltenbach *et al.*, 1977). It may represent the placental response to oxygen deficiency or supersaturation with carbon dioxide in smokers.

The maternal hPL levels were significantly higher in contrast to the oestrogen excretion between the 36th and 40th weeks of gestation with increasing cigarette consumption, in accordance with Spellacy *et al.* (1977). A high hPL concentration in smokers can be interpreted as the placental reaction to the poor metabolic conditions of the fetoplacental unit.

To decide if the percentage of pregnancies with lower oestrogen excretion is higher in smokers, a greater number of patients should be studied (Targett *et al.*, 1973).

REFERENCES

Adelstein, P. and Frerrick, J. (1978). Paper presented at the 1st Congress of the International Society for the Study of Hypertension in Pregnancy, Dublin.

Aherne, W. and Dunnill, S. (1966). *Journal of Pathology and Bacteriology* **91**, 123.

Asmussen, I. (1977). *Acta obstetrica et gynecologia scandinavica* **56**, 119.

Baur, R. (1973). *Acta anatomica Basel* **8**, 75.

Bender, H. G. (1974). *Archiv für Gynäkologie* **216**, 289.

Fox, H. (1970). *American Journal of Obstetrics and Gynecology* **107**, 1058.

Fox, H. (1978). "Pathology of the Placenta", W. B. Saunders, Philadelphia, p.158 *ff.*

Goecke, C. (1970). *Medizinische Klinik* **65**, 1957.

Hennig, A. (1956). *Mikroskopie* **11**, 1.

Hennig, A. (1958). *Zeiss-Werkzeitschrift* **6**, 78.

Hölzl, M. (1973). *Zentralblatt für Gynäkologie* **95**, 1481.

Ittrich, G. (1958). *Zentralblatt für Gynäkologie* **80**, 771.

Josimovich, J. B. (1970). *Obstetrics and Gynecology* **36**, 244.

Kaltenbach, F. J., Fettig, O. and Krieger, M. L. (1974). *Archiv für Gynäkologie* **369**, 216.

Kaltenbach, F. J., Schmitt, R. and Dieterich, W. (1977). *Archiv für Gynäkologie* **222**, 249.

Klopper, A., Masson, G. and Wilson, G. (1977). *British Journal of Obstetrics and Gynaecology* **84**, 648.

Krauss, A., Schlegel, L. and Canzler, E. (1968). *Gynecologia* **166**, 455.

Russel, S., Taylor, C. R. and Law, C. E. (1968). *British Journal of Preventative and Social Medicine* **22**, 11.

Saxena, B. N. (1969). *New England Journal of Medicine* **281**, 225.

Sciarra, J. J. (1968). *American Journal of Obstetrics and Gynecology* **101**, 413.

Sciarra, J. J., Kaplan, S. L. and Grumbach, M. M. (1963). *Nature, London* **199**, 100.

Simpson, W. J. (1957). *American Journal of Obstetrics and Gynecology* **73**, 808.

Singer, W. (1970). *Obstetrics and Gynecology* **36**, 222.

Spellacy, W. N. (1966). *American Journal of Obstetrics and Gynecology* **96**, 116.

Spellacy, W. N., Buhi, W. C. and Birk, S. A. (1977). *American Journal of Obstetrics and Gynecology* **127**, 232.

Targett, Ch. S., Gunsee, H., McBride, F. and Beischer, N. A. (1973). *Journal of Obstetrics and Gynaecology of the British Commonwealth* **80**, 815.

Targett, Ch. S., Ratten, G. J., Abell, D. A. and Beischer, N. A. (1977). *Australian and New Zealand Journal of Obstetrics and Gynecology* **17**, 126.

Wingerd, J., Christianson, R. and Lowitt, W. V. (1976). *American Journal of Obstetrics and Gynecology* **124**, 671.

THE MORPHOLOGICAL BASIS OF PLACENTAL
ENDOCRINE ACTIVITY

M. Sideri[1], G. Fumagalli[1], G. De Virgiliis and G. Remotti

I Clinica Ostetrico Ginecologica Dell'Universita di Milano, and
[1]C.N.R. Centre of Cytopharmacology, Milan, Italy

INTRODUCTION

The morphological basis of placental endocrine activity is not well defined. At present, it has not been established whether only the syncytiotrophoblast (STB) or both STB and the cytotrophoblast (CTB) secrete placental hormones, nor what are the morphological steps in the secretion of protein hormones. Conflicting results have been obtained by immunohistoenzymological, immunofluorescence and immunocytochemical studies, by *in vitro* culture and by electron microscopic studies. Some authors (De Ikonikoff and Cedard, 1973), by using the peroxidase bridge technique, have localized hCG and hPL from the sixth week of gestation to term in the syncytial villi and in some cells of the amniotic epithelium, but not in Langhans' cells. Immunofluorescence (Midgley and Pierce 1962; Thiede and Choate, 1963) and immunocytochemical techniques (Dreskin *et al.*, 1970) also localized hCG in the STB, but not in the Langhans' cells. On the other hand, other authors (Loke *et al.*, 1972) demonstrated, by mixed agglutination, that in monolayer cultures both CTB and STB produce hCG. Transmission electron microscopic studies also suggested (Wynn, 1972; De Virgiliis *et al.*, 1978) that the differentiation of the trophoblast is correlated with its elaboration of protein hormones, because both STB and the specialized CTB contain an abundance of organelles associated with hormonal secretion. Although these electron microscopic studies have shown a connection between the trophoblastic fine structure and the protein secretory activity, no particular

Serono Symposium No. 35, "The Human Placenta", edited by A. Klopper,
A. Genazzani and P. G. Crosignani, 1980. Academic Press, London and New York.

attention has been given to the morphological aspects of synthesis, storage and release or the trophoblastic protein hormones. This paper reports our observations on the morphological aspects of trophoblastic protein hormone secretion by means of transmission electron microscopy and "freeze-fracture" techniques.

MATERIALS AND METHODS

Our study was based on the examination of 20 placentae of 10–13 weeks obtained from voluntary interruptions of pregnancy and 10 placentae of 38–40 weeks obtained by vaginal delivery. In all cases histological controls and normal biochemical data (hCG, hPL and, at term, oestriol) were available. Biopsies of villous trophoblast were performed (1) at random in the early placentae; (2) in the central zone in the term placentae; (3) in the central zone in the chorion laeve at term. Biopsies were fixed in 2.5% glutaraldehyde, post-fixed in 1% osmium tetroxide and embedded in epon. Thin sections were cut with a diamond knife. The biopsies for freeze-fracture examination were fixed with 1.5% glutaraldehyde + 1% paraformaldehyde in 0.12 M phosphate buffer, pH 7.3, then infiltrated with glycerol (at concentrations increasing from 10 to 30%) in the same buffer. Samples were frozen in Freon 22, cooled at $-150\,^{\circ}$C in liquid nitrogen, then freeze-fractured according to Moor and

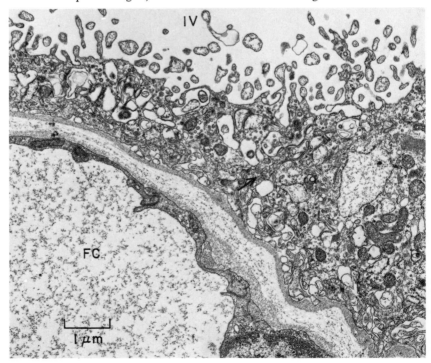

Fig. 1. Term placenta: alpha zone. The arrows indicate osmiophilic cytoplasmatic granules. No exocytosis is evident into the intervillous space. FC, fetal capillary; IV, intervillous space.

Mühlethaler (1973) in a Balzers freeze-etching device (Balzers AG, Balzers, Liechtenstein). The fracturing temperature was −100 °C. Platinum–carbon replicas were washed in sodium hypochlorite solution to remove organic material, then in distilled water, and finally recovered on 200 mesh copper grids. The observations were carried out with a Philips EM 200 electron microscope.

RESULTS

Transmission Electron Microscopic Results

The early villous trophoblast shows the well-known ultrastructural pattern. The syncytium appears as a high layer with some nuclei and many microvilli, while the cytotrophoblast appears as a continuous cellular layer. Some dense granules are present beneath, or inside, the trophoblastic basement membrane. Many differences are evident in the fine structure of the syncytial and cellular cytoplasm. The syncytium shows a well-developed endoplasmic reticulum with many cisternae, a small Golgi apparatus and few osmiophilic granules. On the other hand, CTB shows a rough, membraneous endoplasmic reticulum, a larger Golgi apparatus and few, very dense, cytoplasmic granules. All the inter-

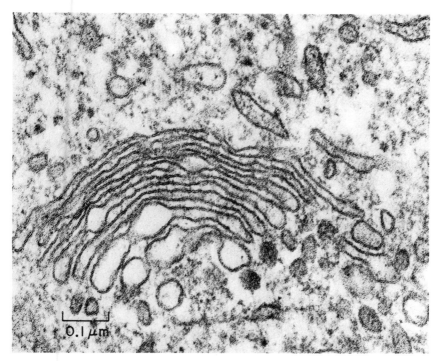

Fig. 2. Term placenta. The Golgi apparatus shows no evidence of condensation of protein matter.

cellular surfaces create a canalicular network in contact with the trophoblastic basement membrane. We observed that osmiophilic granules were seldom released into this canalicular network, and never into the intervillous space (Remotti *et al.*, 1979). In the term placenta the villous trophoblast is generally differentiated into the alpha and the beta zones (Fig. 1). Alpha zones are characterized by a thin cytoplasmic strip, without any nuclei, in close relation

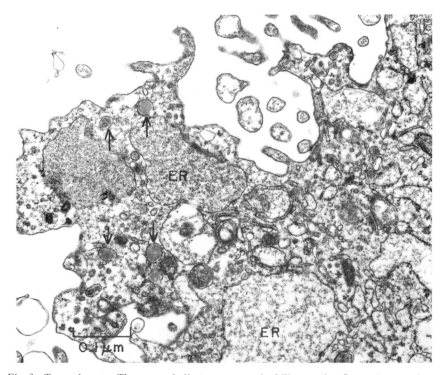

Fig. 3. Term placenta. The arrows indicate many osmiophilic granules. Some pinocytotic vesicles are present. No evidence of granular exocytosis. IV, intervillous space; ER, endoplasmic reticulum.

with the fetal capillary. This scarce cytoplasm presents an endoplasmic reticulum constituted by many cisternae, no evidence of Golgi apparatus and some dense granules varying in size and osmiophility; no granular release into the intervillous space can be seen. Beta zones have a higher cytoplasm and some nuclei; the endoplasmic reticulum appears as a complex membranous system, and the Golgi apparatus is evident (Fig. 2). Also in this syncytial zone, although many dense granules are present in the cytoplasm, no exocytosis is evident (Fig. 3). In the term placenta Langhans' CTB is not well developed, while the CTB of the chorion laeve shows interesting aspects (De Virgiliis *et al.*, 1973). In fact it presents a rich membranous endoplasmic reticulum, a large Golgi apparatus and some dense osmiophilic granules. Nevertheless, we were unable to observe a release of these granules.

Freeze-fracture Results

The same structures observed by transmission electron microscopy can be seen in Fig. 4. The P-face of the microvillar surface (Fig. 5) shows the cross-sections of the microvilli and a uniform distribution of the intramembraneous particles. Particle-free areas are not evident. In studying this syncytial membrane by the freeze-fracture method, the most striking observations are the low number of

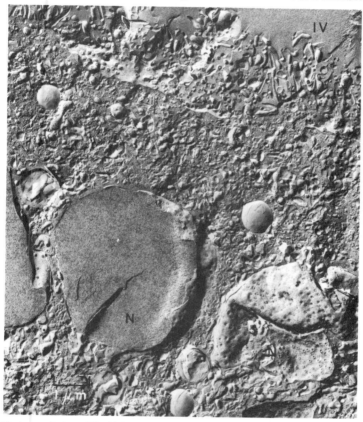

Fig. 4. Early trophobast. The high syncytium with many microvilli and some nuclei. IV, intervillous space; N, nuclei.

pinocytotic vesicles and the presence of some small, tight junctions. Tight junctions are also present between the cellular and syncytial membranes of the trophoblastic tissue, but they do not show a perfect organization (Fig. 6) as seen in other secretory epithelia (Staehelim, 1974; Meldolesi *et al.*, 1978).

DISCUSSION

Our observations on the fine structure of the placental trophoblast are in agreement with the previous reports on early and term placental ultrastructure.

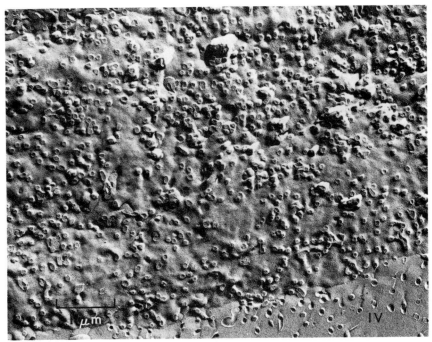

Fig. 5. Term placenta: P-face of the microvillar surface. Note the cross-section of microvilli and the uniform distribution of the intramembranous particles. No particle-free areas are evident. IV, intervillous space.

Nevertheless, these works offered few details on the morphological basis of the secretory processes. Our observations emphasize the following findings: (a) the Golgi apparatus does not show evidence of condensation of protein material; (b) many dense granules are present in the cytoplasm of both cellular and syncytial trophoblast; (c) no exocytosis into the intervillous space is evident.

Up to now, immunocytochemical studies have been especially directed at localizing hCG and hPL (De Ikonikoff and Cedard, 1973). hCG was found in the endoplasmic reticulum and on the microvillar surface, while no reaction for hCG was found in the Golgi apparatus, nor in the granules (Dreskin *et al.*, 1970). Nevertheless, one must be cautious in suggesting that these data can define a model for hCG secretion. Some considerations, in our opinion, are important. First of all, protein glycolysis is carried out only partially in the endoplasmic reticulum, most of it taking place in the Golgi apparatus. Secondly, it is well known that protein secretion is carried out by the Golgi apparatus even if the secretory product is not condensed in the Golgi nor stored in the granules, as is the case for antibodies in plasma cells (Murphy *et al.*, 1972). Further research is necessary for investigating the meaning and content of these syncytial osmiophilic granules that resemble secretory ones. At present, it is possible to speculate that in these granules are stored (a) a modified form of hCG that does not react immunocytochemically; (b) other protein hormones or other placental matter; (c) substances which have different functions as compared to the common secretory granules.

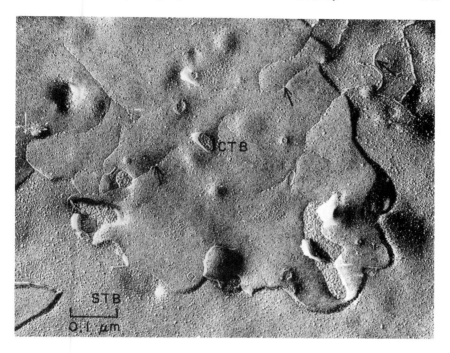

Fig. 6. Early trophoblast. The arrows indicate tight junctions between the cytotrophoblast (CTB) and the syncytiotrophoblast (STB). Note their lack of organization.

Our transmission electron microscopic observation that granular extrusion does not take place, or is not a prominent event, could have a technical explanation: in fact, it is possible that our observations were not sufficiently extensive or that we did not cut enough serial sections. Our freeze-fracture study showed that the microvillar surface has a minimal rate of pinocytosis and that, always considering the above-mentioned technical limitations, this seems to confirm that exocytosis is a rare event on the luminal syncytial membrane. This fact would support the hypothesis that hCG secretion is probably a continuous and slow event (Martin *et al.*, 1973).

The problem of the protein placental hormone secretion is complicated by the role the cytotrophoblast may play. Although it is possible to observe the extrusion of some dense granules from Langhans' cells, we have suggested that these features are related to placental transfer rather than to protein endocrine placental activity (Remotti *et al.*, 1979). However, it is well known that there is a parallel reduction in hCG secretion and the volume of cytotrophoblast in the early placenta. Nelson *et al.* (1978) have recently demonstrated an active incorporation of labelled galactose into the Golgi apparatus of the CTB. According to other authors (Hustin *et al.*, 1979), the assumption that the CTB is involved in the production of only a part (α-hCG) of the complete, final hormone is supported by the ultrastructural observation of an abundance of organelles associated with the secretory process in CTB.

REFERENCES

De Ikonicoff, L. K. and Cedard, L. (1973). *American Journal of Obstetrics and Gynecology* **116**, 1124.

De Virgiliis, G., Carinelli, S. and Remotti, G., (1973). *Annali di Ostetricia Ginecologia e Medicina Perinatale* **4**, 239.

De Virgiliis, G., Zaninetti, P. and Remotti, G., (1978). *Annali di Ostetricia Ginecologia e Medicina Perinatale* **4**, 218.

Dreskin, R. B., Spicer, S. S. and Green, W. B. (1970. *Journal of Histochemistry and Cytochemistry* **18**, 862.

Loke, Y. W., Wilson, D. V. and Borland, R. (1972). *American Journal of Obstetrics and Gynecology* **7**, 875.

Martin, B. J., Spicer, S. S. and Smythe, N. M., (1973). *Anatomical Record* **178**, 769.

Meldolesi, J., Castiglioni, G., Parama, R., Nassivera, N. and De Camilli, P. (1978). *Journal of Cell Biology* **79**, 156.

Midgley, A. R. and Pierce, G. B. (1962). *Journal of Experimental Medicine* **115**, 289.

Moor, H. and Mühlethaler (1973). *Journal of Cell Biology* **17**, 609.

Murphy, M. J., Hay, J. B., Morris, B. and Bessis, M. C. (1972). *American Journal of Pathology* **66**, 25.

Nelson, D. M., Enders, A. C. and King, B. F. (1978). *Journal of Cell Biology* **76**, 418.

Remotti, G., De Virgiliis, G. and Bianco, V. (1979). (In press).

Staehelim, L. A. (1974). *International Review of Cytology* **39**, 191.

Thiede, H. A. and Choate, J. W. (1963). *Obstetrics and Gynecology* **22**, 433.

Wynn, R. M. (1972). *American Journal of Obstetrics and Gynecology* **114**, 339.

Section Six

PROLACTIN

PHYSIOLOGY OF THE MAMMARY GLAND AND OF THE MAMMOTROPIC HORMONES DURING PREGNANCY AND LACTATION

C. Robyn

Human Reproduction Research Unit, Université Libre de Bruxelles, Hôpital Saint-Pierre, 322 rue Haute, 1000-Brussels, Belgium

INTRODUCTION

In all mammals lactation is essential for the survival of the species. The mammary gland is the umbilical cord of the newborn: it assumes the entire nutritional responsibility until the young are autonomous and capable of providing for their own nutritional needs. Furthermore, lactation is associated with a neuroendocrine balance that suppresses fertility so that delivery of a new baby does not compromise the chances of survival of a preceding offspring, or so that a new pregnancy would not dry up the mother's milk supply before the preceding offspring is adequately grown. It is very likely that in most mammals such a natural birth spacing method is a major factor in preventing a demographic explosion.

A few centuries of civilization were enough to provide human societies with substitutes for these two processes governing the survival of the species. Bottled milk replaced breast feeding and active methods of contraception compensated for the birth spacing effect of lactation. The use of bottled milk makes the child less dependent on his mother for his elementary development in life; this, however, was at first associated with considerable mortality during the neonatal period and early childhood. Modern methods of contraception are much more efficient than the natural fertility control associated with lactation. However, if

Serono Symposium No. 35, "The Human Placenta", edited by A. Klopper,
A. Genazzani and P. G. Crosignani, 1980. Academic Press, London and New York.

this natural regulation of birth spacing is relatively ineffective at the level of the individual, it is very effective at the level of the population in preventing excessive population growth. Furthermore, lactational infertility does not require the basic motivations for the active use of modern methods of contraception.

The mammary gland is characterized by a discontinuous development. After a first wave of growth at puberty in girls, the gland remains unchanged until the first pregnancy. At this time, the mammary gland undergoes further growth and differentiation for milk secretion. Lactation is controlled by an interplay of hormones, among which prolactin is essential for both the nutritional and birth spacing effect.

MAMMARY GLAND

Morphological Changes during Pregnancy and Lactation

As with the uterus, the mammary gland undergoes striking changes during pregnancy. In early pregnancy, the predominant change is growth, while in late gestation the most striking feature is cellular differentiation. Growth mainly consists in proliferation or hyperplasia of the distal epithelial elements of the ductal tree. The lobules grow in size: the number of tubular elements in each lobule increases markedly. These changes are maximum during the first trimester of pregnancy. Not all the lobules proliferate and develop at the same time. (*See* Salazar and Tobon, 1974.)

In most species, the glandular acini formed during the proliferative phase develop into a true lobulo-alveolar system during mid-gestation. From then on, cell proliferation is reduced and cell differentiation is the predominant feature: enlargement of the cytoplasm, accumulation of organelles and secretory products, dilatation of the alveoli. The intralobular space becomes more vascularized. Cytoplasmic enlargment with signs of intense protein synthesis progresses with vacuolation of the apical region. Colostrum appears in the lumen of the acini.

Just before delivery, there is a new wave of mitotic activity: it continues during the first days *post partum*. In women, true milk secretion starts some 2 days after delivery. Initiation of lactation is associated with specific morphological changes: the alveoli are dilated and full of secretory material, the epithelial cells have a clear vacuolated cytoplasm, cell borders are ragged toward the luminal pole.

At weaning, involutional changes occur in the mammary gland. Cells decrease in size and the signs of secretory activity regress. Active phagocytosis of stagnant secretory material becomes apparent. The stroma is more dense, less vacuolized and infiltrated with fat. Lysosomes increase in numbers and grow in size.

Endocrine Control of Growth and Secretion

Mammogenesis

In hypophysectomized animals, e.g. rats and mice, complete lobuloalveolar growth can only be obtained by complex hormonal interplay including sex steroids (oestrogen and progesterone), a lactogenic hormone (prolactin or growth hormone) and corticoids (Cowie, 1966). However, hypophysectomy dramatically changes the metabolic and nutritional states of the animal; this affects mammary growth too. Insulin increases the responsiveness of the mammary gland of hypophysectomized rats to ovarian hormones. But this effect is limited to the ducts and the end buds. It was also found to be enhanced by thyroxine. Even *in vitro*, insulin appears to be essential for mammogenesis. The relative importance of sex steroids and prolactin on mammogenesis seems to vary from one species to another. In some mammalia, prolactin is interchangeable with growth hormone in the hormonal combination evoking lobulo-alveolar growth. Human mammary gland tissue, obtained by biopsy of a mass at the 6th month of pregnancy, degenerated within a week when cultured in the absence of hormones (Flaxman *et al.*, 1976). Insulin, cortisol and low prolactin concentration could not prevent such degeneration. High prolactin concentration greatly improved the survival of the tissue and the continuation of DNA synthesis (Flaxman *et al.*, 1976). In mice, rats and monkeys, the pituitary gland can be removed during gestation, and the mammary development will proceed normally. Thus, the mammogenic hormone produced by the placenta seems to be able to compensate for the suppression of the mammogenic hormones produced by the pituitary gland.

How oestrogen and progesterone cause the mammary gland to proliferate is still unclear. A direct effect is supported by the demonstration of specific cytoplasmic receptors for oestrogens in the mammary epithelium. Complex interactions exist between oestrogens and prolactin at the level of both the mammary and the pituitary gland. Indeed, oestrogens stimulate release and synthesis of prolactin by the lactotrophs. They also have a potent mitogenic activity on these cells (Jacobi *et al.*, 1977). Even *in vitro* (Leung *et al.*, 1976), prolactin enhances oestrogen binding by the mammary tissue (Horrobin, 1977). Hypophysectomy in the rat is followed by a drop in oestrogen receptors in the liver: a single injection of ovine prolactin returns them toward control levels (Chamness *et al.*, 1975).

The relative importance of sex steroids in preparing the mammary gland for lactation is emphasized by the hormonal combination used to induce lactation in non-pregnant animals. In sheep, cows and heifers, lactation is consistently induced by treatment with oestrogen and progesterone, alone or in combination with dexamethasone (Fulkerson and McDowell, 1975; Fulkerson *et al.*, 1976; Erb *et al.*, 1976; Willett *et al.*, 1976; Hart, 1976). As a rule, lactation begins when steroid treatment is stopped. Such steroid treatment results in rising circulating levels of prolactin. Suppressing prolactin secretion by bromocriptine prevents lactation in goats and heifers prepared by sex steroids (Hart, 1976; Schams, 1976).

Self-stimulation of the nipples was reported to be important for mammary development in pregnant rats (Herrenkohl and Campbell, 1976). When self-stimulation during gestation is prevented by collars, the mammary glands were only half of the size seen in controls. Mechanical stimulation of the nipples in rats with collars causes normal mammary development. Thus, if oestrogen and progesterone play a key role in mammogenesis, the lactogenic hormones of pituitary and placental origin seem to be essential for full lobulo-alveolar growth during pregnancy. Furthermore, adequate metabolic and nutritional states are decisive for optimal expression of the specific endocrine control.

Milk Secretion

Cell differentiation leading to the secretion of milk by the mammary epithelium is primarily under the control of prolactin. Prolactin enhances synthesis of milk proteins, lipids and carbohydrates. It preferentially stimulates glucose oxidation by the pentose pathway, and activates pyruvate dehydrogenase activity. Prolactin increases the formation of both components of lactose synthetase: α-lactalbumin and galactosyl transferase. Synthesis of α-lactalbumin is inhibited by progesterone (Horrobin, 1977). Prolactin induces accumulation of casein messenger RNA (mRNA) in rat mammary gland organ culture (Matusik and Rosen, 1978). Prolactin actually increases both the rate of transcription and the half-life of casein mRNA. Hydrocortisone regulates casein mRNA accumulation after casein mRNA transcription. Progesterone blocks prolactin-mediated casein mRNA transcription (Matusik *et al.*, 1979). The regulation of specific gene transcription by a peptide hormone such as prolactin may be mediated by a surface membrane receptor via an indirect mechanism or via the direct interaction of the internalized peptide hormones with the genetic constituents. The binding of prolactin to a membrane receptor has been reported to be a prerequisite for induction of casein synthesis (O'Malley and Means, 1974).

In some species, such as the rabbit, the only hormone required to initiate milk secretion is prolactin (Stricker, 1951). In other species such as mice, rats, and goats a complex of other hormones is needed: corticoids, thyroxin, insulin. However, lactation does not take place during pregnancy despite elevated levels of circulating prolactin. In sheep, the initiation of milk secretion occurs at the very end of gestation after progesterone withdrawal and subsequent high levels of circulating prolactin *ante partum* (Kann *et al.*, 1978). Inhibitory influence of progesterone on the lactogenic effect of prolactin in the rabbit was also reported (Assairi *et al.*, 1974). It has already been mentioned that progesterone can suppress prolactin-mediated casein mRNA transcription and α-lactalbumin production. Progesterone can also block the biosynthesis of lactose (Yokoyama *et al.*, 1969; Kuhn, 1970). Before delivery, in women, guinea-pigs and mares, circulating levels of progesterone change little or not at all. They partially decline in ewes, cows and rats. Complete withdrawal of progesterone occurs at the time of delivery in cows, goats and bitches (Stabenfeldt, 1974). In women, onset of lactation takes place 2–3 days after delivery. To what extent progesterone withdrawal after delivery is effective in triggering lactation in women also remains to be clarified. At least in women, oestrogens also seem to contribute to the suppression of the lactogenic effect of prolactin during pregnancy.

Progesterone suppresses prolactin secretion as stimulated by oestrogens (March *et al.*, 1979; Labrie and Veilleux, 1979; Libertum *et al.*, 1979).

It has been proposed that human placental lactogen (hPL) may also contribute to the suppression of the lactogenic effect of prolactin during pregnancy. The affinity of hPL for prolactin binding sites is similar to that of prolactin, although its biological activity is considerably lower than that of prolactin. Since there is much more hPL (± 40 times) than prolactin in the circulation at the end of pregnancy, the binding sites for lactogenic hormones may be occupied by hPL, biologically a comparatively inactive hormone.

That prolactin is essential in lactogenesis is well documented. Suppression of prolactin secretion by bromocriptine in ewes 1 week *ante partum* causes the onset of lactation to be completely abolished or delayed (Kann *et al.*, 1978). Similar data were obtained in cows (Schams, 1976). Contrarily, treatment with thyroid hormone releasing hormone (THRH) before parturition increased the milk yield (Schams, 1976). In women, as in ewes and cows, the onset of lactation is abolished when prolactin secretion is suppressed by bromocriptine immediately after delivery. However, partial inhibition of prolactin secretion as obtained by ergot alkaloids other than bromocriptine (ergobasine maleate; Perez-Lopez *et al.*, 1975) does not alter the lactation performance in women (Jolivet *et al.*, 1978). Thus, if prolactin appears to be essential for lactogenesis in women, major hyperprolactinaemia is not a prerequisite.

Maintenance of an established lactation or galactopoeisis, as with lactogenesis, is controlled by an interplay of several hormones: prolactin, growth hormone, corticoids, thyroid hormones and insulin. The relative importance of these hormones in such a control varies from one species to another. In addition, the mechanical stimulation of the breast (or teat) is of decisive importance in the maintenenace of established lactation. In some species, such as cows (Schams, 1976) and goats (Hart, 1973), the mechanical stimulation of the gland seems to be the dominating factor. Maintenance of milk secretion is observed with very low levels of circulating prolactin: inhibition of prolactin secretion by bromocriptine does not affect the milk yield much in cows and goats. In some other species, such as sheep, rats, pigs, rabbits, dogs and humans (Billeter and Flückiger, 1968; Shaar and Clemens, 1972; Flückiger, 1972; del Pozo and Flückiger, 1973; Kann *et al.*, 1978; Hooley *et al.*, 1978), inhibition of prolactin secretion by bromocriptine significantly suppresses galactopoiesis. However, even in women, significant hyperprolactinaemia is not necessary for maintenance of milk secretion. In a population of mothers from Kivu (Zaïre) nursing for more than 2 years, serum prolactin levels are within the normal range for non-pregnant and non-lactating women from the same region; but, they still produce an average of 300 ml of milk per day (Ph. Hennart *et al.*, in preparation). It is also known that galactorrhoea can occur in women with normal circulating levels of prolactin. Treatment with bromocriptine would suppress such pathological lactation in most of the cases. It is quite likely that the threshold level of circulating prolactin required for maintaining milk secretion varies according to the balance of all other hormones involved; oestrogens, corticoids, thyroid hormones and growth hormone.

Blocking prolactin release, which would normally occur in response to suckling, does not influence the amount of milk synthesized during the subsequent 8 h (Grosvenor and Mena, 1973) but greatly reduces the amount of prolactin which reaccumulates during the 8 h interval following the next suckling episode, even when the prolactin release is not suppressed during this second suckling episode (Grosvenor and Mena, 1973). Thus, there is a rather long time lag between the suckling-induced release of prolactin and its galactopoietic effect. It is conceivable that such a time lag is conditioned by a phasing effect of other hormones (corticosteroids) on prolactin responsiveness (Nicoll, 1973). The attempts to improve lactation by the use of drugs which stimulate prolactin secretion (THRH or neuroleptics) were disappointing in animals (Kelly *et al.*, 1973; Convey *et al.*, 1973; Schams, 1976) or contradictory in women. Tyson *et al.* (1976) reported positive results with THRH in mothers with lactational insufficiency, while Zarate *et al.* (1972) reported negative results using the same drug.

Experiments conducted to restore milk secretion in hypophysectomized ruminants revealed the importance of growth hormone in the control of galacto-poeisis. Prolactin in the absence of growth hormone, and growth hormone in the absence of prolactin, both exert only minor effects in the maintenance of milk secretion in hypophysectomized goats. Only the combination of the two hormones exerts major effects (Cowie, 1966; Cowie and Tindal, 1971). In man, however, dwarfs with isolated growth hormone deficiency were reported to be able to breastfeed their babies normally (Rimoin et al., 1968).

Breast Development and Cancer

In women from industrialized countries, the development of the breast is characterized by a rather long time lag, several years, between puberty and com-plete growth and differentiation of the mammary epithelium resulting from the first pregnancy. This is in sharp contrast with the development of the breast in developing countries, where the first pregnancy almost immediately follows puberty. McMahon et al. (1973) reported that women who are delivered of their first child before the age of 18 have about one-third the breast cancer risk of those whose first delivery is delayed until age 35 or older. Protection is exerted only by the first full-term pregnancy. Subsequent births even at an early maternal age do not convey additional protection. Therefore, it seems that complete growth and differentiation of the mammary epithelium, occurring soon after puberty as a result of the first pregnancy, protects the mammary epithelium against carcino-genic factors. The greater incidence of breast cancer in industrialized countries as compared to developing countries may be related, at least partly, to a longer time lag between puberty and the first pregnancy. A more complete study of the endocrine factors involved in such a protective effect of the first pregnancy is essential before investigating whether significant prevention of breast cancer can be obtained with an adequate prophylactic endocrine treatment.

LACTOGENIC HORMONES DURING PREGNANCY

In man there are three lactogenic hormones: growth hormone, prolactin, and human chorionic somatomammotrophin (or human placental lactogen) (hCS or hPL). Various molecular forms of growth hormone have been described; some exerting much more lactogenic activity than others (Lewis et al., 1976).

Maternal Compartment

Circulating levels of prolactin increase progressively during pregnancy (Hwang et al., 1971; Friesen et al., 1972; L'Hermite and Robyn, 1972; Daughaday and Jacobs, 1972; Rigg et al., 1977). At term they are some 10 times higher than before pregnancy. This results from the stimulation of the lactotrophs by the massive amounts of oestrogens produced by the fetoplacental unit during preg-nancy. Actually in most mammals (rat, sheep, Rhesus monkey), circulating levels of prolactin rise only during late gestation and sometimes only just before delivery; in these species massive oestrogen production does not occur before the terminal stage of gestation (Morishige *et al.*, 1973; Davis *et al.*, 1971; Weiss *et al.*, 1976).

Oestrogens exert three distinct effects on the lactotrophs. They stimulate prolactin release by antagonizing the inhibitory influence of dopamine at the level of the lactotrophs, as shown by *in vitro* and *in vivo* experiments (Labrie *et al.*, 1978; Ferland and Beaulieu, 1979). Oestrogens increase the synthesis of prolactin and also have a strong mitogenic effect on the lactotrophs (Jacobi *et al.*, 1977). In women, during pregnancy, the weight of the pituitary gland increases by some 50% (Romeis, 1940). This is mostly due to hyperplasia and hypertrophy of the lactotrophs. That both the release and the pituitary reserve of prolactin are increased during pregnancy is shown by the prolactin response to TRH and dopamine antagonists: the maximum value is much higher, but the relative increase in circulating levels of prolactin is much less, than in non-pregnant women (L'Hermite *et al.*, 1975; Guitelman and Aparicio, 1978).

During late gestation, circadian variations in serum prolactin levels are blunted: the nocturnal peak is of very small amplitude (Robyn *et al.*, 1976).

During parturition, multiphasic changes in prolactin secretion occur (Rigg and Yen, 1977). There is a highly significant decline in circulating levels of prolactin during labour with a maximum about 2 h prior to delivery. Immediately after delivery, a surge of prolactin takes place, with peak levels in serum prolactin within 2 hours *post partum*. Thereafter, prolactin levels fall, reaching a second minimum about 9 h *post partum*. This low level is maintained for 9-24 h. These changes in circulating levels of prolactin are not correlated with changes in concentrations of adrenal or sex steroids. These levels are also unaffected by narcotic analgesic agents or anaesthesia.

No significant changes in circulating levels of prolactin were observed in patients with pathological pregnancies such as pre-eclamptic toxaemia, latent diabetes or premature rupture of the membranes (Sadovsky *et al.*, 1977). Thus, serum prolactin determinations are of no diagnostic value in pathological pregnancies.

Fetal Compartment

Pasteels (1962) detected prolactin by bioassay in cultures of human fetal pituitary glands from fetuses of 5 months. This was confirmed by Silder-Khodr *et al.* (1974), who demonstrated immunoreactive prolactin in culture media of human fetal pituitaries from 5 weeks of gestation until term. The prolactin content of the pituitary gland is low (2 ng/gland) before 115 days. A marked increase to some 1000 ng/gland occurs between 115 and 170 days. Thereafter, no further significant increase is observed (Aubert *et al.*, 1976). The sex of the fetus does not influence the prolactin content of the pituitary.

Serum prolactin is low (20 ng/ml) before 30 weeks of gestation. Then a striking increase takes place: between 30 weeks and term the levels are around 200 ng/ml (Aubert *et al.*, 1976). Badawi *et al.* (1978) reported a progressive increase in circulating levels of prolactin with birthweight from 1048 μIU/ml between 1500 and 1999 g to 1707 μIU/ml between 3500 and 4499 g. There is no significant difference in serum prolactin levels between boys and girls, at the time of delivery (Badawi *et al.*, 1978).

Pituitary prolactin levels are strongly correlated with pituitary growth hormone levels, whereas there is a negative correlation between the serum concentrations of these two hormones (Aubert *et al.*, 1976).

Significant changes in cord serum prolactin levels are found according to the time of the day when the delivery takes place: the highest values are seen between midnight and 04.00. Thus, circadian variation in serum prolactin concentration seems to occur in the neonate without any relationship to sleep (Badawi *et al.*, 1978).

After birth, serum prolactin levels decrease within 1 week to some 30% of their values at the time of delivery. The decline is then slower: at 6 weeks the values are low, as they are during all the prepubertal period (Aubert *et al.*, 1976). The hyperprolactinaemia is more prolonged after birth in pre-term infants than in full-term infants (Perlman *et al.*, 1978).

The increase in circulating levels of oestrogens in the fetus, as reported by Schutt *et al.* (1974), may be a factor controlling fetal hyperprolactinaemia. However, as reported by Martin-Comin and Robyn (1976), there is no major hyperplasia of the pituitary lactotrophs in the fetal pituitary gland. Hyperprolactinaemia is also reported in anencephalic infants (Aubert *et al.*, 1976; Martin-Comin and Robyn, 1976). In most anencephalics, there is a pituitary gland, but no hypothalamus. Thus, it may be postulated that, in late pregnancy and during the first weeks of life, the dopamine inhibitory mechanism controlling prolactin secretion is not completely mature. This is supported by the relatively very small amplitude of the prolactin response to THRH seen in newborn infants (Hiba *et al.*, 1977).

The fall in serum prolactin levels between 2 and 12 weeks of postnatal age in full-term infants, and between 2 and 20 weeks in pre-term infants, may also result from the maturation of the hypothalamic inhibitory control of prolactin secretion. Such maturation is related to postconceptual age and not to postnatal age.

The mechanism inducing milk secretion in newborn children (witch's milk) was studied by Hiba *et al.* (1977). As with milk secretion in their mothers, the onset of milk secretion in neonates coincides with the disappearance of sex steroids from their plasma and elevated plasma prolactin concentration.

The heterogeneity of prolactin molecules in cord serum is similar to that of prolactin molecules in serum of adults (Lopez del Campo and Robyn, 1976), with a possible additional component in the range of "little" prolactin.

Amniotic fluid, at least in primates, contains enormous amounts of prolactin (Friesen *et al.*, 1972); 5–10 times more than maternal and fetal serum (Badawi *et al.*, 1973; Biswas, 1976). There is no correlation between amniotic fluid and maternal plasma levels of prolactin (Biswas, 1976). Somatomedin receptor activity, growth hormone and prolactin reach high levels in amniotic fluid during early gestation: after 26 weeks, all three hormones decrease in concentration (Chochinov *et al.*, 1976). This decrease is correlated with fetal renal maturation.

Radioactive iodine-labelled human pituitary prolactin injected intravenously into the pregnant monkey during the last trimester of gestation is transferred into the amniotic fluid (Josimovich *et al.*, 1974); no passage into the amniotic fluid was detected after injection of radiolabelled prolactin into the fetal circulation. The disappearance rate of prolactin from the amniotic fluid is extremely slow (Friesen *et al.*, 1972). Replacement of some 80% of the amniotic fluid in the monkey results in an immediate fall in amniotic prolactin levels. This is followed by a sharp increase within 20 min (Josimovich, 1976): thereafter the return to normal pre-existing levels is slower.

Friesen *et al.* (1972) reported that explants of chorionic tissue released small amounts of prolactin during a 24 h culture. Explants of chorion-decidual tissue obtained at delivery from normal full-term pregnancies synthesize and secrete prolactin (Golander *et al.*, 1978). This hormone is indistinguishable from pituitary prolactin by chromatographic, electrophoretic, immunologic and receptor assay techniques. Riddick and Kusmik (1977) observed that decidua, and not amnion or chorion, contains significant amounts of prolactin. The amount of prolactin released by the decidual tissue during incubation exceeds by far the initial tissue content. Riddick *et al.* (1978) extended this observation by showing that when preventing *in vitro* protein synthesis by adding cycloheximide to the medium, 90% of the prolactin present in the tissue was released within 3 h. Thereafter, no additional prolactin accumulated either in the medium or the tissue. When ^{3}H-labelled leucine is supplied during incubation, radioactive proteins are detected in the medium at 24 h: 14–20% are specifically precipitated by antiserum to human pituitary prolactin. All these data suggest that the decidua may be the source of the large quantities of prolactin in the amniotic fluid.

Maslar and Riddick (1979) recently reported that immunoreactive prolactin is synthesised and released *in vitro* by the decidualized endometrium of early intra-uterine and even tubal pregnancies. Therefore, this process does not depend upon the presence of intrauterine trophoblastic tissue. All these observations open new ways to the understanding of the role of decidual tissue in reproduction.

There is evidence that prolactin regulates fluid and electrolyte movements through the amniotic epithelium. Manku *et al.* (1976) observed that ovine prolactin hastens the passage of water from fetal to maternal side of guinea-pig amnion. Similarly, an excess of prolactin in the amniotic fluid of the pregnant Rhesus monkey causes some 50% reduction in amniotic fluid within 2 h. It also seems that large amounts of prolactin in the amniotic fluid protect the primate fetus, at least during the last trimester of pregnancy, from sudden changes in fetal extracellular fluid and electrolytes in the face of altered amniotic fluid tonicities (Josimovich, 1976).

Prolonged bromocriptine treatment of the ovine fetus results in decreased fetal growth and in lower birthweight than in controls (Takahashi *et al.*, 1979). These preliminary data suggest that prolactin may play a role in normal ovine fetal growth.

PROLACTIN SECRETION DURING LACTATION

Effects of Suckling

Suckling is at the origin of a neuroendocrine reflex of vital importance in mammals. It actively contributes to maintain lactation and promote prolonged lactational infertility. Nerve endings responsible for this neuroendocrine reflex are concentrated in the nipple or teats. Breast stimulation outside the nipple area is ineffective (Noel *et al.*, 1974). The neuroendocrine reflex is suppressed after anaesthesia of the nipple by a bland ointment of xylocaine or in women with transplanted nipples resulting from mammoplasty (Tyson *et al.*, 1976).

The suckling stimulus causes a rapid and marked rise in circulating levels of prolactin in rats (Grosvenor *et al.* 1965), cows (Johke, 1969), ewes (Fell *et al.*, 1972, goats (Johke, 1970), mice (Sela and Fuchs, 1979) and women (Hwang *et al.*, 1971) with a parallel release of oxytocin (Folley and Knaggs, 1966; Coch *et al.*, 1968). However, there may be a distinct mechanism for each of the two hormonal releases since suckling of an anaesthetized nipple blunts the prolactin release but not the milk ejection from the contralateral non-anaesthetized breast (Tyson *et al.*, 1976). Prolactin and oxytocin are also released when teats are stimulated without milk withdrawal (Schams, 1976).

The milk ejection reflex is not essential for removal of milk in some species such as goats, sheep and cows (Cowie and Tindal, 1971; Schans, 1976). It seems that oxytocin does not stimulate prolactin secretion. In rats, oxytocin injection through an atrial cannula does not change prolactin secretion (Shani *et al.*, 1976). This is in contrast to arginine and vasotocin, which, both *in vitro* and *in vivo*, stimulate prolactin secretion. There is no correlation between prolactin and oxytocin surges during suckling (Burnet and Wakerley, 1976). In urethane-anaesthetized rats, the threshold stimulus for the suckling-induced oxytocin release is different from the threshold for the release of prolactin (Wakerley *et al.*, 1978). Oxytocin may be released without prolactin during suckling, but the reverse does not occur. Thus, some of the factors associated with oxytocin release could be essential for triggering prolactin release. This is confirmed by the observation that, in animals responding to suckling by both oxytocin and prolactin releases, there is a linear relationship between the amplitudes of the two endocrine responses (Wakerley *et al.*, 1978). The releases of prolactin and oxytocin are inversely related to the intensity of the preceding suckling stimulus (Wakerley *et al.*, 1978). Suckling is associated with either a small rise or no change in circulating levels of TSH (Grosvenor, 1964; Sar and Meites, 1969; Blake, 1974). In cows, during maximal stimulation with THRH, milking causes a further prolactin rise (Vines *et al.*, 1976). These observations do not support the idea that the prolactin response to suckling is mediated by THRH (Meites, 1973; Jeppson *et al.*, 1976). There is increasing evidence that serotonin is an important mediator in suckling-induced prolactin secretion. Suckling depletes hypothalamic serotonin and increases the hypothalamic levels of its metabolite, 5-hydroxyindoleacetic acid (Mena *et al.*, 1976). Blockade of serotonin secretion or action has little effect on basal levels of circulating prolactin but prevents prolactin release in response to suckling (Enjalbert *et al.*, 1978). Suckling-induced prolactin release seems, therefore, to be mediated by activation of a serotoninergic pathway terminating in the hypothalamus (Enjalbert *et al.*, 1978). Serotonin can be assumed to sensitize the hypothalamus to the prolactin releasing effect of suckling. The median forebrain bundle contains most of the serotoninergic ascending projections. The bundle of Schutz seems to transit the specific triggering signal resulting from mammary stimulation (Enjalbert *et al.*, 1978). It is well documented that serotonin is a prolactin releaser. However, as shown by *in vitro* experiments, these effects, in contrast to those of dopamine, are not exerted directly at the level of the lactotrophs (McLeod and Lamberts, 1978).

In monkeys, elevation of serum prolactin is blocked by bromocriptine or apomorphine. Both drugs are potent dopamine antagonists (Gala *et al.*, 1976). There are contradictory data on the possible role of dopamine itself in the stimulation of prolactin secretion during nursing. The dopamine content in hypophysial blood has been shown to be reduced in lactating rats just after delivery and to increase, but only slightly, when the pups are removed from their mother (Ben Jonathan *et al.*, 1978). Dopamine concentration in stalk plasma first progressively decreases during electric stimulation of a mammary nerve trunk but then increases after the end of stimulation (Plotsky *et al.*, 1979). Furthermore, dopamine turnover in the tubero-infundibular region of the hypothalamus is markedly increased during lactation, as in all other hyperprolactinaemic states (Fuxe and Hökfelt, 1975). Such activation of dopamine turn-over in the median eminence is considered to be a mechanism by which prolactin inhibits its own secretion (Fuxe *et al.*, 1978; McLeod and Robyn, 1977). However, this mechanism cannot account for transient, or more permanent, hyperprolactinaemia during lactation. Another explanation would be that nursing stimulates the release of a prolactin releasing factor different from THRH: this may even act by antagonizing dopamine effects at the pituitary level. Such a prolactin releasing factor with direct effects at the pituitary level has been found in serum of women with non-tumoural hyperprolactinaemia (Garthwaite and Hagen, 1978).

Prolactin release induced by suckling depends on the duration of the stimulation: prolonged teat stimulation results in refractoriness to the neuroendocrine pathway. The time interval for optimal stimulation of prolactin release appears to be 2 h (Schams, 1976). The amplitude of prolactin release caused by suckling decreases with the stage of lactation in all species tested: cows (Koprowski and Tucker, 1973), goats (Hart, 1975) and women (Noel *et al.*, 1974). In Caucasian populations, the prolactin response to suckling was reported to be barely significant after 3 months *post partum* (Tyson *et al.*, 1972). In Central Africa, where mothers nurse for more than 2 years, the prolactin response to suckling is quickly blunted during the first year *post partum*. However, during the second year the increase of circulating prolactin levels in response to suckling is relatively greater than during the first year, the basal levels being relatively lower. During the first year *post partum* the release of prolactin by the lactotrophs is almost maximal: THRH does not increase the already high basal levels of serum prolactin (Delvoye *et al.*, 1978a). During the second year of lactation, the hypothalamic inhibition progressively recurs: basal levels of serum prolactin are lower and THRH is again as effective as suckling in raising these levels.

In addition to suckling, exteroceptive stimuli can also release prolactin in lactating mammals. When lactating rats are separated from their litters for 10 h, prolactin accumulates in their pituitary glands. When the pups are with their mothers again, the concentration of prolactin in the pituitary glands falls. When the pups are prevented from suckling by means of a wire screen, the fall in pituitary prolactin concentration is the same as that induced by nursing (Grosvenor, 1965). Terkel *et al.* (1978) reported that ultrasonic vocalizations of infant rats specifically stimulate prolactin release in lactating females. This is the first report on a naturally occurring communication that involves the release of an anterior pituitary hormone.

Lactational Hyperprolactinaemia

In mammals, basal levels of serum prolactin remain high during the lactation period: they decline very rapidly when the young are removed or after weaning (Terkel *et al.*, 1978; Bevers *et al.*, 1978; Concannon *et al.*, 1978). In most species, suckling by the infants is almost permanent, at least during the first stage of lactation. In non-lactating mothers, serum basal prolactin levels decrease very rapidly after delivery: they return to pre-pregnancy levels within 7–15 days (Tyson *et al.*, 1972).

In women too, hyperprolactinaemia persists during lactation. This was first observed during a few weeks in Caucasian populations where lactation is of very short duration (Tyson *et al.*, 1976; Rolland *et al.*, 1975). Delvoye *et al.* (1976, 1977a) reported that in Central Africa, long-lasting lactation is associated with persistent hyperprolactinaemia. Mothers nursing for 2 years or more remain hyperprolactinaemic during the first 15–18 months *post partum*: thereafter, basal levels of serum prolactin progressively decline to reach pre-pregnancy levels after 21 months *post partum*. Bunner *et al.* (1978) confirmed this observation in Californian mothers nursing for 1 year.

In women, maintenance of permanent hyperprolactinaemia is directly related to the number of suckling episodes per day. When mothers give the breast more than six times per day, basal levels of serum prolactin remain high for more than 1 year (Delvoye *et al.*, 1977c). When mothers give the breast less than six times per day their serum prolactin levels rapidly return to the range of values seen in non-lactating and non-pregnant women. Thus, persistence of hyperprolactinaemia during lactation requires that mothers breastfeed their baby on demand, i.e. the baby, being always with the mother, has free access to the breast. In Kivu (Central Africa), the average number of feedings per day is 13. This is in contrast with a maximum of six in industrialized countries (Vis and Hennart, 1978).

It is not yet established how long the hyperplasia of the lactotrophs, as seen during pregnancy, persists during lactation. As early as a few weeks after delivery, the maximum serum prolactin levels obtained after THRH are much lower than those obtained during pregnancy and almost equivalent to those obtained in non-pregnant and non-lactating women.

Prolonged lactational hyperprolactinaemia is associated with amenorrhoea (Delvoye *et al.*, 1977a, 1978b), with anovulatory cycles and with luteal insufficiency (Delvoye *et al.*, 1978b). Pathological hyperprolactinaemia (pituitary adenoma or inadequate dopaminergic inhibition) and pharmacological hyperprolactinaemia are also associated with amenorrhoea, anovulation and infertility (Robyn *et al.*, 1976). Lactation is associated with similar infertility in non-human primates too (Altmann *et al.*, 1978).

It is established that prolactin interferes, at the hypothalamic and at the ovarian level, with the mechanisms regulating ovulation and corpus luteum function (for a review, *see* Robyn *et al.*, 1976). Thus, infertility associated with prolonged lactation is likely similar to that associated with the other two types of hyperprolactinaemia. Furthermore, Delvoye *et al.* (1978b) reported that the endocrine pattern of lactational hyperprolactinaemia is very similar to that of both pathological and pharmacological hyperprolactinaemia: basal levels of serum follicle stimulating hormone (FSH) are moderately elevated as during the early follicular phase of a normal cycle and the FSH response to luteinizing hormone releasing hormone (LHRH) is excessive, the positive feedback of oestrogen on luteinizing hormone (LH) secretion is suppressed, basal levels of serum oestradiol are low, and basal levels of serum LH are normal (within the range of values seen during the follicular phase of a normal cycle).

However, it remains to be clarified to what extent malnutrition of mothers who are lactating for a long time, as in Africa and in other developing countries, contributes to lactational infertility. Indeed, in countries where lactation is of long duration, proteocaloric malnutrition is often endemic. Lactation even more than gestation is an energy-demanding process: additional energy is required for synthesis of milk by the mother and for its digestion and resorption by the child. It seems that the newborn baby has priority over its mother for the satisfaction of its energy demand and thus the mother may lose weight as lactation proceeds while the baby continues to grow (Smith, 1947; Rao and Rao, 1974; Crawford and Hall, 1975). In Central Africa, Delvoye *et al.* (1978a) did not observe any significant difference in body weight and in serum albumin levels between amenor-rhoeic and non-amenorrhoeic nursing mothers during the two first years *post partum*. It would be of great interest to investigate the consequence of the endo-crine changes resulting from lactation and particularly of prolactin on the energy balance of the mother.

Another factor that may influence fertility during lactation is suckling itself. Indeed, during early lactation in rats, the suckling stimulus more than prolactin contributes to the suppression of the postcastration rise in LH, but not in FSH (Smith, 1978). Only during the later part of lactation does the inhibition of prolactin lead to maximum postcastration response and the administration of exogenous prolactin completely prevent any increase in LH and FSH after ovari-ectomy. Thus, at that time, prolactin alone accounts for the decrease in gonado-trophin secretion. In addition, Smith (1978) reported that, at least in this experi-mental model, the suckling stimulus is permissive to the action of prolactin in suppressing gonadotrophin secretion.

Significant amounts of prolactin are excreted by the mammary gland and found in the milk of rats (McMurtry and Malven, 1974; Grosvenor and Withworth, 1976), goats, sheep (Malven and McMurtry, 1974) and women (Gala *et al.*, 1975).

Immunohistochemical demonstration of prolactin in the alveolar lumen and in apical region of epithelial cells in lactating mammary gland was reported by Nolin and Witorsch (1976). Infusion of prolactin is followed by considerable increase in milk concentration of prolactin. Prolactin is sequestered in milk for several hours. Thus, at least in rats, the offspring consumes significant amounts of maternal prolactin during each nursing period. Radioiodinated prolactin is found in the plasma of 9–14 day old rats after being nursed by mothers previously injected with radioiodinated prolactin (Whitworth and Grosvenor, 1978). Such transfer through the gastrointestinal mucosa also occurs when radioiodinated rat prolactin is given to the pups by gastric incubation: some 16% of the radioiodinated prolactin is found in the plasma of the offspring. Such transfer of prolactin from the mother's milk to the circulation of the young does not take place in 23 day old rats: the capacity for intestinal resorption of this protein hormone is associated with the stage of neonatal development during which the intestine is permeable to large molecules, even much larger than prolactin (Halliday, 1955; Clarke and Hardy, 1969). The immunoreactivity of prolactin transferred to pups with the milk is similar to that of the native hormone. Also, extensive degradation of the hormone upon entering milk is not observed in chromatographic studies: milk prolactin in women consists of a single component similar to "little" prolactin, the predomi-nent molecular form in serum (Gala and van de Walle, 1977). Nothing is known yet concerning the biological integrity of milk prolactin and of that of prolactin after absorption into the circulation of the young. However, this is essential before considering more extensively the physiological significance of such transfer of maternal prolactin to the young, via milk ingestion.

Circulating levels of prolactin are very labile (Robyn *et al.*, 1976). Most commonly, emphasis is put on variation in the secretion rate of that hormone under hypothalamic influence. But, one should consider that the half-life of circulating prolactin is very short, 15–20 min in man. In rats, the metabolic clearance rate of prolactin, as assessed by continuous infusion to equilibrium, increases as the infusion rate increases (Grosvenor *et al.*, 1977). This implies that plasma prolactin concentration does not necessarily mirror the rate of prolactin secretion from the lactotrophs. The metabolic clearance rate is slightly higher in lactating rats than in non-lactating rats (Grosvenor *et al.*, 1977). These data confirm the observation by Kwa *et al.* (1970) that bovine prolactin disappears from plasma of rats more rapidly when higher doses of that hormone were administered or when the animal was hyperprolactinaemic. An explanation might be that prolactin stimulates cardiac output. Indeed, in lactating rats, the cardiac output is higher than in non-lactating rats (Chatwin *et al.*, 1969; Hanwell and Linzell, 1973). This effect of lactation can be mimicked by injection of ovine prolactin (Hanwell and Linzell, 1972). Thus the increase of metabolic clearance rate in response to higher levels of the hormone in the circulation may result from the increased blood flow induced by prolactin itself (Grosvenor *et al.*, 1977). An alternative explanation is that the circulating levels of prolactin alter the clearance of prolactin in various organs directly.

REFERENCES

Altmann, J., Altmann, S. A. and Hausfater, G. (1978). *Science, New York* **201**, 1028.

Assairi, L., Delouis, C., Gaye, P., Houbedine, L. M., Ollivier-Bousquet, M. and Denamur, R. (1974). *Biochemical Journal* **144**, 245.

Aubert, M. L., Sizonenko, P. C., Kaplan, S. L. and Grumbach, M. M. (1976). *In* "Prolactin and Human Reproduction" (P. G. Crosignani and C. Robyn, eds), pp. 9–20, Academic Press, London and New York.

Badawi, M., Perez-Lopez, F. R. and Robyn, C. (1973). *Acta endocrinologia, Copenhagen* Suppl. 177, 237.

Badawi, M., Van Exter, C., Delogne-Desnoeck, J., Van Meenen, F. and Robyn, C. (1978). *Acta endocrinologia, Copenhagen* **87**, 241.

Ben Jonathan, N., Neill, M. A., Arbogast, L. A., Peters, L. L. and Hoefer, M. T. (1978). Paper presented at the 60th annual Endocrine Society Meeting (abstract no. 238).

Bevers, M. M., Willemse, A. H. and Kruip, T. A. M. (1978). *Biology of Reproduction* **19**, 628.

Billeter, E. and Flückiger, E. (1968). *Experientia* **27**, 464.

Biswas, S. (1976). *Clinica chimica acta* **73**, 363.

Blake, C. A. (1974). *Endocrinology* **94**, 503.

Bunner, D. L., Vanderlaan, E. E. and Vanderlaan, W. P. (1978). *American Journal of Obstetrics and Gynecology* **131**, 250.

Burnet, F. R. and Wakerley, J. B. (1976). *Journal of Endocrinology* **70**, 429.

Chamness, G. C., Costlow, M. E. and McGuire, W. L. (1975). *Steroids* **26**, 363.

Chatwin, A. L., Linzell, J. L. and Setchell, B. P. (1969). *Journal of Endocrinology* **44**, 247.

Chochinov, R. H., Ketupanya, A., Mariz, I. K., Underwood, L. E. and Daughaday, W. H. (1976). *Journal of Clinical Endocrinology and Metabolism* **42**, 983.

Clarke, R. M. and Hardy, R. N. (1969). *Journal of Physiology, London* **204**, 113.

Coch, J., Fielitz, C., Brovetto, J., Cabot, H. M., Coda, H. and Fraga, A. (1968). *Journal of Endocrinology* **40**, 137.

Concannon, P. W., Butler, W. R., Hansel, W., Knight, P. J. and Hamilton, J. M. (1978). *Biology of Reproduction* **19**, 1113.

Convey, E. M., Thomas, J. W., Tucker, H. A. and Gill, J. L. (1973). *Journal of Dairy Science* **56**, 484.

Cowie, A. T. (1966). *In* "The Pituitary Gland" (G. W. Harris and B. T. Donovan, eds), Vol. 2, pp. 412–443. Butterworth, London.

Cowie, A. T. and Tindal, J. S. (1971). *In* "Monographs of the Physiological Society" (H. Dawson, A. D. M. Greefiled, R. Whittam and G. S. Brindley, eds), Vol. 22, p. 105. Edward Arnold, London.

Crawford, M. A. and Hall, B. (1975). *British Medical Journal iii*, 232.

Daughaday, W. H. and Jacobs, L. S. (1972). *In* "Ergebnisse der Physiologie", Vol. 67, pp. 169–194, Springer Verlag, Berlin.

Davis, S. L., Reichert, L. E. and Niswender, G. D. (1971). *Biology of Reproduction* **4**, 145.

del Pozo, E. and Flückiger, E. (1973). *In* "Human Prolactin" (J. L. Pasteels and C. Robyn, eds), International Congress Series No. 308, pp. 291–301, Excerpta Medica, Amsterdam.

Delvoye, P., Desnoeck-Delogne, J. and Robyn, C. (1976). *Lancet ii*, 288.

Delvoye, P., Badawi, M., Demaegd, M. and Robyn, C. (1977a). *In* "Progress in Prolactin Physiology and Pathology" (C. Robyn and M. Harter, eds), pp. 213–232, Elsevier/North Holland Biomedical Press, Amsterdam.

Delvoye, P., Delogne-Desnoeck, J., Uwaytu-Nyampeta and Robyn, C. (1977b). *Clinical Endocrinology* **7**, 257.

Delvoye, P., Demaegd, M., Delogne-Desnoeck, J. and Robyn, C. (1977c). *Journal of Biosocial Science* **9**, 447.

Delvoye, P., Demaegd, M., Uwayitu-Nyampeta and Robyn, C. (1978a). *American Journal of Obstetrics and Gynecology* **130**, 635.

Delvoye, P., Delogne-Desnoeck, J. and Robyn, C. (1978b). *American Journal of Obstetrics and Gynecology* in press.

Enjalbert, A., Ruberg, M. and Kordon, C. (1978). *In* "Progress in Prolactin Physiology and Pathology" (C. Robyn and M. Harter, eds), pp. 83–94. Elsevier/North Holland Biomedical Press, Amsterdam.

Erb, R. E., Malven, P. V., Monk, E. L., Mollett, T. A., Smith, K. L., Schanbacher, F. L. and Willett, L. B. (1976). *Journal of Dairy Science* **59**, 1420.

Fell, L. R., Beck, C., Brown, J. M., Cumming, I. A. and Goding, J. R. (1972). *Journal of Reproduction and Fertility* **28**, 133.

Ferland, L. and Beaulieu, M. (1979). Paper presented at the 61st Annual Society Meeting (abstract no. 873).

Flaxman, B. A., Dyckman, J. and Feldman, A. (1976). *In vitro* **12**, 467.

Flückiger, E. (1972). *In* "Prolactin and Carcinogenesis" (A. R. Boyns and K. Griffiths, eds), pp. 162–171, Alpha Omega Alpha Publishing, Cardiff.

Folley, S. J. and Knaggs, G. S. (1966). *Journal of Endocrinology* **34**, 197.

Friesen, H., Hwang, P., Guyda, H., Tolis, G., Tyson, J. and Myers, R. (1972). *In* "Prolactin and Carcinogenesis" (A. R. Boyns and K. Griffiths, eds), pp. 64–97, Alpha Omega Alpha Publishing, Cardiff.

Fulkerson, W. J. and McDowell, G. H. (1975). *Australian Journal of Biological Science* **28**, 521.

Fulkerson, W. J., Hooley, R. D., McDowell, G. H. and Fell, L. R. (1976). *Australian Journal of Biological Science* **29**, 357.

Fuxe, K. and Hökfelt, T. (1975). *In* "Some Aspects of Hypothalamic Regulation of Endocrine Functions", Symposia Medica Hoechst 7, pp. 51–61, F. K. Schattauer Verlag, Stuttgart.

Fuxe, K., Andersson, K., Hökfelt, T., Agnati, L. F., Ogren, S. O., Eneroth, P., Gustafsson, J. A. and Skett, P. (1978). *In* "Progress in Prolactin Physiology and Pathology" (C. Robyn and M. Harter, eds), pp. 95–109, Elsevier/North Holland Biomedical Press, Amsterdam.

Gala, R. R. and van de Walle, C. (1977). *Life Sciences* **21**, 99.

Gala, R. R., Singhakowinta, A. and Brennan, M. J. (1975). *Hormone Research* **6**, 310.

Gala, R. R., Subramanian, M. G., Peters, J. A. and Jacques, S. (1976). *Experientia* **32**, 941.

Garthwaite, T. L. and Hagen, T. C. (1978). *Journal of Clinical Endocrinology and Metabolism* **47**, 4.

Golander, A., Hurlet, T., Barrett, J., Hizi, A. and Handwerger, S. (1978). *Science, New York 4365*, 311.

Grosvenor, C. E. (1964). *Endocrinology* **74**, 548.

Grosvenor, C. E. (1965). *Endocrinology* **76**, 340.

Grosvenor, C. E. and Mena, F. (1973). *Journal of Endocrinology* **70**, 1.

Grosvenor, C. E. and Whitworth, N. S. (1976). *Journal of Endocrinology* **70**, 1.

Grosvenor, C. E., McCann, S. M. and Nalbar, R. (1965). *Endocrinology* **76**, 883.

Grosvenor, C. E., Mena, F. and Whitworth, N. S. (1977). *Journal of Endocrinology* **73**, 1.

Guitelman, A. and Aparicio, N. J. (1978). *Fertility and Sterility* **29**, 26.

Halliday, R. (1955). *Proceedings of the Royal Society* **143**, 408.

Hanwell, A. and Linzell, J. L. (1972). *Journal of Endocrinology* **53**, IVII.

Hanwell, A. and Linzell, J. L. (1973). *Journal of Physiology, London* **233**, 93.

Hart, I. C. (1973). *Journal of Endocrinology* **57**, 179.

Hart, I. C. (1975). *Journal of Endocrinology* **64**, 1.

Hart, I. C. (1976). *Journal of Endocrinology* **71**, 412P.

Herrenkohl, L. R. and Campbell, C. (1976). *Hormonal and Behavior* **7**, 183.

Hiba, J., del Pozo, E., Genazzani, A., Pusterla, E., Lancranjan, I., Sidiropoulos, D. and Gunti, J. (1977). *Journal of Clinical Endocrinology and Metabolism* **44**, 973.

Hooley, R. D., Campbell, J. J. and Findlay, J. K. (1978). *Journal of Endocrinology* **79**, 301.

Horrobin, D. F. (ed.) (1977). "Prolactin 1977", Churchill Livingstone, Edinburgh.

Hwang, P., Guyda, H. and Friesen, H. (1971). *Proceedings of the National Academy of Sciences of the U.S.A.* **68**, 1902.

Jacobi, J., Lloyd, H. M. and Meares, J. D. (1977). *Journal of Endocrinology* **72**, 35.

Jeppson, S., Nilsson, K. O., Rannevik, G. and Wide, L. (1976). *Acta endocrinologia, Copenhagen* **82**, 246.

Johke, T. (1969). *Endocrinologia Japonica* **16**, 179.

Johke, T. (1970). *Endocrinoligia Japonica* **16**, 393.

Jolivet, A., Robyn, A., Huraux-Rendu, C. and Gautray, J. P. (1978). *Journal de gynécologie obstétrique et biologie de la reproduction* **7**, 129.

Josimovich, J. B. (1976). *In* "Prolactin and Human Reproduction" (P. G. Crosignani and C. Robyn, eds), pp. 27–36, Academic Press, London and New York.

Josimovich, J. B., Weiss, G. and Hutchinson, D. L. (1974). *Endocrinology* **94**, 1367.

Kann, G., Carpentier, M.-C., Feure, J., Martinet, J., Maubon, M., Meusnier, C., Paly, J. and Vermeire, N. (1978). *In* "Progress in Prolactin Physiology and Pathology (C. Robyn and M. Harter, eds), Elsevier/North Holland Biomedical Press, Amsterdam.

Kelly, P. A., Bedirian, K. N., Baker, R. R. D. and Friesen, H. G. (1973). *Endocrinology* **92**, 1289.

Koprowski, J. A. and Tucker, H. A. (1973). *Endocrinology* **93**, 645.

Kuhn, N. J. (1970). *In* "Lactation" (I. R. Falconer, ed.), p. 161, Butterworth, London.

Kwa, H. G., Feltkamp, C. A., Van der Gugten, A. A. and Verhofstad, F. (1970). *Journal of Endocrinology* **61**, 211.

Labrie, F. and Veilleux, R. (1979). Paper presented at the 61st Annual Endocrine Society Meeting (abstract no. 872).

Labrie, F., Beaulieu, M., Caron, M. G. and Raymond, V. (1978). *In* "Progress in Prolactin Physiology and Pathology" (C. Robyn and M. Harter, eds), pp. 21-136, Elsevier/North Holland Biomedical Press, Amsterdam.

Leung, B. S., Jack, W. M. and Reiney, C. G. (1976). *Journal of Steroid Biochemistry* **7**, 89.

Lewis, U. J., Singh, R. N. P., Peterson, S. M. and Vanderlaan, W. P. (1976). *In* "Growth Hormone and Related Peptides" (A. Pecile and E. E. Müller, eds), International Congress Series no. 381, pp. 64-74, Excerpta Medica, Amsterdam.

L'Hermite, M. and Robyn, C. (1972). *Annales d'endocrinologie* **33**, 357.

L'Hermite, M., Degueldre, M., Caufriez, A., Delvoye, P. and Robyn, C. (1975). *Pathologie Biologie* **23**, 769.

Libertum, C., Kaplan, S. E. and De Nicola, A. F. (1979). *Neuroendocrinology* **28**, 64.

Lopez del Campo, G. J. and Robyn, C. (1976). Paper presented at the Vth International Congress of Endocrinology, Hamburg (abstract no. 327).

McLeod, R. M. and Robyn, C. (1977). *Journal of Endocrinology* **72**, 273.

McLeod, R. M. and Lamberts, S. W. J. (1978). *In* "Progress in Prolactin Physiology and Pathology" (C. Robyn and M. Harter, eds), pp. 111-119, Elsevier/North Holland Biomedical Press, Amsterdam.

McMahon, B., Cole, P. and Brown, J. (1973). *Journal of the National Cancer Institute* **50**, 21.

McMurtry, J. P. and Malven, P. V. (1974). *Journal of Endocrinology* **61**, 211.

Malven, P. V. and McMurtry, J. P. (1974). *Journal of Dairy Science* **57**, 411.

Manku, M. S., Mtabaji, J. P. and Horrobin, D. F. (1976). *Journal of Endocrinology* **68**, 13P.

March, C. M., Marrs, R. P., Nakamura, R. M. and Mishell, D. R. (1979). Paper presented at the 61st Annual Endocrine Society Meeting (abstract no. 856).

Martin-Comin, J. and Robyn, C. (1976). *Journal of Histochemistry and Cytochemistry* **24**, 1012.

Maslar, I. A. and Riddick, D. H. (1979). Paper presented at the 61st Annual Society Meeting (abstract no. 349).

Matusik, R. J. and Rosen, J. M. (1978). *Journal of Biological Chemistry* **253**, 2343.

Matusik, R. J., Guyette, W. A. and Rosen, J. M. (1979). Paper presented at the 61st Annual Endocrine Society Meeting (abstract no. 173).

Meites, J. (1973). *In* "Human Prolactin" (J. L. Pasteels and C. Robyn, eds), International Congress Series no. 308, pp. 105-118, Excerpta Medica, Amsterdam.

Mena, F., Enjalbert, A., Carbonell, L., Priam, M. and Kordon, C. (1976). *Endocrinology* **99**, 445.

Morishige, W. K., Pepe, G. J. and Rothchild, I. (1973). *Endocrinology* **92**, 1527.

Neill, M. A., Abrogast, L. A., Peters, L. L. and Hoefer, M. T. (1978). Paper presented at the 60th Annual Endocrine Society Meeting (abstract no. 238).

Nicoll, C. S. (1973). *In* "Human Prolactin" (J. L. Pasteels and C. Robyn, eds), International Congress Series no. 308, pp. 119–136, Excerpta Medica, Amsterdam.

Noel, G. L., Suh, H. G. and Frantz, A. G. (1974). *Journal of Clinical Endocrinology and Metabolism* **38**, 413.

Nolin, J. M. and Witorsch, R. J. (1976). *Endocrinology* **99**, 949.

O'Malley, B. W. and Means, A. R. (1974). *Science, New York* **183**, 610.

Pasteels, J. L. (1962). *Comptes rendus hebdomadaires des séances de l'Académie des sciences* **254**, 4083.

Perez-Lopez, F. R., Delvoye, P., Denayer, P., Roncero, M. C. and Robyn, C. (1975). *Acta endocrinologia, Copenhagen* **79**, 644.

Perlman, M., Schenker, J., Glassman, M. and Ben-David, M. (1978). *Journal of Clinical Endocrinology and Metabolism* **47**, 894.

Plotsky, P. M., de Greef, W. J. and Neill, J. D. (1979). Paper presented at the 61st Annual Endocrine Society Meeting (abstract no. 449).

Rao, C. N. and Rao, B. S. N. (1974). *Indian Journal of Medical Research* **62**, 1619.

Riddick, D. H. and Kusmik, W. F. (1977). *American Journal of Obstetrics and Gynecology* **127**, 187.

Riddick, D. H., Luciano, A. A., Kusmik, W. E. and Maslar, I. A. (1978). *Life Sciences* **23**, 1913.

Rigg, L. A., Lein, A., Yen, S. S. C. (1977). *American Journal of Obstetrics and Gynecology* **129**, 454.

Rigg, L. A. and Yen, S. S. C. (1977). *American Journal of Obstetrics and Gynecology* **128**, 215.

Rimoin, D. L., Holzman, G. B., Merimee, T. J., Rabinowitz, D., Barnes, A. C., Tyson, J. E. A. and McKusick, V. A. (1968). *Journal of Clinical Endocrinology* **28**, 1183.

Robyn, C., Delvoye, P., Van Exter, C., Vekemans, M., Caufriez, A., Denayer, P., Delogne-Desnoeck, J. and L'Hermite, M. (1976). *In* "Prolactin and Human Reproduction" (P. G. Crosignani and C. Robyn, eds), pp. 71–96, Academic Press, London and New York.

Rolland, R., Lequin, R. M., Schellekens, L. A. and De Jong, F. H. (1975). *Clinical Endocrinology* **4**, 15.

Romeis, B. (1940). *In* "Handbuch der Mikroskopischen Anatomie des Menschen", Teil 3 (W. von Möllendorff, ed.), Verlag von Julius Springer, Berlin.

Sadovsky, E., Weinstein, D., Ben David, M. and Polishuk, W. Z. (1977). *Obstetrics and Gynecology* **50**, 559.

Salazar, H. and Tobon, H. (1974). *In* "Lactogenic Hormones, Fetal Nutrition and Lactation" (J. B. Josimovich, M. Reynolds and E. Cabo, eds), pp. 221–277, Wiley, New York.

Sar, M. and Meites, J. (1969). *Neuroendocrinology* **4**, 25.

Schams, D. (1976). *In* "Breast-feeding and the Mother", Ciba Foundation Symposium no. 45, pp. 27–43, Elsevier/North Holland, Amsterdam.

Schutt, D. A., Smith, L. D. and Shearman, R. P. (1974). *Journal of Endocrinology* **60**, 333.

Sela, H. and Fuchs, A. R. (1979). Paper presented at the 61st Endocrine Society Meeting (abstract no. 874).

Shaar, C. J. and Clemens, J. A. (1972). *Endocrinology* **90**, 285.

Shani, J., Urbach, L., Terkel, J. and Goldhaber, G. (1976). *Archives internationales de pharmacodynamie et de therapie* **221**, 323.

Siler-Khodr, T. M., Morgenstern, L. L. and Greenwood, F. C. (1974). *Journal of Clinical Endocrinology and Metabolism* **39**, 891.

Smith, C. A. (1947). *American Journal of Obstetrics and Gynecology* **54**, 599.

Smith, M. S. (1978). *Biology of Reproduction* **19**, 77.

Stabenfeldt, G. H. (1974). *In* "Avortement et Parturition provoqués" (M. J. Bosc, R. Palmer and Cl. Sureau, eds), pp. 97–122, Masson, Paris.

Stricker, P. (1951). *Colloques Internationales de la Centre Nationale de Recherche Scientifique* **32**, 15.

Takahashi, K., Burd, L. I., Scommegna, A. and Auletta, F. J. (1979). Paper presented at the 61st Annual Endocrine Society Meeting (abstract no. 610).

Terkel, J., Damassa, D. A. and Sawyer, C. H. (1978). Paper presented at the 61st Annual Endocrine Society Meeting (abstract no. 232).

Tyson, J. E. (1976). *In* "Prolactin and Human Reproduction" (P. G. Crosignani and C. Robyn, eds), pp. 97–108, Academic Press, London and New York.

Tyson, J. E., Hwang, P., Guyda, H. and Friesen, H. G. (1972). *American Journal of Obstetrics and Gynecology* **113**, 14.

Tyson, J. E., Freedman, R. S., Perez, A., Zacur, H. A. and Zanartu, J. (1976). *In* "Breast-feeding and the Mother", Ciba Foundation Symposium no. 45, pp. 49–62, Elsevier/North Holland, Amsterdam.

Vines, D. T., Tucker, H. A. and Convey, E. M. (1976). *Journal of Animal Science* **42**, 681.

Vis, H. L. and Hennart, Ph. (1978). *Acta paediatrica, Belgium* **31**, 195.

Wakerley, J. B., O'Neill, D. S. and Ter Haar, M. B. (1978). *Journal of Endocrinology* **76**, 493.

Weiss, G., Butler, W. R., Hotchkiss, J., Dierschke, D. J. and Knobil, E. (1976). *Proceedings of the Society of Experimental Biology and Medicine* **151**, 113.

Whitworth, N. S. and Grosvenor, C. E. (1978). *Journal of Endocrinology* **79**, 191.

Willett, L. B., Smith, K. L., Schanbacher, F. L., Erb, R. E. and Malven, P. V. (1976). *Journal of Dairy Science* **59**, 504.

Yokoyama, A., Shinde, Y. and Ota, K. (1969). *In* "Lactogenesis: The Initiation of Milk Secretion at Parturition" (M. Reynolds and S. J. Foley, eds), pp. 65–71, University of Pennsylvania Press, Philadelphia.

Zarate, A., Canales, E. S., Soria, J., Ruiz, F. and McGregor, C. (1972). *American Journal of Obstetrics and Gynecology* **112**, 1130.

PROLACTIN FROM HUMAN DECIDUA: SPECIFIC
PRODUCTION AND BIOLOGICAL ACTIVITY

M. Bigazzi, G. Pollicino, E. Nardi, F. Petrucci, R. Ronga and G. F. Scarselli

*The RIA Section, Prosperius Institute and the Endocrine Unit,
Poggiosecco Hospital, Florence, Italy*

INTRODUCTION

The prolactin (PRL) present in high levels in the amniotic fluid (AF) shows
biological and biochemical properties similar to pituitary PRL (Ben-David *et al.*,
1973), but there is accumulating evidence that its source is neither the maternal
nor the fetal pituitary. In fact, it has been shown that amniotic prolactin has a
chromatographic distribution among small, medium and big fractions which is
different from the maternal and the fetal pituitary PRL (Fang and Kim, 1975).

The increase of PRL in AF which occurs as pregnancy progresses anticipates
the rise of PRL in the mother and in the fetus (Tyson *et al.*, 1972). Furthermore,
in normal pregnancies the concentration of PRL in AF is always higher than in the
mother or in the fetus (Fang and Kim, 1975), and it is maintained at elevated levels
even when prolactin concentrations in maternal or fetal blood are depressed by
bromocryptine therapy during pregnancy (Bigazzi *et al.*, 1976, 1977, 1979;
Bigazzi and Del Pozo, 1978).

From the clinical observations we postulated a chorionic origin for amniotic
fluid PRL (Bigazzi *et al.*, 1977, 1979). Recently it has been proved that during *in
vitro* cultures a significant release of PRL occurs from human decidua and not
from placenta and amnion (Riddick and Kusmik, 1977; Bigazzi *et al.*, 1978).

Serono Symposium No. 35, "The Human Placenta", edited by A. Klopper,
A. Genazzani and P. G. Crosignani, 1980. Academic Press, London and New York.

These observations raise the possibility that decidua could be considered as an endocrine organ involved in the production of PRL during pregnancy; perhaps being the source of the PRL found in amniotic fluid.

To reinforce this hypothesis it would be helpful to demonstrate that the release of PRL from decidua is specific and occurs following active protein synthesis and that it is not due to a passive release of a hormone adsorbed to the decidual cells. Furthermore, the material released from decidua *in vitro* should be similar to pituitary PRL also in its biological properties, since there is the possibility that the findings result from a contamination by human placental lactogen (hPL).

Finally, if AF prolactin is produced by decidua, the release of this hormone *in vitro* should not be influenced by bromocryptine exposure, as happens when bromocryptine is administered *in vivo* (Bigazzi *et al.*, 1979; Bigazzi and Del Pozo, 1978).

MATERIALS AND METHODS

The experiments were done on human tissues obtained from normal pregnancies at term following spontaneous delivery. Placenta and associated membranes were washed three times in buffered saline, pH 7.4, to eliminate the contamination from blood and amniotic fluid. Amnion was separated carefully from chorion by delamination. Fragments of decidua capsularis were separated from chorion by scraping the maternal side of the chorionic membrane with a blade. (Histological control of the preparations showed that decidua was contaminated by some chorionic cells, and the chorion preparation could contain decidual residues.) Samples of placenta were cut from the basal portion of the villus. The tissues were minced, weighed and approximately 300 mg were incubated separately, in duplicate, in Ehrlenmeyer flasks, with 10 ml of medium. The incubation medium was composed of oxygenated Gey's solution (Porterfield, 1960), pH 7.4, modified by addition of HEPES (20 mM), penicillin (50 IU/ml) and calf serum (10%). The cultures were placed in a metabolic incubator at 37 °C for 19–45 h.

Samples of the medium were taken at various times.

PRL, hPL, chorionic gonadotrophin (hCG) and growth hormone (GH) were measured in the samples by radioimmunoassay (RIA) using a double antibody method with material kindly given by Biodata (Rome). The results were expressed as total quantity of hormone released in the median per 300 mg of tissue. Statistics were done by paired t-test.

The experiments done to test for inhibition of the release of PRL from decidua with inhibitors of the protein synthesis and with the dopamine agonist, bromocryptine, were carried out in the following manner. The decidua, coming from the same subject, was divided into several similar fractions, in such a manner that the same tissue was used for the control and for the experiment. Puromycin (10 μg/ml), actinomycin (5 μg/ml) or bromocryptine (1, 5 and 10 μg/ml), respectively, were added to the medium.

The biological activity of the PRL-like material released from decidua was assessed with the local "micro" pigeon crop sac method of Nicoll (1967).

The incubation media of the decidua cultures were pooled, lyophilized and resuspended in a different volume to obtain concentrations of PRL of 100, 200 and 400 ng/ml. One millilitre of the solution was injected intradermally over 2 days (0.250 ml every 12 h) on one side of the crop sac of a pigeon: the contralateral side was used for control and injected with the same quantity of "blank" medium. Hydrocortisone succinate (Solu-Cortef, Upjohn, Milano) (5 mg) was injected intradermally, after the first injection of medium, to minimize the inflammatory reaction. The animals were killed and the crop sac was carefully dissected. Each hemi-crop sac was placed over the special holding apparatus as described by Nicoll (1967) and a disk of mucosa of 4 cm around the injection site was cut and lyophilized. The percentage increase of the dry weight of the disk of crop sac, over the control, was used to measure the biological activity of decidual PRL.

RESULTS AND COMMENTS

The separate *in vitro* cultures of placenta and associated membranes show a great increase in the medium of PRL, hCG and hPL, but not of GH (Fig. 1). The release of the hormones is clearly specific; in fact hCG and hPL are produced only by the placenta and not by the decidua, and conversely PRL is released only from the decidua and not from the placenta. No significant increase of any hormone is found in the medium of amnion cultures. A smaller release of PRL can

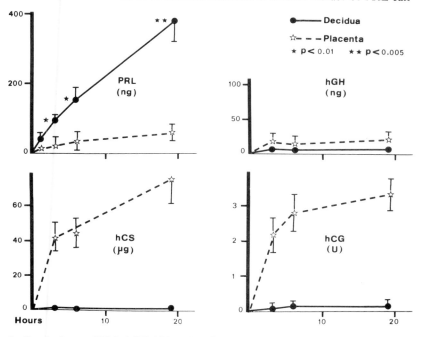

Fig. 1. Total release of PRL, hGH, hPL and hCG from decidua capsularis and placenta during *in vitro* cultures. The figures show the complete separation in the release of PRL and of hPL and hCG.

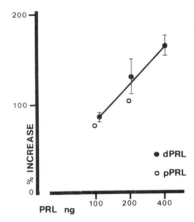

Fig. 2. Percentage increase of the dry weight of the pigeon crop sac in the local micro bioassay for PRL. The solid circles show a progressive increase in the doses of decidual PRL. The response to increasing doses of pituitary PRL (from a male patient with a prolactinoma) are shown by open circles.

sometimes be found during the culture of chorion, but it is probable that it derives from contamination of the chorion preparations by decidual residues.

The material released from decidua and measured in RIA as PRL seems to possess the same biological properties as pituitary PRL also. The experiments done by the crop sac local microassay are reported in Fig. 2. It is evident that there is a clear dose–response curve of the dry weight of the crop sac to increasing amounts of decidual PRL which is similar to the reponse obtained by injecting analogous quantities of pituitary PRL from a subject with prolactinoma.

The complete separation that we have described in the release of PRL and in

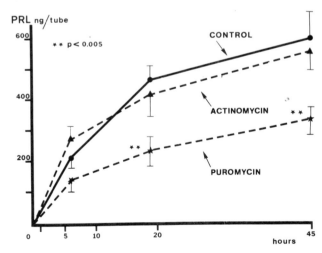

Fig. 3. Effect of protein synthesis inhibitors added to the cultures of decidua capsularis. Puromycin shows highly significant inhibition of the PRL release.

the release of the placental hormones rules out both the possibility of a cross-reaction between these hormones in the radioimmunoassay and also the possibility that the bioactivity comes from a contamination of hPL in the cultures of decidua.

From the experiments with the use of inhibitors of the protein synthesis it may be concluded that the production of PRL from the decidual cells requires an active synthetic process. As shown in Fig. 3, the addition of puromycin, which inhibits the synthesis at the level of cytoplasmatic RNA (Korbosky, 1967), produces, after a 6 h interval, a 50% inhibition of the release of PRL in the medium as compared to the controls. The delay we found in the effect may indicate that some amount of this hormone is stored in the decidual cells. Conversely, actinomycin, which affects RNA polymerase at the nuclear level (Korbosky, 1967), does not significantly influence the release of PRL. The different behaviour of the two inhibitors may be explained by supposing that the decidual cell is rich in preformed RNA, so that newly synthesized RNA is not necessary for the production of the PRL during the interval of our experiments.

The physiological meaning of PRL secretion from decidua is unknown, but it is likely that this plays an important role in the origin of this hormone in the amniotic fluid. In fact the experiments done by the addition to decidua cultures of increasing doses of bromocryptine, which strongly inhibits *in vitro* secretion of PRL from the pituitary, show that this tissue is not influenced by the potent dopamine agonist (Fig. 4). *In vivo* we found that amniotic PRL is not inhibited by bromocryptine while maternal and fetal levels of this hormone are suppressed (Bigazzi and Del Pozo, 1978; Bigazzi *et al.*, 1979), and we postulated that the eventual source of amniotic PRL (different from pituitary) would not possess dopamine receptors.

The finding that *in vitro* the decidua does not respond to bromocryptine strongly supports the hypothesis that this organ is the structure responsible for the production of the amniotic fluid PRL.

From our results is appears that both placenta and decidua in the human have distinct and characteristic endocrine activities and that the decidua seems specialized for the production of PRL, even if it is not yet fully comprehensible why, in women, part of the brain functions are shared with the uterus.

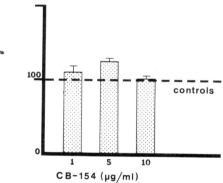

Fig. 4. Effect of addition of bromocryptine (CB-154) in increasing doses on the release of PRL from decidua capsularis. The drug did not show any inhibition of the PRL levels in the culture medium.

ACKNOWLEDGEMENTS

The authors wish to acknowledge the assistance provided by Professor Bani of the Institute of Histology of the University of Florence in the histological control of the tissue preparation and of the pigeon crop sac responses.

REFERENCES

Ben-David, M., Rodbard, D., Bates, R. W., Bridson, W. E. and Chrambach, A. (1973). *Journal of Clinical Endocrinology and Metabolism* **36**, 951.

Bigazzi, M. and Del Pozo, E. (1978). *Triangolo* **16**, Suppl., 89.

Bigazzi, M., Scarselli, G., Zurli, A., De Luca, V., Marrucci, G., Di Lollo, S. and Ronga, R. (1977). *Giornate Endocrinologiche Pisane* **1**, 27.

Bigazzi, M., Zurli, A., Branconi, F., Martorana, G., Buzzoni, P., Ronga, R. and Del Pozo, E. (1976). Paper presented at the 16th National Meeting of the Endocrine Society, Bari, May 1976 (Abstract C21).

Bigazzi, M., Ronga, R., Lancranjan, I., Ferraro, S., Branconi, F., Buzzoni, P., Martorana, G., Scarselli, G., and Del Pozo, E. (1979). *Journal of Clinical Endocrinology and Metabolism* **48**, 9.

Fang, V. S. and Kim, M. H. (1975). *Journal of Clinical Endocrinology and Metabolism* **41**, 1030.

Korbosky, T. (1967). *In* "Antibiotics: Origin, Nature, and Properties", Pergamon Press, Oxford.

Nicoll, C. S. (1967). *Endocrinology* **80**, 641.

Porterfield, J. S. (1960). *Bulletin of the World Health Organization* **22**, 373.

Riddick, D. H. and Kusmik, W. F. (1977). *American Journal of Obstetrics and Gynecology* **127**, 187.

Tyson, J. E., Hwang, P., Guyda, H. and Friesen, H. (1972). *American Journal of Obstetrics and Gynecology* **113**, 14.

PLASMA AND AMNIOTIC FLUID PROLACTIN LEVELS IN PRE-ECLAMPSIA

C. Nappi, F. Mercorio and G. Russo

Cattedra di Fisiopatologia, Ostetrica e Ginecologica, II Facoltà di Medicina e Chirurgia, Università degli Studi di Napoli, Naples, Italy

INTRODUCTION

An increased pressor response to angiotensin II characterizes pre-eclampsia (Assali and Vaughn, 1977); Gant *et al.* (1973) have devised a method to identify the hypertensive pregnancies in the preclinical stage. The factors involved in the heightened response of the blood vessels to pressor substances in pre-eclampsia are not yet clearly understood, but it seems that the renin–angiotensin system can be excluded.

Plasma concentrations of renin, renin substrate, angiotensin II and aldosterone have been reported to be normal or reduced in pre-eclampsia (Weir *et al.*, 1973); moreover, the blood pressure elevation which persists in the immediate post-partum period does not respond to compounds blocking the renin–angiotensin system, as demonstrated by Jay *et al.* (1978).

There is evidence of serum factors modulating the pressor response in pregnancy. Prostaglandins (Everett *et al.*, 1978a), progesterone (Everett *et al.*, 1978b) and glucocorticoids (Edelstone *et al.*, 1978) have been inculpated.

Stumpe *et al.* (1977) reporting successful treatment of hypertensive hyperprolactinaemic men with bromocriptine (CB-154), stressed the relationship between prolactin, hypertension and central dopaminergic control of blood pressure. The

Serono Symposium No. 35, "The Human Placenta", edited by A. Klopper, A. Genazzani and P. G. Crosignani, 1980. Academic Press, London and New York.

role of prolactin in salt and water balance and the supposed direct action of prolactin on the vessel wall itself are open to question. Although prolactin levels do not change with the sodium intake, and there is no evidence of prolactin-induced release of aldosterone (Holland *et al.*, 1977), nevertheless recent reports of the premenstrual syndrome associated with elevated levels of prolactin (Horrobin *et al.*, 1973) emphasize the fact that the role of this hormone in salt and water metabolism has not yet been clarified.

In addition, as demonstrated by Muriuki *et al.* (1974), the antagonist action of prolactin on the pressor effect of norepinephrine on the isolated rat mesenteric arterial tree underlines the role of this hormone as a modulator of the pressor response to hypertensive agents.

We have measured plasma and amniotic prolactin levels in pre-eclamptic women to examine a possible role of prolactin in pregnancy-induced hypertension.

PATIENTS AND METHODS

Nineteen pre-eclamptic and three eclamptic women were studied They ranged in stage of gestation from 32 to 40 weeks. All patients were primiparas, aged between 18 and 24 years. A control group, matched for age, parity and time of gestation, was chosen from normal pregnant women. Diet and activity were not restricted; no patient was receiving diurectic or hypotensive drugs.

All blood pressure measurements were recorded in the supine position with a standard sphygmomanometer after a period of recumbency of at least 30 min.

Pre-eclampsia was defined by the following criteria: a rise of blood pressure above 150/90 mm Hg after the 24th week of gestation; a proteinuria of at least 0.3 g/l, as measured by a turbidometric method; and oedema of face and hands with body weight increase greater than 500 g/week. These features were present in all the patients studied.

Maternal venous blood was collected between 09.00 and 10.00 every day, placed into tubes containing ethylenediamine tetraacetic acid (EDTA) as anticoagulant and the plasma separated and stored at $-30\,^{\circ}$C for prolactin assay.

Samples of amniotic fluid were obtained at the time of diagnostic amniocentesis.

In the eclamptic women, the serum and amniotic fluid samples were obtained at the time of caesarean section performed for fetal distress.

Prolactin was assayed by a specific double antibody radioimmunoassay (Cea-Ire-Sorin).

RESULTS

The results are summarized in Table I. The mean plasma prolactin levels in patients with mild or severe EPH gestosis were consistently higher than controls. The concentration in the amniotic fluid was also significantly raised. In the case of the eclamptic women plasma and amniotic fluid prolactin, measured at the time of caesarean section, was still higher than in pre-eclampsia.

Table I. Mean plasma and amniotic prolactin values (in nanograms per millilitre) from the 32nd to the 40th week of pregnancy in 25 controls and 22 patients with mild or severe EPH gestosis.

	Plasma values	Amniotic fluid values
Controls (n = 25)	112 ± 19	890 ± 115
Pre-eclampsia (n = 19)	167 ± 26	1780 ± 278
Eclampsia (n = 3)	240 ± 37	2645 ± 315

DISCUSSION

The role of prolactin in pregnancy is uncertain. The increased plasma and amniotic prolactin levels which we found in pre-eclamptic women suggest a role for prolactin in pregnancy-induced hypertension. Redman *et al.* (1975) also reported elevated prolactin levels; the author correlated the elevated prolactin levels with the major features of pre-eclampsia and found a significant association between the higher prolactin values and the raised plasma urate levels, strongly suggesting the early involvement of the kidney in pre-eclampsia. This statement is underlined by the association of raised prolactin levels in non-pregnant patients with chronic renal failure (Turkington, 1972).

Dubowitz *et al.* (1975) and Ho Yuen *et al.* (1978) reported normal and lowered plasma prolactin concentration respectively in pre-eclampsia, with no differences in the amniotic fluid levels. The lowered prolactin levels may be caused by an altered hypothalamic function; indeed Genazzani *et al.* (1971) first noted raised levels of adrenocorticotropic hormone and thyroid stimulating hormone in pre-eclampsia, and it is likely that the lowered circulating levels of prolactin, reported by Ho Yuen *et al.*, are at least partly due to decreased oestrogen production (Frantz *et al.*, 1972).

Our study reports an increased amniotic fluid prolactin level too, contrasting with the data reported by Ho Yuen *et al.* (1978). It is very difficult to provide an explanation because the source of the amniotic fluid prolactin has yet to be determined.

Because of the lack of equilibrium between the plasma and amniotic fluid prolactin, further studies are required to elucidate the role that prolactin plays in pre-eclampsia.

REFERENCES

Assali, N. S. and Vaughn, D. L. (1977). *American Journal of Obstetrics and Gynecology* **129**, 355.

Dubowitz, L., Strang, F., Hawkins, D., Blair, C. M. and Mashiter, K. (1975). *British Medical Journal* i, 445.

Edelstone, D. I., Botti, J. J., Mueiler-Heubach, E. and Caritis, S. N. (1978). *American Journal of Obstetrics and Gynecology* **130**, 689.

Everett, R. B., Worley, R. J., MacDonald, P. C. and Gant, N. F. (1978a). *Journal of Clinical Endocrinology and Metabolism* **46**, 1007.

Everett, R. B., Worley, R. J., MacDonald, P. C. and Gant, N. F. (1978b). *American Journal of Obstetrics and Gynecology* **131**, 352.

Frantz, A. G., Kleinberg, D. L. and Noel, G. L. (1972). *Recent Progress in Hormone Research* **28**, 527.

Gant, N. F., Daley, G. L., Chand, S., Whalley, P. S. and MacDonald, P. C. (1973). *Journal of Clinical Investigation* **52**, 2682.

Genazzani, A. R., Fioretti, P. and Lemarchand-Beraud, Th. (1971). *Journal of Obstetrics and Gynaecology of the British Commonwealth* **78**, 117.

Holland, O. B., Celso, E., Kem, D. C., Weinberger, M. H., Kramer, N. J. and Higgins, J. R. (1977). *Journal of Clinical Endocrinology and Metabolism* **45**, 1064.

Horrobin, D. F., Manku, M. S., Nassar, B. and Evered, D. (1973). *In* "Prolactin and Human Reproduction. International Symposium of Human Prolactin" (I. L. Pasteels and C. Robyn, eds), Excerpta Medica, Amsterdam.

Ho Yuen, B., Cannon, W., Woolley, S. and Charles, E. (1978). *British Journal of Obstetrics and Gynaecology* **85**, 293.

Jay, M. S., Edmund, T. P., Schoeneberger, A. A., Jennings, J. C., Morrison, J. C. and Ratts, T. E. (1978). *American Journal of Obstetrics and Gynecology* **131**, 707.

Muriuki, P. B., Mugambi, M., Thairu, K. *et al.* (1974). *East African Medical Journal* **51**, 232.

Redman, C. G., Bonnar, J., Beilin, L. J. and McNeilly, A. S. (1975). *British Medical Journal* **i**, 304.

Stumpe, K. O., Kolloch, R., Higughi, M., Kruck, F. and Vetter, H. (1977). *Lancet* **ii**, 211.

Turkington, R. W. (1972). *American Journal of Medicine* **53**, 389.

Weir, R. S., Brown, S. S., Fraser, R. *et al.* (1973). *Lancet* **i**, 291.

PROLACTIN VARIATION IN MATERNAL BLOOD AND IN AMNIOTIC FLUID DURING VAGINAL DELIVERY AND ELECTIVE CAESAREAN SECTION

G. C. Di Renzo, V. Mazza and A. Volpe

*Istituto di Clinica Ostetrica e Ginecologica,
Policlinico Universitario, Via del Pozzo 71, 41100 Modena, Italy*

INTRODUCTION

It has been shown that at term the levels of prolactin in maternal and fetal blood and in amniotic fluid are generally elevated (Schenker *et al.*, 1975; Aubert *et al.*, 1977; Di Renzo *et al.*, 1978). On the other hand, little is known about the pattern of prolactin secretion during labour. In this investigation we intend to evaluate the effect of labour and delivery on prolactin levels in maternal blood and in amniotic fluid at term gestation. 17β-Oestradiol was also measured to determine its relationship to prolactin.

MATERIALS AND METHODS

We have examined 67 patients between 38 and 41 weeks of normal pregnancy: 51 were delivered vaginally of liveborn normal infants, and 16 underwent elective caesarean section before the onset of labour because of presentation by the breech, previous caesarean section or cephalopelvic disproportion. Full and informed consent was obtained from all women. Thirteen patients, who delivered vaginally, had an induction of labour with oxytocin infusion (5 IU in 500 ml of saline

Serono Symposium No. 35, "The Human Placenta", edited by A. Klopper,
A. Genazzani and P. G. Crosignani, 1980. Academic Press, London and New York.

solution), the drip being continued up to delivery. In 21 patients oxytocin was administered during the second stage of labour; in the other 17, no drug was administered during labour. In 27 cases, the rupture of membranes happened 4–8 h before delivery. In the mother, the samples were taken from an antecubital vein every hour from the beginning of labour to 2 h before delivery; every 30 min from this moment to 2 hours after delivery; and, again, every hour up to 10 h of puerperium. In two cases samples were taken every 10 min from 2 h before delivery to 2 h after. In all these samples prolactin and 17β-oestradiol were measured.

During caesarean section, the samples from the mother were taken as in vaginal delivery, but in these cases only prolactin was measured. Moreover, in three cases, to evaluate possible effects due to intervention and/or to anaesthesia, samples were taken just before preanaesthesia and anaesthesia and 5, 10, 15 and 30 min thereafter. In all patients undergoing caesarean section preanaesthesia was performed with atropin (0.25 mg) and prometazine (50 mg) and anaesthesia with thiopentane (250 mg), succinyl choline (50 mg), nitrous oxide (60%) and enfluranum (Ethrane). For the amniotic fluid the samples were taken through the myometrium after the abdomen was opened at caesarean section or in the vaginal deliveries via an amnioscope after spontaneous rupture of the membranes. During labour fluid was taken every 2 h and at delivery by a catheter inserted into the posterior of the uterine cavity via the vagina. Samples were used only if free from contamination with blood or meconium after centrifugation at 3000 r.p.m. for 10 min. Moreover, in all the newborns, prolactin levels were measured in the fetal circulation by sampling the cord vein at delivery.

Prolactin and 17β-oestradiol measurements were performed by radioimmuno-assay: prolactin is quoted in nanograms per millilitre of NIH human prolactin standard, oestradiol is quoted in picograms per millilitre.

RESULTS

In maternal and fetal blood, prolactin levels are significantly higher in elective caesarean sections as compared with levels in vaginal deliveries; in amniotic fluid the difference is not statistically significant (Table I). During the first stage of labour, maternal prolactinaemia shows mean values similar to those observed

Table I. Prolactin (in nanograms per millilitre) in maternal and cord blood and in amniotic fluid at term (38–41 weeks) in relation to vaginal delivery and caesarean section.

	Amniotic fluid	Maternal blood[a]	Fetal blood[b]
Vaginal delivery (51 cases)	482.2 ± 187.9	162.2 ± 85.1	206.1 ± 76.0
Elective caesarean section (16 cases)	561.9 ± 255.8	297.9 ± 121.1	284.3 ± 101.3

[a]$p < 0.005$.
[b]$p < 0.01$.

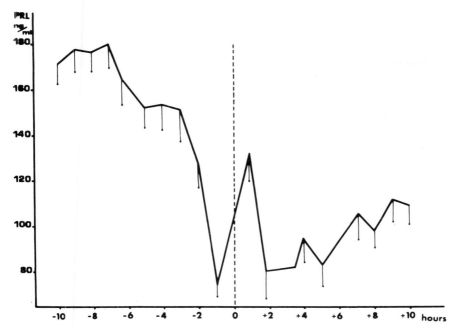

Fig. 1. Maternal prolactinaemia during labour (vaginal delivery at term).

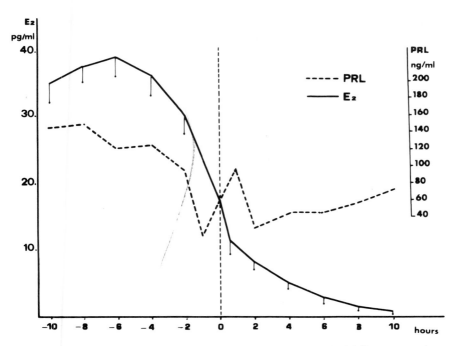

Fig. 2. E$_2$ and prolactin levels during labour in maternal blood (vaginal delivery at term).

during the last week of pregnancy. From 2 h before delivery, hormone levels
decrease, reaching the lowest value an hour before delivery (Fig. 1). From this
moment there is a remarkable rise, with a maximum an hour after delivery; then
prolactin levels decrease slowly for 2–3 h and remain nearly constant, even if at
low values as compared to the first stage of labour. The differences between levels
at the various stages of labour are all statistically significant ($p < 0.01$). In two
patients in whom samples were taken every 10 min, the lowest prolactin level was
reached 10 min before delivery, the highest 15 min after. The pattern of oestradiol
during labour was not related to the prolactin concentration (Fig. 2). Moreover,
the patients were divided into three groups according to whether oxytocin has
been administered during labour or not. Prolactin levels do not show statistically
significant differences between the three groups (Fig. 3). In patients undergoing
elective caesarean section, prolactin does not show any significant variation. The
prolactin concentration decreases a little, and slowly, from about 30 min before
delivery up to 1 h after; then hormone levels remain nearly constant (Fig. 4). But
in the three cases in which samples were also taken during surgery, prolactin levels
show a sharp increase after induction of anaesthesia and rise during the operation,
reaching the highest value 10 min after skin incision. From this moment prolactin
decreases to levels similar to those observed in vaginal delivery (Fig. 5). In
amniotic fluid, prolactin does not show any significant variation during labour,
it even decreases a little in 66% of cases (Table II).

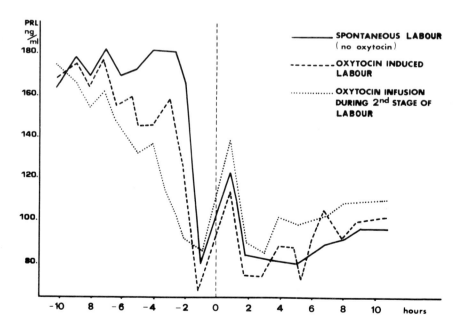

Fig. 3.   Maternal prolactinaemia during labour with and without oxytocin infusion (vaginal
delivery at term).

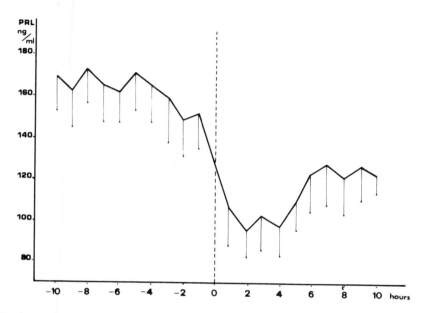

Fig. 4. Maternal prolactinaemia before and after delivery (elective caesarean section at term).

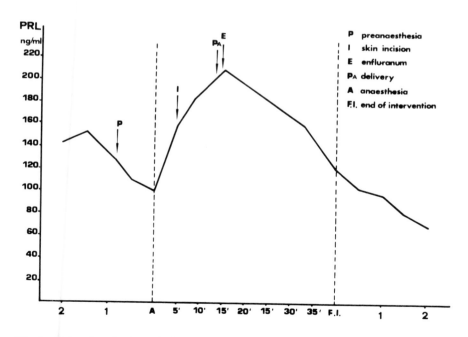

Fig. 5. Maternal prolactinaemia during caesarean section.

Table II. Prolactin in amniotic fluid (in nanograms per millilitre) before and after labour.

	Mean ± S.D.
Before labour	521.3 ± 177.6
At delivery	482.2 ± 187.9

$p > 0.1$.

DISCUSSION

Amniotic, maternal and fetal prolactin levels found in this study confirm our previous data (Di Renzo *et al.*, 1978) and those of others (Schencker *et al.*, 1975; Aubert *et al.*, 1977; Josimovich, 1978). Of particular interest in the present study is the pattern of maternal prolactinaemia during labour. That the hormone decreases before delivery has also recently been described by Rigg and Yen (1977)

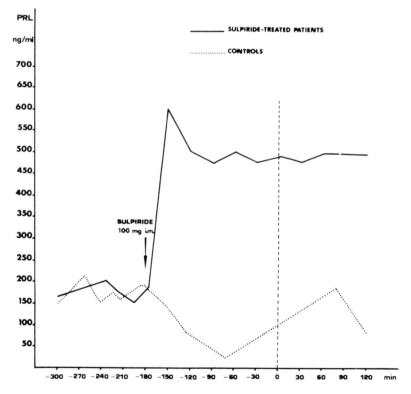

Fig. 6. Maternal prolactinaemia during labour after intramuscular injection of 100 mg sulpiride 3 h before delivery (two cases).

and Gregoriou *et al.* (1979). In the Gregoriou study, the tendency toward lower prolactin concentrations as labour progressed is evident, but the large individual variations and small number of cases (15) probably make the differences not significant statistically. Since labour involves many factors which stimulate prolactin secretion, such as stress (Noel *et al.*, 1972), muscular exercise (Federspil *et al.*, 1976) and psychological tension (Kemeter *et al.*, 1978), the prolactin pattern observed during this event is unexpected. Moreover, during vaginal parturition, prolactin variations are not related to oestrogens. Therefore, the phenomena related to labour and delivery may be definitive in determining prolactin variations. Since dopamine and bromocriptine produce a rapid decrease of prolactin levels, followed by a sharp rise after the end of the drug administration, Rigg and Yen (1977) suggested that there was a transitory rise of dopaminergic activity during labour. In agreement with this hypothesis, even allowing for the large doses used, we observed a sharp rise of prolactin levels in two patients in whom 100 mg of sulpiride were injected intramuscularly 3 h before delivery on account of vomiting, in contrast to the decrease observed in the other cases (Fig. 6).

Prolactin concentration in amniotic fluid does not change significantly during labour and does not seem to be affected by maternal hormone levels. Therefore, it is unlikely that a rapid placental transfer of prolactin takes place at term.

REFERENCES

Aubert, M. L., Sizonenko, P. C., Kaplan, S. L. and Grumbach, M. M. (1977). *In* "Prolactin and Human Reproduction" (P. G. Crosignani and C. Robyn, eds), Academic Press, London and New York.

Di Renzo, G. C., Mazza, V. and Baviera, G. (1978). *In* "Prolattina in Ginecologia" (G. D. Montanari and A. Volpe, eds), pp. 117–129, Piccin Editzione, Padova.

Federspil, G., Franchimont, P. and Hager-Hagelstein, M. T. (1976). *Hormones and Metabolism* 8, 323.

Gregoriou, O., Pitoulis, S., Coutiforis, B., Varonos, D. and Batrinos, M. (1979). *Obstetrics and Gynecology* 53, 630.

Josimovich, J. B. (1978). *In* "Amniotic Fluid" (D. V. I. Fairweather and T. K. A. B. Eskes, eds), pp. 107–133, Excerpta Medica, Amsterdam.

Kemeter, P., Springer-Kremser, M. and Friedrich, F. (1978). Paper presented at the "International Symposium on Pituitary Microadenomas", Milan, 12–14 October 1978.

Noel, G. H., Suh, H. K., Stone, J. G. and Frantz, A. G. (1972). *Journal of Clinical Endocrinology* 35, 840.

Rigg, L. A. and Yen, S. S. C. (1977). *American Journal of Obstetrics and Gynecology* 128, 215.

Schencker, J. G., Ben David, M. and Polishuk, W. Z. (1975). *American Journal of Obstetrics and Gynecology* 123, 834.

Section Seven

MATERNAL PROTEINS

MATERNAL PLASMA PROTEINS

F. Fuchs, L. L. Cederqvist and H. E. Spiegel

*Department of Obstetrics and Gynecology, Cornell University Medical College,
New York, and Department of Clinical Biochemistry, Hoffman-La Roche, Inc.,
Nutley,New Jersey, U.S.A.*

INTRODUCTION

The maternal plasma contains a large number of different proteins which can
be determined accurately by the use of modern immunological methods. The
majority of these plasma proteins are not pregnancy-specific, they are the same
proteins which constitute the bulk of human plasma proteins, but certain quantitative changes are found during pregnancy, such as a lower level of albumin and a
higher level of fibrinogen. With some exceptions, including those just mentioned,
the quantitative aspects of individual plasma proteins during pregnancy have
been subject of surprisingly few studies (Mendenhall, 1970). While it is obvious
that pregnancy-specific plasma proteins of placental or fetal origin are more likely
to reflect the condition of the placenta and fetus, it seemed possible that other
proteins in the maternal plasma could reveal pathological conditions of fetus and
mother. In connection with a screening program for neural tube defects by determination of the AFP levels in maternal serum, we have therefore undertaken a
fishing expedition to examine a number of different proteins in the maternal
blood at various stages of pregnancy. Before one can evaluate the significance of
individual values, however, it is necessary to know the distribution of each of the
proteins under investigation. In this preliminary report we shall present the results
obtained from assays of the following proteins at various stages of pregnancy:
prealbumin, α_1-acid glycoprotein, α_1-antitrypsin, α_2-HS-glycoprotein, haptoglobin,
C-reactive protein, β_2-microglobulin, and α-fetoprotein (AFP).

Serono Symposium No. 35, "The Human Placenta", edited by A. Klopper,
A. Genazzani and P. G. Crosignani, 1980. Academic Press, London and New York.

F. Fuchs et al.

MATERIAL

A total of 138 sera from 136 pregnant patients, who at the time of drawing the blood appeared to have "normal" pregnancies, constitute the main group. All these patients had a normal level of AFP for the time of pregnancy. The sera had been in storage in the frozen state for 2–6 months. Sera from 15 patients with elevated AFP levels were analyzed as a separate group. The data about these patients are shown in Table I. After completion of the protein assays, the charts were reviewed for maternal illness, outcome of pregnancy, and abnormalities in the newborn infants.

Table I. Data on patients whose sera were selected on the basis of high levels of AFP.

New York Hospital No.	Gestation age (weeks)	AFP (ng/ml)	Outcome of pregnancy
146–0801	8	230	Underestimated fetal age; normal
153–6688	13	284	Prostaglandin-induced abortion
149–2642	15	162	Intrauterine death, prostaglandin induction
154–2674	16	180	Repeat AFP normal, normal infant
156–0039	16	151	Prostaglandin-induced abortion, normal fetus
144–9896	16	148	Underestimated fetal age; normal
154–7320	16	322	Anencephalic fetus; prostaglandin induction
136–7044	17	331	Intrauterine death; missed abortion
85–7126	17	201	Twin gestation
158–2777	17	349	Anencephalic fetus; prostaglandin induction
136–2986	18	299	Twin gestation
153–5410	19	205	Intrauterine death later; prostaglandin induction
141–5743	19	576	Intrauterine death; maternal diabetes
158–6497	20	360	Prostaglandin-induced abortion, normal fetus
155–2825	26	664	Intrauterine death; prostaglandin induction, multiple malformations of Potter type

METHODS

The serum glycoproteins, prealbumin, α_1-acid glycoprotein, α_1-antitrypsin, haptoglobin, α_2-HS-glycoprotein, and C-reactive protein, were all determined with the radial immunodiffusion technique described by Mancini *et al.* (1965). Commercially available kits from Behring Diagnostics (American Hoechst Corporation, Somerville, N. J.) were used. Serum albumin was determined by colorimetric reaction (Gindler and Westgard, 1973).

β_2-Microglobulin was determined with a radioimmunoassay developed by Pharmacia (Phadebas β_2-microtest, Pharmacia Diagnostic AB, Uppsala, Sweden).

AFP was measured by a radioimmunoassay developed by Hoffmann-La Roche, Inc.

RESULTS

Albumin

Albumin represents more than half of the total protein present in serum and it is the major protein produced by the liver. Only 30-40% of the body's total exchangeable albumin pool is circulating in the plasma, the remainder is found in the interstitial spaces. It is well known that the average albumin level shows a fall during pregnancy. This is confirmed by our results, as shown in Fig. 1. The range is variously given as 3.5-4.5% (Kawai, 1973) and 3.0-5% (Ritzmann and Daniels, 1975). Most of our values fall within the wider of the two ranges. The albumin levels in the sera with elevated AFP are all below the regression line for the "normal" sera. We have no explanation for this unexpected finding, which deserves further study, but a methodological error must be ruled out first.

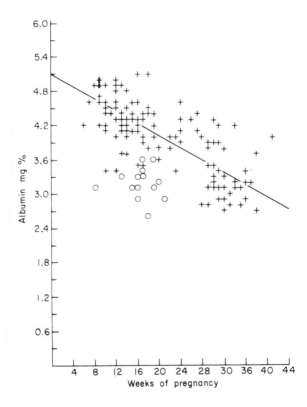

Fig. 1. Albumin concentrations in 138 sera from 136 patients at various stages of pregnancy (+) with regression line. Superimposed is the albumin concentration in 14 sera from patients with high levels of AFP (○).

Prealbumin

Several minor serum components migrate electrophoretically ahead of the albumin fraction and constitute the prealbumin fraction. One protein in this fraction serves as a carrier protein for about one-third of the circulating thyroxin and is referred to as thyroxin-binding prealbumin. The mean value for prealbumin in non-pregnant adults (Kawai, 1973) with the assay used is 25 mg/100 ml with a range of 10–40 mg/100 ml. As seen in Fig. 2, the regression line is almost horizontal. All the values are well within the normal range, including those from patients with abnormally high levels of AFP.

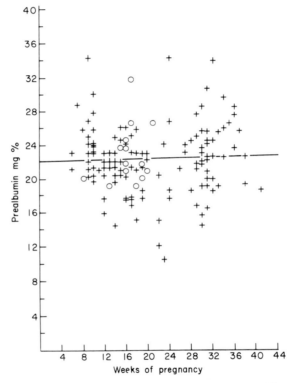

Fig. 2. Prealbumin concentrations in the main group of 138 sera (+), with regression line, and in 14 sera with high AFP levels (○). The patients with values above 32 mg/100 ml or below 14 mg/100 ml had uncomplicated pregnancies.

α_1-Acid Glycoprotein

The α_1 fraction follows the albumin fraction in its electrophoretic migration. It contains several proteins, of which we have determined two, α_1-acid glycoprotein and α_1-antitrypsin. The α_1-acid glycoprotein, also called orosomucoid, is a small protein, composed of 204 amino acids. The normal serum concentration in nonpregnant adults is 75–100 mg/100 ml with a range of 55–140 mg (Becker *et al.*, 1968). Our results, shown in Fig. 3, indicate that the values are slightly lower in pregnancy and decrease moderately with advancing gestation. The levels in the sera with high AFP concentration do not differ from the levels in the main group.

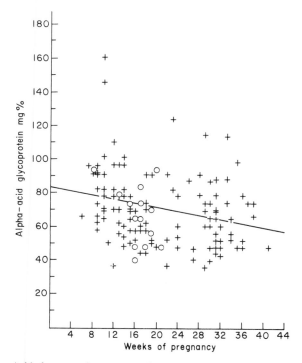

Fig. 3. α_1-Acid glycoprotein concentrations in the main group of 138 sera (+), with regression line, and in 14 sera with high AFP levels (o). The two patients with high values had normal pregnancies.

α_1-Antitrypsin

This protein is larger than the α_1-acid glycoprotein; it inhibits the action of trypsin and chymotrypsin. The normal adult levels are variously given as 200–400 mg/100 ml (Kawai, 1973) and 210–500 mg/100 ml (Ritzmann and Daniels, 1975). The latter range seems to apply during pregnancy (Fig. 4), but in contrast to pre-albumin, albumin and α_1-acid glycoprotein, there seems to be a marked increase with advancing gestation. The sera with high AFP tend to have high levels, although within the normal range.

Haptoglobin

The α_2-fraction contains as many as 12 minor components, of which we measured haptoglobin and α_2-HS-glycoprotein. There are three types of hapto-

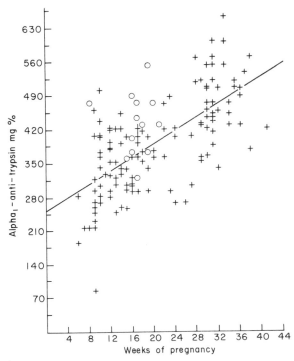

Fig. 4. α_1-Antitrypsin concentrations in the main group of 138 sera (+), with regression line, and in 14 sera with high AFP levels (○).

globin, which are designated Hp 1-1, Hp 2-2 and Hp 2-1. They are expressions of two autosomal genes (Fink *et al.*, 1967). The haptoglobins bind hemoglobin released into the circulation by intravascular hemolysis. This binding constitutes an "iron trap" which allows re-utilization of iron in the synthesis of new hemoglobin for erythrocyte production (Ritzmann and Daniels, 1975), a function which is particularly important during pregnancy. The ranges are variously given as 30-290 mg/100 ml (Kawai, 1973) and 100-300 mg/100 ml (Ritzmann and Daniels, 1975). The wide range apparently also applies in pregnancy, as shown in Fig. 5. The sera with high AFP have haptoglobin levels within the normal, wide range, though mostly in the lower part of the range. The regression line is essentially horizontal.

α_2-HS-Glycoprotein

α_2-HS-Glycoprotein is another protein included in the α_2 fraction. It has a molecular weight of 49 000 daltons and is composed of 402 amino acids. In the

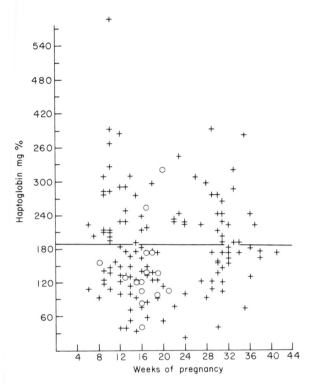

Fig. 5. Haptoglobin concentrations in the main group of 138 sera (+), with regression line, and in 15 sera with high AFP levels (○). No information is available about the patient with a very high level.

normal, nonpregnant adult the mean is 60 mg/100 ml with a range of 40–85 mg/100 ml (Schultze and Heremans, 1966). The levels in pregnancy (Fig. 6) appear to be higher than in nonpregnant subjects and seem to increase with advancing gestation. Sera with high AFP have α_2-HS-glycoprotein levels in the same range.

β_2-Microglobulin

The β_2-microglobulin has a molecular weight of only 11 600 daltons and the concentration in sera from nonpregnant subjects is 0.1–0.2 mg/100 ml (Ritzmann and Daniels, 1975). It is related to the Fc fragments of immunoglobulins and to HL-A antigens. The levels in pregnancy appear to be considerably higher, with a slight tendency to increase with advancing gestation (Fig. 7), but the level has only been determined in 103 sera of the main group, with a preponderance of sera from the first half of pregnancy.

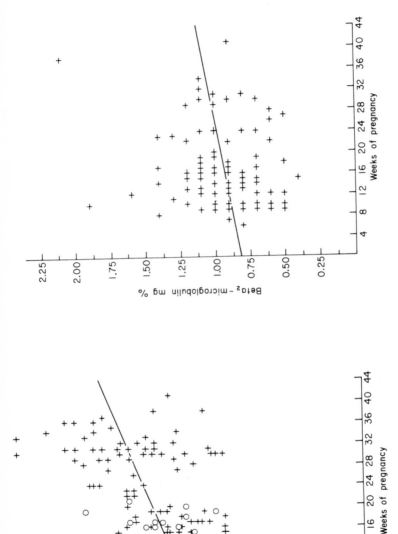

Fig. 6. α₂-HS-Glycoprotein concentrations in the main group of 138 sera (+), with regression line, and in 15 sera with high AFP levels (○). The patient with the low value had congenital heart disease.

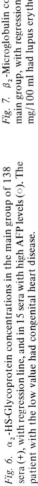

Fig. 7. β₂-Microglobulin concentrations in 102 of the 138 sera in the main group, with regression line. The patient with more than 2.06 mg/100 ml had lupus erythematosis.

C-Reactive Protein

The acute-phase proteins constitute an electrophoretically heterogeneous group of glycoproteins that migrate between the albumin and the α-globulin fractions. They include α_1-antitrypsin, haptoglobin, α_1-acid glycoprotein and C-reactive protein. These acute-phase proteins are valuable in the detection, diagnosis, prognosis and therapeutic monitoring of diseases involving tissue damage and inflammation. C-Reactive protein is unique among the acute-phase proteins in that it is usually not found in normal individuals. It was first thought to be specific for patients with pneumococcal infections, but it was subsequently found to be relatively unspecific. As shown in Fig. 8, the majority of our patients

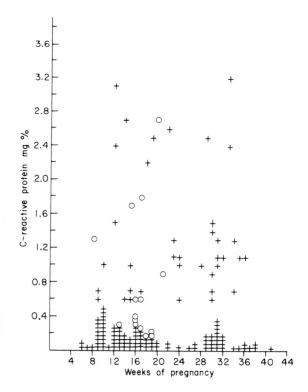

Fig. 8. C-Reactive protein concentrations in the main group of 138 sera (+) and in 15 sera with high AFP levels (○). The limit of detection of the assay is 0.6 mg/100 ml.

had non-detectable levels (below 0.6 mg/100 ml), but as many as 22% had measurable concentrations. A review of the charts has revealed that some patients with manifest infections fall in this group, but otherwise there is no explanation. About half of the patients with high AFP have measurable C-reactive protein.

DISCUSSION

The proteins in the plasma form a fascinating panorama. While a large number of individual proteins have been isolated and characterized, there is only a limited knowledge of their individual purpose and function. Some general functions are known, including the maintenance of the osmotic pressure in the plasma, the role in immunology, and the carrier function in the transport of hormones, pigments and other compounds. In addition, the proteins serve as a reservoir of amino acids which, after degradation of the protein, can be used for synthesis of other proteins. This function may be particularly important in pregnancy.

During pregnancy, the maternal organism must undergo a number of changes to provide the optimal nutrition for the growing conceptus. Since the conceptus grows exponentially, the maternal organism must provide nutrients at an exponentially increasing rate and it must do this without disturbing the homeostatic balance which is necessary to maintain its own vital functions. To complicate matters, the exponential curves for individual nutrients vary considerably. Thus, the concentrations of calcium and phosphorus in the fetus increase with advancing gestation (Fuchs, 1957), which means that the supply curves for these two elements are steeper than the growth curve. There is also an increase in the protein concentration with advancing gestation; thus the supply curves for amino acids must be steeper than the average growth curve, too. In addition, placental transfer of certain substances takes place against a gradient and thus requires active transport mechanisms; this, too, applies to calcium, phosphorus and amino acids. Much attention has been paid to the mechanisms of placental transfer of blood gases, water, ions, and nutrients. Much less attention has been paid to the mechanisms by which the maternal organism satisfies the ever-increasing demand from the fetus without disturbing her own homeostasis. Toward the end of gestation, the quantities of nutrients given off to the fetus from the blood during its passage through the intervillous space are considerable and the mother must rapidly replenish the nutrients lost from the blood from her own body stores.

Maternal malnutrition is known to result in underweight infants with impaired brain development. The relationship between the maternal proteins and amino acids and fetal growth and mental development has been demonstrated by Moghissi et al. (1975) and others. Thus, we have proof that the maternal supply system can become deficient—and considering the demands on this system, it should come as no surprise. A study of the sources from which, and the mechanisms by which, the maternal organism mobilizes the exponentially increasing amount of amino acids and other vital building stones is badly needed.

Since the demonstration that the pregnancy-specific hormone discovered by Aschheim and Zondek (1927) was not, as they first thought, a pituitary hormone but was produced by the trophoblast, there has been a search for pregnancy-specific substances in the mother which can give information about the condition of the fetus and or the placenta. As a result we have chorionic gonadotrophin (hCG), placental lactogen (hPL), AFP and the new pregnancy-specific proteins discussed in this book. To provide optimal information, such compounds should be easy to measure accurately, have a fairly narrow range during pregnancy, and show a distinct correlation between abnormal values and specific pathological conditions in the fetus or placenta. So far, the ideal marker for specific fetal conditions has eluded us, although AFP comes close. Theoretical considerations make it unlikely that highly specific markers exist, except maybe for very rare conditions. It should be noted, though, that markers need not be pregnancy-specific, as evidenced by the use of estriol and estetrol.

This preliminary study has shown the range of a number of well-characterized proteins in the maternal serum at various stages of pregnancy. With the exception of C-reactive protein, the levels of the proteins studied are not materially different from the levels in normal nonpregnant adults and the ranges are quite wide. These proteins, therefore, show no great promise as indicators of pregnancy-related pathology. It is quite interesting, however, that some tend to fall, some remain unchanged, and some go up markedly during gestation. The C-reactive protein does not show any specific disease correlation either, but the high proportion of measurable levels may justify further study.

Does it serve any purpose, then, to look at plasma proteins which are not pregnancy specific? If the sole purpose is to identify markers of fetal pathology, then perhaps the present study could be characterized as fishing in the wrong waters. But let me remind you that the queen of the fishes, the salmon, is caught both in fresh and in salty waters. The plasma proteins do have something to tell about the maternal condition of relevance to the fetus, and who knows where a detailed analysis of the maternal protein pool may lead us. When we started to look into the characteristics of amniotic fluid cells in 1955, we did not know whether it would have any practical value, but just a year later the perspectives began to dawn upon us (Fuchs *et al.*, 1956).

REFERENCES

Aschheim, S. and Zondek, B. (1927). *Klinische Wochenschrift* **6**, 1322.

Becker, W., Rapp, W., Schwick, H. G. and Störiko, K. (1968). *Zeitschrift für Klinische Chemie* **6**, 113.

Fink, D. J., Petz, L. D. and Black, M. B. (1967). *Journal of the American Medical Association* **199**, 615.

Fuchs, F. (1957). "Studies on the Passage of Phosphate between Mother and Foetus in the Guinea Pig," Munksgaard, Copenhagen.

Fuchs, F., Freiesleben, E., Knudsen, E. E. and Riis, P. (1956). *Acta genetica* **6**, 261.

Gindler, E. M. and Westgard, J. O. (1973). *Clinical Chemistry* **19**, 647.

Kawai, T. (1973). "Clinical Aspects of the Plasma Proteins", Igaku Shoin, Tokyo.

Mancini, G., Carbonara, A. O. and Heremans, J. F. (1965). *Immunochemistry* **2**, 235.

Mendenhall, H. W. (1970). *American Journal of Obstetrics and Gynecology* **106**, 388.

Moghissi, K. S., Churchill, J. A. and Kurrie, B. (1975). *American Journal of Obstetrics and Gynecology* **123**, 398.

Ritzmann, S. E. and Daniels, J. C. (eds) (1975). "Serum Protein Abnormalities. Diagnostic and Clinical Aspects", Little, Brown and Co., Boston.

Schultze, H. E. and Heremans, J. F. (1966). "Molecular Biology of Human Proteins", Vol. 1, Elsevier, Amsterdam.

THE ROLE OF MATERNAL CIRCULATING LOW DENSITY LIPOPROTEIN IN REGULATING PLACENTAL CHOLESTEROL METABOLISM AND PROGESTERONE BIOSYNTHESIS*

C. A. Winkel, P. C. MacDonald and E. R. Simpson

Cecil H. and Ida Green Center for Reproductive Biology Sciences and the Departments of Obstetrics and Gynecology and Biochemistry, The University of Texas Southwestern Medical School, Dallas, Texas, U.S.A.

The human placenta has an extraordinary capacity for steroidogenesis; indeed, the production of progesterone by the human placenta at term is 250 mg or more per day (Pearlman, 1957 Lin *et al.*, 1972). This amount of steroid biosynthesis necessitates the utilization of a quantity of cholesterol equivalent to one-fourth to one third of the total daily cholesterol turnover in nonpregnant adults (Grundy and Ahrens, 1969). Thus, the source of cholesterol for placental progesterone biosynthesis is an important physiologic issue.

Bloch (1945) demonstrated that circulating maternal cholesterol was the principal precursor for placental progesterone biosynthesis. In addition, Woolever *et al.* (1968) and Van Leusden and Villee (1965) found that *de novo* synthesis of cholesterol from C_2 units (acetate) by human placental tissue was negligible. We sought to ascertain (a) which form of maternal plasma cholesterol is taken up by the placenta; (b) what mechanism of uptake is involved; and (c) does the rate of uptake of cholesterol serve to regulate the rates of *de novo* synthesis and metabolism of cholesterol by the human placenta?

In these studies we employed term human placentas obtained aseptically at the time of repeat caesarean section performed on women not in labor and with fetal membranes intact. Primary cultures of placental trophoblastic cells were

Serono Symposium No. 35, "The Human Placenta", edited by A. Klopper,
A. Genazzani and P. G. Crosignani, 1980. Academic Press, London and New York.

prepared in the following manner. Trophoblastic tissue was separated from vascular stroma and a fine mince of the placental tissue was prepared. Following trypsin digestion and erythrocyte lysis, the dispersed trophoblastic cells were placed in culture in medium containing fetal bovine serum (10% v/v). After 2 days the culture medium was changed to one that contained no lipoproteins. This was accomplished by using medium which contained lipoprotein-poor human serum (10% v/v) prepared according to the method described by Goldstein and Brown (1974) from blood obtained from adult men who had fasted overnight. After 3 days in the latter medium, experiments were begun.

To evaluate the role of low density lipoprotein (LDL) in the regulation of placental progesterone biosynthesis, we investigated the rate of secretion of progesterone by trophoblastic cells maintained in medium containing LDL in various concentrations ranging from 0 to 420 μg lipoprotein protein/ml (Fig. 1). The 24 h progesterone secretion rates for the first, second, and third 24 h are presented in Fig. 1, panels A, B, and C, respectively. The cumulative 72 h progesterone secretion by these cells is shown in panel D. Progesterone secretion by cells maintained in culture medium containing no LDL declined progressively, possibly the result of declining endogenous cholesterol content in these cells. Progesterone secretion was stimulated by LDL in a dose-related manner at lower concentrations of LDL. The shape of each curve (Fig. 1) suggests that stimulation of progesterone secretion by LDL was mediated by a saturable process.

The rate of progesterone secretion by human trophoblastic cells as a function of the concentration of high density lipoprotein (HDL) in the culture medium was also investigated. The findings of this study are presented in Fig. 2. Maximal

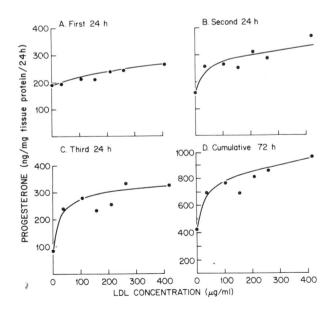

Fig. 1. Progesterone secretion rates by human trophoblastic cells maintained in media containing LDL at various concentrations.

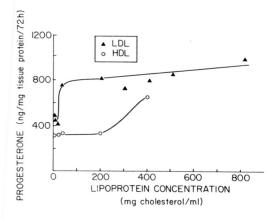

Fig. 2. Progesterone secretion rates by human trophoblastic cells maintained in media containing LDL or HDL at similar concentrations.

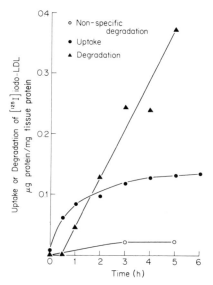

Fig. 3. Uptake and degradation of [^{125}I]iodo-LDL by human trophoblastic cells as a function of incubation time.

progesterone secretion by trophoblastic cells was achieved when LDL cholesterol concentrations were between 50 and 150 μg/ml, whereas, even at HDL cholesterol concentrations of 400 μg/ml, similar progesterone secretion rates were not attained. At equal cholesterol concentrations, LDL appeared to be more effective than HDL in supplying cholesterol for progesterone biosynthesis.

The kinetics of uptake and degradation of LDL by trophoblastic cells were examined utilizing [^{125}I]iodo-LDL, employing techniques described by Simpson *et al.* (1979). Trophoblastic cells were incubated for various lengths of time in the presence of [^{125}I]iodo-LDL in order to determine the time course of LDL processing by these cells. The results obtained during the first 6 h of this study are illustrated in Fig. 3. Uptake of [^{125}I]iodo-LDL was initially rapid and steady state conditions were attained within 5–6 h. Degradation of [^{125}I]iodo-LDL, which did not commence for 30 min, increased progressively thereafter for the entire 32 h of this study.

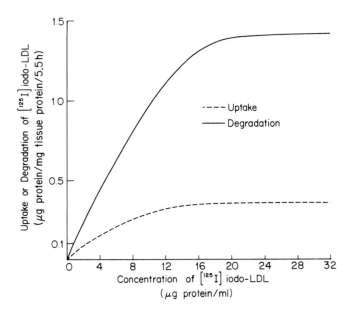

Fig. 4. Uptake and degradation of [^{125}I]iodo-LDL by human trophoblastic cells maintained in media containing [^{125}I]iodo-LDL at various concentrations.

The uptake and degradation of [^{125}I]iodo-LDL as a function of [^{125}I]iodo-LDL concentration in the culture medium was examined. The incubation time employed was 5.5 h (Fig. 4). The shape of each curve is indicative of a population of low capacity binding sites. These data were analyzed by linear transformation employing the method of double reciprocals. Assuming an LDL particle weight of 3×10^6 daltons and a protein content of 25%, we calculated the apparent dissociation constants to be 10×10^{-9} M for [^{125}I]iodo-LDL uptake and 7×10^{-9} M for [^{125}I]iodo-LDL degradation. The similarity of these values for the uptake and degradation of LDL suggests that both processes are causally related and mediated by a common population of high affinity receptors.

In order to evaluate the mechanism of LDL degradation, we investigated the effect of chloroquine, a known inhibitor of lysosomal enzyme activity, on the degradation of [^{125}I]iodo-LDL by trophoblastic cells (Table I). In the presence of chloroquine, [^{125}I]iodo-LDL degradation was inhibited in a dose-dependent fashion. We interpret this to mean that the degradation of LDL by these cells is mediated by the activity of lysosomal enzymes.

Table I. The effect of chloroquine on degradation of [^{125}I]iodo-LDL[a] by human trophoblastic cells.

Conditions	Elapsed time, (h)							
	2	3	4	5	6	8	12	24
Degradation (without chloroquine)	–	6	8	10	15	30	55	125
Degradation (with chloroquine)	5	2	3	5	–	15	10	20

[a]Degradation of LDL is expressed as nanograms of [^{125}I]iodo-LDL degraded/mg cellular protein. The results have been corrected for non-specific degradation.

To evaluate the role of LDL on *de novo* synthesis of cholesterol by human placental trophoblastic cells, we examined the rate of incorporation of ^{14}C-labelled acetate into cellular steroids, principally cholesterol and progesterone. In the absence of LDL these cells incorporated ^{14}C-labelled acetate at a rate of 290 pmol/mg protein per 20 h period. In the presence of LDL the rate of ^{14}C-labelled acetate incorporation was reduced to only 20 pmol/mg protein per 20 h period. Thus, in the absence of lipoprotein, human trophoblastic cells do synthesize cholesterol *de novo*, albeit at a low rate, but in the presence of LDL *de novo* synthesis of cholesterol was negligible.

Based on the results of these studies, we propose that maternal circulating LDL is the principal source of cholesterol for progesterone synthesized by the human placenta. The contribution of cholesterol synthesized *de novo* to progesterone biosynthesis is minimal and, moreover, is further decreased in the presence of LDL.

LDL is bound to high affinity cell membrane receptors, internalized, and degraded by lysosomal enzymes. The liberated cholesterol becomes available for pregnenolone and progesterone biosynthesis. Progesterone is secreted principally into the maternal circulation. Since progesterone secretion by trophoblastic cells appears to be regulated by the rate of uptake and degradation of LDL, it seems likely that the rate of progesterone secretion is dependent largely on the number of LDL receptors on the trophoblastic cell surfaces. Maternal plasma LDL cholesterol concentrations are such that under physiologic conditions the LDL receptor population is saturated. This may explain the observation that placental secretion of progesterone appears to be largely independent of uteroplacental blood flow.

ACKNOWLEDGEMENT

This research was supported in part by USPHS Grant no. 5-P50-HD11149.

REFERENCES

Bloch, K. (1945). *Journal of Biological Chemistry* **157**, 661.
Goldstein, J. L. and Brown, M. S. (1974). *Journal of Biological Chemistry* **249**, 5153.
Grundy, S. M. and Abrens, E. H., Jr (1969). *Journal of Lipid Research* **10**, 91.

Lin, T. J., Lin, S. L., Erlenmeyer, F., Kline, I. T., Underwood, R., Billiar, R. B. and Little, B. (1972). *Journal of Clinical Endocrinology and Metabolism* **34**, 287.

Pearlman, W. H. (1957). *Biochemical Journal* **67**, 1.

Simpson, E. R., Bilheimer, D. W., MacDonald, P. C. and Porter, J. C. (1979). *Endocrinology* **104**, 8.

Van Leusden, H. and Villee, C. A. (1965). *Steroids* **6**, 31.

Woolever, C. A., Goldfien, A. and Page, E. W. (1968). *American Journal of Obstetrics and Gynecology* **101**, 534.

PRESENCE OF HIGH LEVELS OF BLOCKED
GONADOTROPHIN-LIKE MATERIALS IN HUMAN SERA

A. Pala and L. Carenza

II Clinica Ostetrica e Ginecologica, Università di Roma, Italy

INTRODUCTION

Previous studies have shown that radioimmunoassayable amounts of human chorionic gonadotrophin (hCG) are present in the blood of patients with a variety of malignancies (Braunstein *et al.*, 1973a,b; Franchimont *et al.*, 1977; Rutanen and Seppälä, 1978) as well as in biological fluids and in tissue extracts of apparently healthy persons (Braunstein *et al.*, 1978; Braunstein, 1979; Pala *et al.*, 1979).

On the other hand Wass *et al.* (1978) were able to demonstrate the presence of antibodies to hCG and luteinizing hormone (hLH) in normal human sera.

We report here that large quantities of "gonadotrophin-like" materials became radioimmunoassayable in human sera after removal of anti-hCG and anti-hLH antibodies by affinity chromatography.

MATERIALS AND METHODS

Protein A Affinity Chromatography

Serum samples were directly chromatographed on protein A-Sepharose CL-4B (Pharmacia) columns. The bound IgG fraction was separated from the serum proteins as described by Hjelm *et al.* (1972).

Serono Symposium No. 35, "The Human Placenta", edited by A. Klopper,
A. Genazzani and P. G. Crosignani, 1980. Academic Press, London and New York.

Sepharose 4B–hCG Affinity Chromatography

Highly purified hCG (12 000 IU/mg), coupled to divinylsulphonyl-Sepharose 4B as described by Sairam and Porath (1976) was used for anti-hCG/LH IgG separation. IgG from 1 ml of serum was placed on the column in a 0.1 M Tris–HCl buffer solution, pH 7.6, containing 0.3 M NaCl. Unabsorbed proteins were eluted with the same buffer until the optical density at 278 nm fell to base levels. The bound IgG fraction was eluted with 1 M NH_4OH and immediate dialysed against 1% NH_4HCO_3 before concentration by ultrafiltration.

Radioimmunoassays

Radioimmunoassays were performed according to the double antibody technique (Midgley, 1966) using the immunochemicals described previously (Pala *et al.*, 1979).

Ultrafiltration

Ultrafiltration dialysis of the sera was carried out in stirred cells (Amicon) using Diaflo PM-30 membrane with a nominal molecular weight cut-off of 30 000 daltons. Deionized and boiled water was used as diluent.

RESULTS AND DISCUSSION

In preliminary experiments carried out to concentrate the β-hCG-like radio-immunoassayable activity by ultrafiltration before gel chromatography, surprisingly high β-hCG concentrations were found in the Diaflo PM-30 retentate. In subsequent experiments 30 sera from normal men, normally menstruating women and from amenorrhoeic women were submitted to ultrafiltration. Despite the poor reproducibility of the results, the β-hCG concentrations found in most retentates ranged from 15 to hundreds of milliunits per millilitre. The extensive dialysis of the sera against water resulted in a γ-globulin precipitation: quantitative double diffusion tests indicated that some 85% of the serum IgM content and some 15% of the serum IgG content was precipitated on a weight basis.

Since γ-globulin precipitation seemed to enhance the effect of the ultrafiltration, in a subsequent set of experiments normal sera were passed through Sepharose CL 4B-protein A column in order to remove IgG. The serum proteins were eluted as an unabsorbed peak and the column was thoroughly washed with the buffer solution used for protein application. Increased concentrations of β-hCG, hLH and follicle stimulating hormone (FSH) were measured in the eluate by radioimmunoassay. More surprising, however, were the highly increased concentrations of radioimmunoassayable gonadotropins found in the macrosolute fraction of the same eluates after ultrafiltration on Diaflo PM-30 membrane. In some specimens we were unable to detect increased FSH radioimmunoassayable activity.

The typical effect of the ultrafiltration following protein A affinity chromatography is shown in Table I.

Table I. Effect of protein A affinity chromatography and of ultrafiltration on the radioimmunoassayable gonadotrophins from the serum of a normally menstruating woman.

Stage of purification	β-hCG	hLH	FSH
	(mIU/ml of original serum)		
Original serum	n.d.	19.6	11.3
Protein A affinity chromatography (non-retained)	73.8	63.6	77.0
Diaflo PM-30 ultrafiltration			
Macrosolute fraction	1351	3812	1584
Ultrafiltrate	450	613	332

n.d., not detectable.

The IgG fraction eluted from the Sepharose CL 4B–protein A column was subsequently immunochromatographed on Sepharose 4B-divinylsulphonyl-hCG and the antigen-bound fraction eluted with 1 M NH_4OH.

The isolated antibodies were checked for binding with ^{125}I-labelled hCH and ^{125}I-labelled hLH. At the highest dilutions tested, corresponding to 2.5 μl of the original serum, 90% of the 200 pg of iodinated tracer was bound: this corresponded to a binding capacity of a minimum of 72 ng tracer/ml serum.

In another experiment 467 mIU/ml hCG and 2604 mIU/ml hLH were found in the PM-30 retentate, whereas 330 mIU/ml hCG and 489 mIU/ml hLH were found in the corresponding ultrafiltrate. The incubation of the two fractions for 15 h before radioimmunoassay resulted in the loss of some 40% of the β-hCG activity and some 32% of the hLH activity. However the addition of the corresponding isolated anti-hCG/hLH fraction to the incubation mixture resulted in a complete disappearance of hCG and hLH radioimmunoactivities.

These preliminary observations suggested the following:

(a) A material affecting radioimmunoassays is present in human sera. Its removal by ultrafiltration seems to be much easier and reproducible after antibody separation.

(b) Radioimmunoassayable β-hCG, hLH and, perhaps, FSH are present in human sera in higher quantities than we thought.

(c) Anti-hormone antibodies seem to provide an example of autoimmunity to self-proteins in physiological conditions.

REFERENCES

Braunstein, G. D. (1979). *In* "Recent Advances in Reproduction and Regulating of Fertility" (G. P. Talwar, ed.), Proceedings of the Symposium held in New Delhi, India, 24–28, October 1978. pp. 389–397. Elsevier/North Holland Biomedical Press, Amsterdam.

Braunstein, G. D., Kamdar, V., Rasor, J., Swaminathan, N. and Wade, M. E. (1978). Paper presented at the 60th Annual Meeting of the Endocrine Society (abstract no. 44).

Braunstein, G. D., Vaitukaitis, J. L., Carbone, P. P., *et al.* (1973a). *Annals of Internal Medicine* **78**, 39.

Braunstein, G. D., Vogel, C. L., Vaitukaitis, J. L., *et al.* (1973b). *Cancer* **32**, 223.

Franchimont, P., Zangerle, P. F. and Hendrick, J. C. (1977). *Cancer* **39**, 2806.

Hjelm, H., Hjelm, K. and Sjöquist, J. (1972). *Federation of European Biochemical Societies Letters* **28**, 73.

Midgley, A. R., Jr (1966). *Endocrinology* **79**, 10.

Pala, A., Donini, P. and Carenza, L. (1979). *In* "Recent Advances in Reproduction and Regulation of Fertility" (G. P. Talwar, ed.), Proceedings of the Symposium held in New Delhi, India, 24–28 October 1978 pp. 439–451. Elsevier/North Holland Biomedical Press, Amsterdam.

Rutanen, E. M. and Seppälä, M. (1978). *Cancer* **41**, 692.

Sairam, M. R. and Porath, J. (1976). *Biochemistry and Biophysics Research Communications* **69**, 190.

Wass, M., McCann, K. and Bagshawe, K. D. (1978). *Nature, London* **274**, 368.

DETERMINATION OF PREGNANCY-ASSOCIATED
α_2-GLYCOPROTEIN (SP$_3$) BY RADIOIMMUNOASSAY IN
MATERNAL PLASMA DURING NORMAL AND
PATHOLOGICAL PREGNANCIES*

H. Würz, W. Geiger, H. J. Künzig, J. Courtail, G. Lüben[1] and H. Bohn[1]

Universitäts-Frauenklinik Köln, and
[1] *Research Laboratories, Behringwerke AG, Marburg, German Federal Republic*

INTRODUCTION

Pregnancy-associated α_2-glycoprotein (α_2-PAG, SP$_3$, pregnancy zone protein, α_2-pregnoglobulin) has been purified and studied by several groups of investigators (Bohn, 1971; Stimson and Eubank-Scott, 1972; Berne, 1973; von Schoultz and Stigbrand, 1973; Straube *et al.*, 1974; Than *et al.*, 1974).

This high molecular weight glycoprotein is present in trace amounts in normal individuals and is markedly raised in the maternal blood during gestation. In this study we tried to establish whether different patterns of SP$_3$ levels can be correlated with various pathological conditions in pregnancy. A Double-antibody radioimmunoassay was devised and applied to c. 800 samples of pregnancy serum. The serum concentrations of patients with abortion, fetal death, Rhesus-incompatibility, diabetes, toxaemia and intrauterine growth retardation (IUGR) were compared with the normal range.

---

*This study was supported by the Deutsche Forschungsgemeinschaft.

Serono Symposium No. 35, "The Human Placenta", edited by A. Klopper,
A. Genazzani and P. G. Crosignani, 1980. Academic Press, London and New York.

411

MATERIALS AND METHODS

Radioiodination

Five micrograms of SP_3 purified from placenta (Bohn and Winkler, 1976; charge no. 14/13 Se 2), was dissolved in 10 μl of phosphate-buffered saline (PBS) and mixed with 10 μl of a Na ^{125}I solution (0.5 mg) (Behringwerke AG, Marburg, Germany; 8–15 Ci ^{125}I/mg I and with a suspension of 1 μg lactoperoxidase (EC 1.11.1.7., Boehringer, Mannheim, Germany). H_2O_2 in 30% solution was used at a 1:10 000 dilution in PBS and 10 μl were added in portions of 1 μl/min. After a further 10 min of stirring at room temperature, the reaction was stopped by 0.2 ml of 1% NaN_3 in PBS containing 1% of bovine serum albumin. The labelled SP_3 was purified by gel filtration on Sephadex G-200 (Pharmacia, Uppsala, Sweden). The immunologically active protein was eluted with the void volume and contained *c*. 50 Ci ^{125}I/g SP_3. A second, smaller protein peak was immunologically unreactive and was not suitable for the assay.

Radioimmunoassay

Serum (0.1 ml) at dilutions of 1:10 to 1:500 in PBS containing 1% BSA, 0.1 ml with 0.5 ng of labelled SP_3 and 0.1 ml of monospecific antiserum were incubated at room temperature for 20 h. (Anti-SP_3 serum was obtained from rabbits, charge no. 224C, and used at a dilution of 1:250 000.)

Precipitation was achieved either by addition of 1 ml "DASP" 1:30 (Organon, Oss, The Netherlands) or by addition of 0.1 ml 0.25% rabbit serum and 0.1 ml of anti-rabbit serum from a donkey (Wellcome, Beckenham, England) at a dilution of 1:16. After 17 h at room temperature the precipitates were centrifuged and washed with the PBS containing 1% of BSA and 0.5% of Tween 20 (Serva, Germany). The standard (charge no. 1025) contained 1.59 mg SP_3/ml and was used at concentrations from 0.02 to 10 μg/ml. The optimal working range of the standard curve reached from 0.1 to 5 μg/ml. No cross-reaction was observed with purified α_2-macroglobulin.

RESULTS AND DISCUSSION

Normal Range

A steep increase in the SP_3 concentration was observed in the first trimester of pregnancy with mean levels rising from 10 to 600 μg/ml. A plateau was reached after the 20th week of gestation with minor changes towards term. Figure 1 shows a scatter diagram of 416 single values assayed in pregnancies from week 3 to week 41, including serial studies in some individuals. There was a widespread distribution of values from 10 to more than 3000 μg/ml in pregnancies which were retrospectively judged to be normal. In normally menstruating women plasma levels of 0.3 to 58 μg/ml were found, with slight variations during individual cycles. The sensitivity of the radioimmunoassay made it possible to measure SP_3 in healthy men and newborn babies (Table I). In the fetal compartment and in amniotic fluid SP_3 was found only in trace amounts (0.1–2.6 μg/ml). The concentrations in umbilical vein and artery were similar in the same individual.

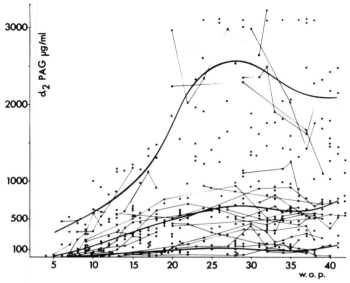

Fig. 1. Serum levels of SP₃ in normal pregnancies. (Curves represent the 10th, 50th and 90th percentiles.)

Table I. Concentrations of SP₃

Collective	No. of assays	Range (μg/ml)	Mean value (μg/ml)
Healthy men	15	0.1–20	3.8
Women with normal cycle	38	0.3–58	15.0
Newborn babies (5 days old)	8	0.1–6.0	1.8
Amniotic fluid, early pregnancy	9	0.1–1.5	0.5
Amniotic fluid, at term	12	0.1–2.5	0.9
Umbilical vein	15	0.2–2.6	0.9
Umbilical artery	15	0.1–2.3	0.9
Normal pregnant women, 3–41 weeks of pregnancy	416	10–3000	

Abortion

Figure 2 demonstrates single values or serial controls of patients with complications in early stages of gestation. The plasma concentrations in most of the cases of threatened abortion and incomplete abortion were found within the normal range and equally distributed above and below the median. Four cases of recurrent abortion were associated with elevated levels. These results are in contrast to the findings of other authors (Beckman *et al.*, 1974b; Than *et al.*, 1975), who reported decreased serum levels in cases of abortion. Significantly increased concentrations (above the 90th percentile) were observed in six cases of intrauterine fetal death (Table II).

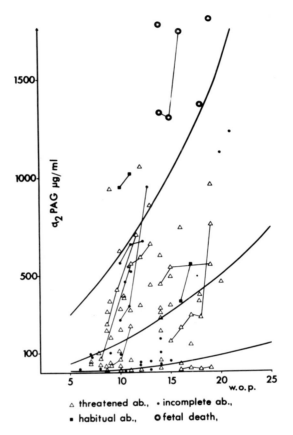

Fig. 2. Serum concentrations in cases of abortion.

Table II. Serum levels of SP₃ in pathological pregnancies.

Patients	No. of single assays	Percentage above mean	Percentage below mean
Diabetes	78	53	47
Gestosis	181	53	47
Rh-incompatibility	26	65	35
Threatened abortion	65	51	49
Incomplete abortion	26	46	54
Recurrent abortion	4	100	
Intrauterine death	6	100	
Small for date babies	62	95	5
Stillborn babies	7	86	14

Rhesus-incompatibility, Diabetes

Serum concentrations of patients with Rh-hyperimmunization and diabetes mellitus (Fig. 3) were determined in the second half of pregnancy. The assay exhibited a widespread distribution within the normal range. No tendency to elevated or decreased values was detected.

Toxaemia

Follow-ups of 13 patients with severe gestosis (oedema, proteinurea, hypertension) in the third trimester of pregnancy are presented in Fig. 4. The assay values are superimposed on the median, the 10% and the 90% confidence limits. No differences between these findings and the analogous serial controls of normal pregnant women could be observed since most of the concentration values fell within the normal range. In contrast to cases of fetal death in early pregnancy, in which SP_3 levels were significantly elevated, the serum level of SP_3 in a case of fetal death in the 30th week of gestation due to severe toxaemia was found below the 10th percentile (curve no. 9).

From the same patients, the plasma concentrations of placental lactogen (hPL) and pregnancy-specific β_1-glycoprotein (PSβG, SP_1) were determined at the same time (Würz *et al.*, 1978). Both placental proteins reflect the pathological condition better than SP_3. In the majority of cases their levels were found below the median or even below the 10th percentile.

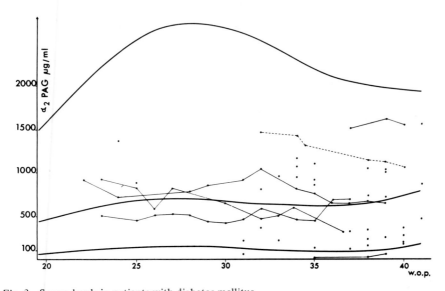

Fig. 3. Serum levels in patients with diabetes mellitus.

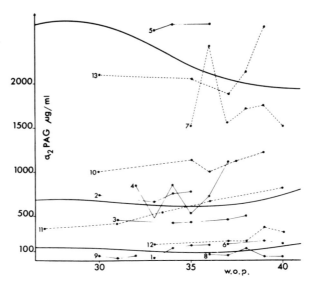

Fig. 4. Serial assays of SP₃ in patients with severe gestosis (EPH).

Fetal Growth Retardation

In intrauterine growth retardation with or without signs of dystrophia, 95% of the assay values were elevated above the mean (Fig. 5). This is in contrast to analogous serial controls of the placental proteins hPL and SP_1 (Würz *et al.*, 1978) and the steroids oestriol and oestetrol (Künzig *et al.*, 1977).

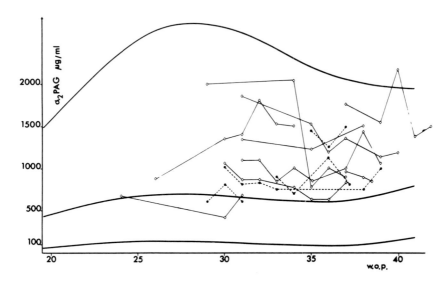

Fig. 5. Maternal plasma concentrations of SP₃ in pregnancies which led to small for date babies: – · – · – · –, with signs of malnutrition; ◇——◇, without signs of malnutrition.

Comparison of SP_3 and Oestradiol Levels

Oestradiol increases the SP_3 concentration in the plasma of non-pregnant individuals. In normal and in a variety of pathological pregnancies we could not establish any correlation between the quantity of SP_3 and that of oestradiol in maternal blood.

From the results so far obtained it appears that the determination of the pregnancy-associated α_2-glycoprotein (SP_3) is less valuable in supervising complicated pregnancies than steroids or placental proteins. As shown in Table II differences from the normal were detected only in cases of habitual abortion, fetal death and retarded fetal growth. It is interesting that in these conditions of pregnancy the SP_3 level in the maternal blood is elevated in contrast to decreased concentrations of the other biochemical parameters such as hPL, SP_1 and oestrogens.

It has been suggested (Beckman *et al.*, 1974a) that.in cases of mother–child incompatibility the production of SP_3 can be stimulated. A feedback was considered between reactive and suppressive mechanisms in the maternal-fetal immunological interplay. It may be that our findings of elevated concentrations of SP_3 under certain pathological conditions are to be explained by similar disturbances in the mother–child relationship.

ACKNOWLEDGEMENTS

The technical assistance of Mrs M. Hoffmann, Mrs B. Schmitz-Röckerath and Miss E. Spangenberg is gratefully appreciated. We thank Dr H. Kuhn for the documentation of numerous case reports.

This study was supported by the Deutsche Forschungsgemeinschaft.

REFERENCES

Beckman, G., Beckman, L. and von Schoultz, B. (1974a). *Human Heredity* **24**, 558.

Beckman, G. Beckman, L., Magnusson, S. S. and von Schoultz, B. (1974b). *Acta obstetrica et gynecologia scandinavica* **53**, 177.

Berne, B. H. (1973). *Federation Proceedings. Federation of American Societies for Experimental Biology* **32**, 677.

Bohn, H. (1971). *Archiv für Gynäkologie* **210**, 440.

Künzig, H. J., Geiger, W., Kuhn, H. and Schütt, A. (1977). *In* "Poor Intrauterine Fetal Growth" (B. Salvadori and A. Bacchi Modena, eds), Edizione Minerve Medica.

Stimson, W. H. and Eubank-Scott, L. (1972). *Federation of European Biochemical Societies Letters* **23**, 298.

Straube, W., Hofmann, R., Klausch, B., Kücken, G. and Brock, I. (1974). *Archiv für Gynäkologie* **217**, 415.

Than, G. N., Csaba, I. F. and Szabó, D. G., (1974). *Lancet ii*, 1578.

Than, G. N., Csaba, I. F., Karg, N. I., Szabó, D. G. and Novák, P. F. (1975). *IRCS Medical Science* **3**, 94.

von Schoultz, B. and Stigbrand, T. (1973). *Acta obstetrica et gynecologia scandinavica* **52**, 51.

Würz, H., Geiger, W., Künzig, H. J., Jabs-Lehman, A. and Hoffmann, M. (1978). Paper presented at the 6th European Congress of Perinatal Medicine, Vienna.

Section Eight

ABORTION

FAILURE OF HORMONAL TREATMENT IN THREATENED ABORTION. A COLLABORATIVE DOUBLE-BLIND STUDY IN A GROUP OF LOMBARDY HOSPITALS

L. Ferrario, M. Inzalaco, G. Tognoni and P. G. Crosignani[1]

Istituto di Ricerche Farmacologiche, 'Mario Negri'.
Via Eritrea, 62-20157 Milan and [1] IV Department of Obstetrics and Gynaecology,
University of Milan, Milan, Italy

INTRODUCTION

Hormonal treatment of threatened abortion in early pregnancy has long been prescribed in medical practice without ever having been shown to be effective. On the other hand, data from double-blind controlled clinical trials have repeatedly documented that no differences could be found between groups treated with active or placebo preparations (Goldzieher, 1964; Klopper *et al.*, 1965; Alling Møller and Fuchs, 1965; Govaerts-Videtzky *et al.*, 1965; Berle and Behnke, 1977). The wide popularity the approach enjoyed in general and obstetric practice in most countries, however, came under reconsideration when data were published suggesting a causal association between hormonal exposure during pregnancy and congenital (mainly cardiac) malformations (Anon., 1974; Greenberg *et al.*, 1975; Janerich *et al.*, 1977; Heinonen *et al.*, 1977; World Health Organization, 1977; U.S. Food and Drug Administration, 1977). As the benefit/risk balance could no longer be considered on a neutral basis of no benefit–no risk, the question became how to induce change in medical practice specifically in those countries where epidemiological evidence is known not to be widely read or readily accepted.

Systematic public presentation of the evidence to various clinical audiences in Italy during 1975–76 met, for instance, with marked resistance. A double-blind

Scrono Symposium No. 35, "The Human Placenta", edited by A. Klopper,
A. Genazzani and P. G. Crosignani, 1980. Academic Press, London and New York.

placebo controlled clinical trial was thought to be an effective tool both for checking previous evidence and for producing data from within actual medical practice, where pharmaceutical manufacturers' advertising campaign claims go unchallenged by any public statement of warning or information.

MATERIALS AND METHODS

The research was designed as a double-blind, multicentre trial in which women with clinically diagnosed threatened abortion during the first 14 weeks of pregnancy were randomly allocated to either oral (allystrenol, 10 mg/day) or intramuscular (hydroxyprogesterone capronate, 25 mg every 5 days) hormonal treatment or to the placebo group. This treatment schedule was selected during a pilot phase, which established the prevalent therapeutic practice in participating centres, and provided a check on the reliability of data collection. Clinical and biochemical (human chorionic gonadotrophin, hCG) tests were required on days 1, 7, 15, 21 after admission to the trial. The duration of treatment was set at 8 weeks. Twelve hospital staffs agreed to participate in the trial. Radioimmunoassay of hCG was performed at the end of the trial in a central laboratory under strict quality control conditions.

hCG results were used as reliable markers of the pregnancy status, and in particular to identify subjects who already aborted when entering the trial (12).

The two-way $(2 \times 2) \chi^2$ statistical test was used to assess differences of outcome in the groups; statistical analysis was also made to check for sample size for comparing two proportions, so as to have a high probability of obtaining a significant result.

Table I. Clinical profile of drug-treated (74) and placebo-treated (71) patients.

	Mean age	Parity				Previous abortions				Weeks of gestation			
		0	1	2	>2	0	1	2	≥3 ?	4-6	7-9	10-12	13-14
Drug	28.8	33	19	13	9	48	20	3	3 5	2	23	37	7
Placebo	26.7	32	27	7	5	50	15	3	3 5	5	25	26	10

Table II. Matching for other factors (%).

	Groups	
	Drug	Placebo
Medical history	2.4	2.3
Oral contraceptives within previous 2 years	21.5	20.4
Concomitant treatments (mainly antimetics and vitamins)	54.9	53.1

Table III. Clinical results.

	Length of treatment (weeks)				Outcome		
	1	1–3	4–8	N.D.	–	+	N.D.
Drug	9	17	32	16	26 (35.1%)	45 (60.8%)	3 (4.0%)
Placebo	4	21	33	13	21 (29.5%)	47 (66.1%)	3 (4.2%)

Abbreviations: –, patients who aborted; +, successful pregnancies; N.D., information not specified in medical records.

Table IV. Biochemical tests (99 out of 145 patients).[a]

	Plasma hCG within normal range ($\pm$ 2 S.D.)		Plasma hCG below -2 S.D.
Drug	36	– 8 (22.2%) + 28 (77.8%)	12
Placebo	46	– 9 (19.5%) + 37 (80.5%)	5

[a] 46 samples were excluded for the following reasons: 19 were examined outside central quality control; 17 appeared to have been inadequately stored; 10 were of doubtful attribution.
Abbreviations: –, patients who aborted; +, successful pregnancy.

RESULTS

Of the 145 women admitted to the trial, 74 received hormonal preparations and 71 placebos. The clinical data on these patients are given in Table I, which documents the close comparability of the two populations. They were also matched for other factors (Table II). No difference in pregnancy outcome could be documented between the two groups (Table III); the results still overlap closely when pregnancy status is checked against hCG values in two-thirds of women where biochemical parameters were actually measured (Table IV).

Statistical analysis obviously confirmed the absence of any significant difference between the two groups.

DISCUSSION

The present trial confirms the lack of beneficial effect of hormonal treatment in early threatened abortion with results which closely reproduce those reported by other authors (Goldzieher, 1864; Klopper *et al.*, 1965; Alling Møller and Fuchs, 1965; Govaerts-Videtzky *et al.*, 1965; Berle and Behnke, 1977). Market data, however, show that there was no decline in sales over the last few years, at least in Europe (with the notable exception of the U.K.). The lack of effect of official warnings (World Health Organization, 1977; Crosignani *et al.*, 1974) seems all the more impressive when the two drawbacks (no therapeutic effects and increased risk) are considered together.

The importance of avoiding ineffective treatments cannot be overemphasized. Even when they are not associated with a real risk, their continuation in medical practice (and particularly in pregnancy) implies a disregard for real clinical needs and for potentially useful supportive measures. In addition, there may be a carry-over effect favouring new but not necessarily better treatments. This may, for instance, apply to betamimetics in early pregnancy despite the fact that their use is increasing in many countries.

The indiscriminate use of hormonal treatment in unselected populations of pregnant women would also thwart attempts to identify subgroups (if any) which might possibly benefit from hormonal treatment. Although current knowledge, which suggests that genetic defects are the causal factor in the overwhelming majority of early abortion cases, does not leave much space for this possibility, testing for responsive subgroups was beyond the scope of our trial.

Controlled trial methodology has proved on this occasion to be an appropriate part of a more general policy for improving drug therapy in hospital and outpatient practice (Tognoni, 1978; Tognoni *et al.*, 1978) by creating a body of evidence which appears more convincing to practising doctors than the data available only through literature, where information may be biased.

ACKNOWLEDGEMENTS

Supported by C.N.R. Program of Reproductive Biology and Convention on Clinical Pharmacology. We are grateful to the clinicians in the various centres who collaborated with us in this trial.

REFERENCES

Alling Møller, K. J. and Fuchs, F. (1965). *Journal of Obstetrics and Gynaecology of the British Commonwealth* 72, 1022.

Anon. (1974). *British Medical Journal iv*, 485.

Berle, P. and Behnke, K. (1977). *Geburtshilfe und Frauenheilklinik* 37, 139.

Crosignani, P. G., Trojsi, L., Attanasio, A. E. M. and Lombraso Finzi, G. C. (1974). *Obstetrics and Gynecology* 44, 673.

Goldzieher, J. W. (1964). *Journal of the American Medical Association* 188, 651.

Govaerts–Videtzky, M., Martin, L. and Hubinot, P. O. (1965). *Journal of Obstetrics and Gynaecology of the British Commonwealth* 72, 1034.

Greenberg, G., Inman, W. H. W., Weatherall, J. A. C. and Adelstein, A. M. (1975). *British Medical Journal ii*, 191.

Heinonen, O. P., Slone, D., Monson, R. R., Hook, E. B. and Shapiro, S. (1977). *New England Journal of Medicine* 296, 67.

Janerich, D. T., Dugan, J. M., Standfast, S. J. and Strite, L. (1977). *British Medical Journal ii*, 1058.

Klopper, A. and MacNaughton, M. (1965). *Journal of Obstetrics and Gynaecology of the British Commonwealth* **72**, 1022.

Tognoni, G. (1978). *Lancet i*, 1352.

Tognoni, G., Bellantuono, C., Columbo, F., Farina, M. L., Ferrario, L., Franzosi, M. G., Mancini, M. and Mandelli, M. (1978). *Advances in Pharmacology and Therapeutics* **6**, 101.

U.S. Food and Drug Administration (1977). *Federal Register* **42**, 37643.

World Health Organization (1977). Drug information sheet PDT/D1/77.3.

PLASMA HORMONE CHANGES INDUCED BY
15(S),15-METHYL-PROSTAGLANDIN F₂ IN EARLY
PREGNANCY

A. Nasi, M. De Murtas, G. Parodo, P. Manca, B. Carcangiu, U. Lecca and
F. Caminiti

*Department of Obstetrics and Gynaecology, University Medical School,
Cagliari, Italy*

INTRODUCTION

The name "prostaglandin" was given by von Euler in 1936 to a factor found in human seminal fluid which stimulated smooth muscle and lowered blood-pressure. We now know that prostaglandin is not a single substance but a group of chemically related C_{20} long-chain hydroxyl fatty acids. Thirteen prostaglandins have been isolated from human semen (Bergstrom and Samuelson, 1967). They are widely distributed in mammalian tissues and have a wide range of pharmacological actions (Bergstrom *et al.*, 1968; Karim *et al.*, 1967).

Prostaglandins are efficient as oxytocics, and prostaglandins E_1, E_2, $F_{1\alpha}$, $F_{2\alpha}$ have been used for the induction of labour and abortion in women (Karim, 1969; Lehman *et al.*, 1973; Karim and Filshie, 1970).

The 15(S),15-methyl-prostaglandin $F_{2\alpha}$ (15-ME-PGF$_{2\alpha}$), which is resistant to degradation by the enzyme 15-hydroxydehydrogenase (Bundy *et al.*, 1971; Yanker and Bundy, 1972) has proved to be the most effective for early pregnancy interruption (Wiqvist *et al.*, 1972; Karim and Sharma, 1972; Toppozada *et al.*, 1972); this compound is also 20–100 times more potent than its parent prostaglandin $F_{2\alpha}$ (Karim *et al.*, 1973; Bygdeman *et al.*, 1976). Several studies have

Serono Symposium No. 35, "The Human Placenta", edited by A. Klopper,
A. Genazzani and P. G. Crosignani, 1980. Academic Press, London and New York.

427

been made on its abortifacient effectiveness, but the mechanism of action is still unclear (Leibman *et al.*, 1974; Lauerson and Wilson, 1975, 1976; Powell *et al.*, 1974; Csapo *et al.*, 1974).

The present study was designed to clarify the abortifacient mechanism of 15-ME-PGF$_{2\alpha}$ in 12 early pregnancies. To this purpose, the maternal levels of oestradiol, progesterone, human placental lactogen (hPL), β-subunit of human chorionic gonadotropin (β-hCG) and α-fetoprotein (AFP) were assayed.

MATERIALS AND METHODS

Twelve young women, between 11 and 13 weeks pregnant, who wished termination of their pregnancy, were treated with serial intramuscular injections of 15-ME-PGF$_{2\alpha}$ in doses of 250 μg every 3 h until 12 h after the first injection. In order to minimize the gastrointestinal side-effects, all patients were premedicated with antiemetic and antidiarrhoeic drugs.

Blood samples were collected prior to the first injection of 15-ME-PGF$_{2\alpha}$, and at 3, 6, 9, 12 and 18 h following the beginning of the procedure. Plasma was separated and stored frozen at $-20\,^\circ$C until the assay. Each sample was assayed in triplicate for hPL, β-hCG and AFP by radioimmunoassay (Biodata, Italy); serum oestradiol and progesterone concentrations were measured by a radioimmunoassay following extraction with ether (Cea-Ire-Sorin, Italy). The statistical analysis was performed by Student's *t*-test.

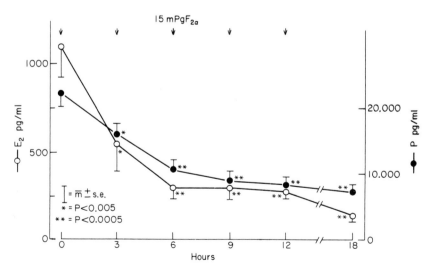

Fig. 1. Oestradiol and progesterone plasma levels during termination of early pregnancy by 15(S),15-methyl-prostaglandin F$_2$. Oestradiol and progesterone show a rapid and significant decrease after the first injection of prostaglandin.

RESULTS

Before the intramuscular injection of 15-ME-PGE$_{2\alpha}$ (time 0), oestradiol, progesterone, hPL, β-hCG and AFP plasma values were in the normal range for the gestational age.

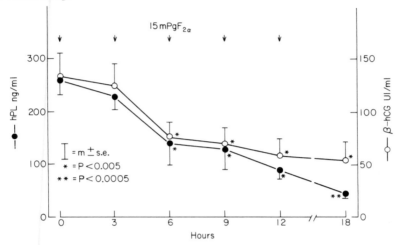

Fig. 2. hPL and hCG serum concentrations during termination of early pregnancy by 15(S),15-methyl-prostaglandin F$_2$. hPL and hCG, unchanged during the first 3 h, show a significant decrease at later times.

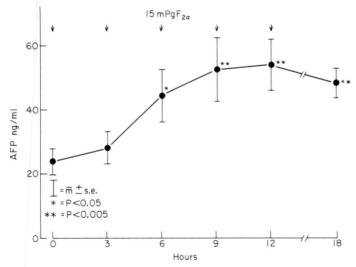

Fig. 3. The AFP plasma concentration shows a significant increase 6 h after the first injection of 15(S),15-methyl-prostaglandin F$_2$. Its plasma values remain significantly higher at the later times.

Serum oestradiol concentrations dropped to 60% of the basal levels at 3 h, to 35% at 6 h, 25% at 9 h, 20% at 12 h and to 10% at 18 h. The statistical analysis showed a significant difference at 3 ($p < 0.005$), 6, 9, 12 and 18 h ($p < 0.0005$) from the initial levels (Fig. 1). Progesterone mean values showed a gradual and consistent decrease during 15-ME-PGF$_{2\alpha}$ treatment, as was found for oestradiol. They dropped to 70% at 3 h, 50% at 6 and 9 h, 35% at 12 h and to 30% at 18 h. The falls in plasma progesterone were statistically significant ($p < 0.005$ at 3 h and $p < 0.0005$ at the following times).

Although virtually unchanged at 3 h, the serum hPL concentrations dropped gradually to 60% at 6 and 9 h ($p < 0.005$), 35% at 12 h ($p < 0.005$) and to 18% at 18 h ($p < 0.0005$) as compared with the initial control levels (Fig. 2).

The β-hCG plasma concentrations decreased similarly to hPL; they remained unchanged at 3 h and dropped significantly at the successive control times ($p < 0.005$).

The AFP plasma levels, unchanged at 3 h, rose progressively later and were significantly higher than the initial mean values at 6 ($p < 0.05$), 9, 12 and 18 h ($p < 0.005$). (Fig. 3).

DISCUSSION

There is disagreement among investigators regarding the moment of the onset of uterine contractions and the significance of the decrease observed in plasma steroid and protein hormones. It is well known that the luteal and placental progesterone production (Karim and Hillier, 1975), is an essential factor for the maintenance of first trimester pregnancy; this is based on the evidence that luteectomy in early pregnancy results in serum progesterone decrease followed by abortion (Csapo et al., 1972). Several studies have been made in order to investigate the abortifacient mechanism of prostaglandins. It is generally agreed that prostaglandins have luteolytic (Csapo et al., 1971) and oxytocic effects and act by suppressing placental steroidogenesis; the subsequent drop in steroid hormones converts the uterus into a more reactive organ (Enkola, 1974; Zoltan et al., 1974) and develops the uterine activity (Csapo et al., 1974). On the other hand, several authors have reported that prostaglandin-induced termination of pregnancy is unrelated to the drop of progesterone but the result of a strong myometrial activity (Lauersen and Wilson, 1975; Lehman et al., 1973; Cantor et al., 1972).

Our results show an important fall in oestradiol and progesterone plasma levels after the first injection of 15-ME-PGF$_{2\alpha}$, while hPL and β-hCG did not show any significant variation. After the second injection a gradual and significant decrease could be found for both the protein and steroid hormones. Serum AFP did not vary during the first 3 h, but a significant increase was noticed later. From these data, we deduce that the abortifacient action of 15-ME-PGF$_{2\alpha}$ is possibly due to an initial luteolytic effect demonstrated by the initial drop in steroid hormones, which could make the uterus more reactive to the oxytocic action of 15-ME-PGF$_{2\alpha}$. The fall of hPL and β-hCG plasma levels can be related to the sustained vasoconstriction of the uteroplacental vessels (Pulkinnen et al., 1975) and to the disruption of the implanted placenta caused by a secondary strong myometrial activity. The delayed rise of plasma values of AFP, which is an index of fetal status (Seppälä and Ruoslahti, 1973; Cohen *et al.*, 1973; Garoff and Seppälä, 1974) could be explained by severe fetal distress or intrauterine death, as a consequence of 15-ME-PGF$_{2\alpha}$-induced placental damage.

REFERENCES

Bergstrom, S. and Samuelsson, H. (1967). *In* "Nobel Symposium 2" (S. Bergstrom and H. Samuelsson, eds), p. 21, Stockholm.

Bergstrom, S., Carlson, L. A. and Weeks, J. H. (1968). *Pharmacological Review* **20**, 1.

Bundy, G., Lincoln, F., Nelson, M., Rike, S. and Schneider, W. (1971). *Annals of the New York Academy of Science* **180**, 76.

Bydgeman, M., Known, S. V., Mukherjee, T. and Wiqvist, N. (1968). *American Journal of Obstetrics and Gynecology* **102**, 317.

Bygdeman, M., Martin, J. M., Leader, A., Lundström, V., Ramadan, M., Eneroth, P. and Green, K. (1976). *Obstetrics and Gynecology* **48**, 221.

Cantor, B., Jewelewicz, R., Warren, N., Dyrenfurth, I., Patner, A. and Van de Wiele, R. L. (1972). *American Journal of Obstetrics and Gynecology* **113**, 607.

Cohen, H., Graham, H. and Lau, H. L. (1973). *American Journal of Obstetrics and Gynecology* **115**, 881.

Csapo, A. I., Pulkkinen, M. O. and Kaihola, M. L. (1974). *American Journal of Obstetrics and Gynecology* **118**, 985.

Csapo, A. I., Sauvage, J. P. and Wiest, W. G. (1971). *American Journal of Obstetrics and Gynecology* **111**, 1059.

Csapo, A. I., Pulkkinen, M. O., Ruttner, B., Sauvage, J. P. and Wiest, W. G. (1972). *American Journal of Obstetrics and Gynecology* **112**, 1061.

Enkola, K. (1974). *Prostaglandins* **5**, 115.

Garoff, L. and Seppälä, M. (1974). *American Journal of Obstetrics and Gynecology* **121**, 257.

Karim, S. M. M. (1969). "Prostaglandins, Amines and Peptides", London.

Karim, S. M. M. and Hillier, K. (1975). *In* "Prostaglandins and Reproduction" (S. M. M. Karim, ed.), M. T. P. Press, Lancaster.

Karim, S. M. M. and Filshie, G. M. (1970). *Lancet* **24**, 157.

Karim, S. M. M. and Sharma, S. D. (1972). *Journal of Obstetrics and Gynaecology of the British Commonwealth* **79**, 737.

Karim, S. M. M., Sandler, M. and Williams, E. D. (1967). *British Journal of Pharmacology and Chemotherapy* **31**, 340.

Karim, S. M. M., Sharma, S. D., Filshie, G. M., Salomon, J. A. and Ganesan, P. A. (1973). *Advances in Biosciences* **9**, 811.

Lauersen, M. M. and Wilson, K. H. (1975). *American Journal of Obstetrics and Gynecology* **121**, 273.

Lauersen, M. M. and Wilson, K. H. (1976). *American Journal of Obstetrics and Gynecology* **124**, 425.

Lehman, F., Peters, F., Breckwoldt, M., Bettendorf, G. (1973). *Advances in Biosciences* **9**, 679.

Leibman, T., Saldoma, L., Shulman, H., Cunningham, M. A. and Radolph, G. (1974). *Prostaglandins* **7**, 443.

Powell, W. S., Hammarstrom, S., Samuelsson, B. and Sjoberg, B. (1974). *Lancet* **i**, 1120.

Pulkinnen, M. O., Pitkanen, Y., Ojala, A., Hannelin, H. (1975). *Prostaglandins*
    9, 61.
Seppälä, M. and Ruoslahti, E. (1973). *American Journal of Obstetrics and Gyne-
    cology* **115**, 48.
Toppozada, M., Beguin, F., Bygdeman, M.and Wiqvist, N. (1972). *Prostaglandins*
    2, 239.
von Euler, U. S. (1936). *Journal of Physiology, London* **88**, 213.
Wiqvist, N., Beguin, F., Bygdeman, M. and Toppozada, M. (1972). *In* "The
    Prostaglandins: Clinical Applications in Human Reproduction" (E. M. Southern,
    ed.), Futura Publishing Co., Mount Kisco, N.Y.
Yanker, E. W. and Bundy, G. L. (1972). *Journal of the American Chemical
    Society* **94**, 3651.
Zoltan, I., Csillag, M., Zsolani, B., Zube, K. L., Moksony, I. and Matanyi, S. (1974).
    Prostaglandins **6**, 211.

Section Nine
MISCELLANEOUS

ENDOCRINE STATUS AT THE END OF PREGNANCY AND THE MECHANISM INVOLVED IN THE INITIATION OF PARTURITION

A. C. Turnbull, M. D. Mitchell and A. B. M. Anderson

Nuffield Department of Obstetrics and Gynaecology, University of Oxford, John Radcliffe Hospital, Oxford OX3 9DU, U.K.

INTRODUCTION

Appropriate timing of parturition is essential for the birth of a mature and healthy infant. In human pregnancy, 95% of infants are born at term, but the remaining 5% of infants, born pre-term, account for 85% of early neonatal deaths not due to lethal deformity (Rush *et al.*, 1976), illustrating the vital importance of a reliable control mechanism for maintaining pregnancy and initiating labour.

There is substantial evidence in many animals implicating the fetus in the timing of the onset of labour (Thorburn *et al.*, 1977), and this applies whether pregnancy is maintained by the placenta, as in the sheep, or by the corpus luteum, as in the goat. In the human, it is difficult to obtain direct evidence because of the inaccessibility of the normal intrauterine fetus in late pregnancy. It therefore seems useful here briefly to review the well-documented cascade of events influencing the onset of labour in the sheep, an animal in which endocrine changes in the fetus lead to changes in placental function which, in turn, initiate parturition. The evidence for and against a similar control mechanism in man will then be presented for comparison.

Serono Symposium No. 35, "The Human Placenta", edited by A. Klopper, A. Genazzani and P. G. Crosignani, 1980. Academic Press, London and New York.

INITIATION OF PARTURITION IN OVINE PREGNANCY

The earliest well-defined event in ovine parturition is a sharp rise in the concentration of cortisol in the fetal circulation 7–10 days before delivery (Bassett and Thorburn, 1969). This reflects mainly an increase in cortisol secretion (Beitins *et al.*, 1970; Liggins *et al.*, 1973), although levels of corticosteroid binding globulin are also raised (Fairclough and Liggins, 1975). Since fetal levels of andrenocorticotrophin (ACTH) rise at the same time as, rather than before, levels of cortisol (Rees *et al.*, 1975; Jones *et al.*, 1977), the increased secretion of cortisol may reflect an increased sensitivity to ACTH (Madill and Bassett, 1973; Liggins *et al.*, 1977a). Recent studies by Silman *et al.* (1979) have shown that there may be qualitative differences between the fetal and adult sheep pituitary corticotrophic stimulus. In the fetal pituitary there are relatively greater proportions of large molecular weight material, thought to be "stem hormones", which could give rise to a family of biologically active peptides. The fact that the "trophic family" engendered varies with the stage of fetal development may explain the different adrenal responses of fetal and adult sheep. Although the exact mechanisms regulating fetal adrenal responsiveness remain to be investigated, it has also been shown that infusion of prostaglandin E (PGE) into the fetus can raise cortisol levels at a time when the fetal adrenal is relatively insensitive to ACTH stimulation (Louis *et al.*, 1976).

The importance of fetal pituitary–adrenal activity in the sheep rests, of course, with the original observations that fetal hypophysectomy prevents the onset of labour (Liggins *et al.*, 1967) while intrafetal infusion of ACTH, cortisol or dexamethasone all induce labour, bringing about all the endocrine changes associated with the spontaneous onset of labour in this species (Liggins, 1969; Currie *et al.*, 1973).

In the sheep fetal placenta, increased fetal cortisol induces both 17α-hydroxylase and C_{17-20} lyase activity (Anderson *et al.*, 1975; Steele *et al.*, 1976). As a result, the production of progesterone falls as that of 17α-hydroxyprogesterone, androstenedione, oestrone and oestrone sulphate increases. The increase in C_{17-20} lyase activity may be an indirect response to cortisol, resulting from a decrease in progesterone concentration, since progesterone inhibits C_{17-20} lyase activity (Mahajan and Samuels, 1975). The C_{19} steroids formed from progesterone and pregnenolone are rapidly converted to oestrogens, so that, under the influence of increased fetal cortisol secretion, the fetal placenta has developed the ability to influence the progesterone and oestrogen biosynthetic pathways (Flint *et al.*, 1975a). Since cortisol may also stimulate aromatase and sterol sulphatase activities (Ash *et al.*, 1973), it can seemingly potentiate all the major enzymatic steps from C_{21} precursors (Fig. 1).

These changes in the steroid environment lead to increased prostaglandin F (PGF) production by the maternal placenta and also the myometrium. This synthesis of PGF may well be stimulated by the raised oestrogens (Liggins *et al.*, 1973), but Mitchell and Flint (1977) have shown that PGF can also be released, and parturition induced without an increase in oestrogen levels, by administration of cyanoketone, an inhibitor of 3β-hydroxysteroid dehydrogenase, which rapidly reduces circulating progesterone concentrations.

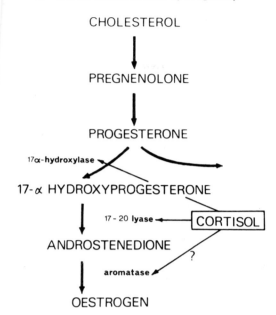

Fig. 1. Pathway of biosynthesis of progesterone and oestrogen in ovine placenta, indicating the possible sites of action of fetal cortisol, after Anderson *et al.* (1975), Steele *et al.* (1976) and Ash *et al.* (1973). (Modified from Liggins *et al.*, 1977a).

As labour progresses, pressure of the fetal presenting part on the cervix and vagina activates a neurohumoral reflex (Ferguson reflex) resulting in maternal secretion of oxytocin (Flint *et al.*, 1975b). Apart from its intrinsic oxytocic activity, oxytocin also stimulates the release of PGF (Mitchell *et al.*, 1975) which in turn stimulates further uterine activity (and further oxytocin release), so that the process of parturition accelerates until the delivery of the fetus is accomplished. Prostaglandins also seem to be involved in the process of cervical dilatation and effacement, although the Oxford experience (D. A. Ellwood *et al.*, in preparation) suggests that PGE may be more involved in bringing about these changes in the cervix than PGF, as suggested by Liggins *et al.* (1977b) and Fitzpatrick (1977).

THE INITIATION OF PARTURITION IN HUMAN PREGNANCY

How does the mechanism in the sheep fit the available data about the initiation of parturition in man? Firstly, does the fetal adrenal play a major role in determining the timing of the onset of human labour? In the absence of hydramnios, anencephaly (a fetal malformation in which the adrenals are hypoplastic), is associated with an increase in the range of gestation at delivery after the spontaneous onset of labour, compared with all pregnancies (Honnebier and Swaab, 1973) (Fig. 2). Although other studies have shown mainly prolongation of

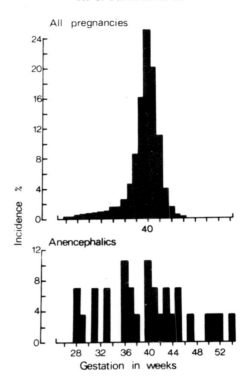

Fig. 2. Incidence of delivery by gestational age; comparison of pregnancy with an anencephalic fetus without hydramnios and "controls". (Adapted from Honnebier and Swaab, 1973).

pregnancy complicated by anencephaly without hydramnios, the study by Honnebier and Swaab provided by far the largest amount of data, and their findings imply that in man, the fetal pituitary–adrenal axis may act as a "fine tuner" of the time of onset of labour, rather than providing an "on/off" switch, which appears to be its role in ovine pregnancy.

Silman *et al.* (1976) have demonstrated maturational events in the human fetal anterior pituitary in the last few weeks of gestation, with secretion of "real" ACTH(1–39) superseding that of fragments similar to α-melanotrophin (α-MSH) and corticotrophin-like intermediate lobe peptide (CLIP). Furthermore, rising concentrations of cortisol have been demonstrated in amniotic fluid during late pregnancy (Gautray *et al.*, 1974; Murphy *et al.*, 1975; Fencl and Tulchinsky, 1975; Turnbull *et al.*, 1977) and higher cortisol levels have been found in cord blood of infants born after the spontaneous onset of labour than after induced labour or elective caesarean section (Murphy, 1973; Cawson *et al.*, 1974; Leong and Murphy, 1976). Although this evidence appears to suggest that increased fetal cortisol secretion precedes the spontaneous onset of labour in man, the fact that Gennser *et al.* (1977) have found no difference between the levels of cortisol in human fetal blood samples obtained before and after the spontaneous onset of labour, at term, is strong evidence against any sudden surge of fetal cortisol preceding labour in man.

Although there is some evidence that intra-amniotic administration of corticosteroids can initiate labour in women past term (Mati *et al.*, 1973; Nwosu *et al.*, 1976), Liggins *et al.* (1977a) have found this effect to be marginal, and there is no evidence for induction of labour before term by administration of corticosteroids.

In fact, we have been unable to demonstrate any evidence of 17α-hydroxylation in the human placenta delivered following the spontaneous onset of labour (A. P. F. Flint, unpublished observation). Administration of potent synthetic glucocorticoids to the mother in late human pregnancy simply suppresses maternal and fetal adrenal activity and reduces the levels of cortisol, dehydroepiandrosterone (DHEA) and oestriol in the mother (Anderson, 1976). There is no suggestion of a fall in progesterone or an increase in oestrogens, as in the sheep.

If increased fetal adrenal activity is a "trigger' for parturition in man, its mechanism of action remains unknown. Dehydroepiandrosterone sulphate (DHEAS), which is an oestrogen precursor, is a major secretory steroid of the fetal adrenal and could be considered as having a potential role in human labour. DHEAS of maternal origin contributes equally with that of fetal origin to oestrogen biosynthesis by the placenta. During pregnancy the metabolic clearance rate of DHEAS increases (Gant *et al.*, 1971) and there is a progressive fall in plasma DHEAS levels during gestation (Siiteri and Macdonald, 1966; Turnbull *et al.*, 1977), although amniotic fluid levels tend to increase (Turnbull *et al.*, 1977).

All these findings suggest gradually increasing fetal adrenal activity and possibly also changes in placental biosynthetic activity in the last few weeks of human pregnancy. Determination of peripheral plasma concentrations of progesterone and oestrogens in recent studies (Turnbull *et al.*, 1974) (Fig. 3) led us to suggest that the changes in their concentration might play a facilitatory, rather than a stimulatory, role in the onset of human labour (Turnbull *et al.*, 1977). Decreased plasma levels of progesterone before labour have only been demonstrated twice

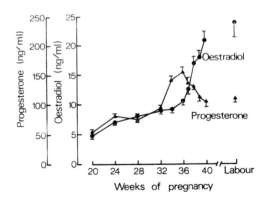

Fig. 3. Concentrations of peripheral plasma progesterone and 17β-oestradiol (mean ± S.E.M.) measured serially in 33 primigravidae between the 20th week of pregnancy and the spontaneous onset of labour at term. Concentrations found in these patients in second-stage labour are also shown. (Adapted from Turnbull *et al.*, 1974.)

(Csapo *et al.*, 1971; Turnbull *et al.*, 1974) in studies in primigravidae chosen with the strictest possible criteria of patient selection for normality. Even then, progesterone "withdrawal" did not occur in every case before labour and was certainly never as complete as that found in sheep before delivery. Similarly, the rise in oestradiol levels was never so dramatic as that seen in relation to ovine parturition. Furthermore, the oestradiol and progesterone levels in labour were the same as those in the week before labour. It must be concluded that the endocrine changes which occur prior to parturition in man do not necessarily include an acute fall in plasma progesterone.

MYOMETRIAL "GAP JUNCTIONS"

Recent studies by Garfield *et al.* (1979) have revealed cell-to-cell contacts, termed gap junctions, and these are thought to be sites of a low resistance pathway to current flow in excitable tissues. These studies were done on myometrium obtained from guinea-pigs and sheep at delivery or *post partum*. In human tissues, they were present in a much higher proportion of samples obtained from women after spontaneous labour than before it. Garfield *et al.* (1979) propose that gap junctions between myometrial cells are essential for effective uterine muscle contraction leading to termination of pregnancy in all animals, including man. In rats and sheep, progesterone withdrawal appears necessary for the formation of gap junctions, raising the possibility that, in some subtle way, progesterone withdrawal actually does occur in the human myometrium with labour.

Alternatively, prostaglandins may stimulate gap junction formation, according to Garfield *et al.* (1979). They also mention that oxytocin does not have this ability, nor can it stimulate myometrial contractions in the absence of gap junctions.

PROSTAGLANDINS

Perhaps the greatest similarity between the mechanism of parturition in man and sheep (and many other species) is the crucial role played by prostaglandins. Turnbull (1978) quotes the many workers who have shown that administration of prostaglandins will stimulate labour or abortion, and that administration of prostaglandin synthetase inhibitors will delay labour and delivery in both species, although the sensitivity of the human uterus to prostaglandins is greater than in the sheep, in which the response to prostaglandins increases markedly as parturition approaches (Mitchell *et al.*, 1977a). What, then, are the trends in prostaglandin concentration in plasma and amniotic fluid in late pregnancy and labour, where do they originate from, and what controls their production?

Measurements of prostaglandins E and F (PGE and PGF) in peripheral plasma are hampered by the low concentrations present due to rapid clearance, especially in the lungs, and also because of prostaglandin production by platelets.It has therefore been suggested by Samuelsson (1974) that measurement of 13,14-dihydro-14-keto-prostaglandin F (PGFM) in peripheral plasma is the best monitor of prostaglandin production. Measurement of PGEM remains technically very difficult because of its instability (Mitchell *et al.*, 1977b).

Peripheral blood levels of PGFM apparently increase slightly in late human pregnancy, with a sharp rise during labour (Gréen *et al.*, 1974; Mitchell *et al.*, 1978a). We have been unable to demonstrate significant changes in peripheral plasma concentrations of PGE and PGF during labour (Mitchell *et al.*, 1978b), which suggests that the lungs are capable of metabolizing the large amount of prostaglandins secreted from the uterus during labour.

Amniotic fluid is not in contact with tissues containing high concentrations of prostaglandin-metabolizing enzymes (Keirse and Turnbull, 1975) and has been the fluid of choice for measuring prostaglandins in relation to labour. The concentrations of prostaglandins are higher in amniotic fluid during labour than before labour and increase rapidly as labour progresses (Karim and Devlin, 1967; Keirse and Turnbull, 1973; Salmon and Amy, 1973; Keirse *et al.*, 1974; Hillier *et al.*, 1974). Although it was suggested that prostaglandin levels in amniotic fluid may increase progressively from 36 weeks onwards (Salmon and Amy, 1973; Hibbard *et al.*, 1974), we could not demonstrate this trend when samples obtained by amniotomy were separated from those obtained by amniocentesis (Mitchell *et al.*, 1977c) (Fig. 4).

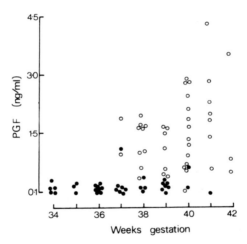

Fig. 4. Concentrations of prostaglandin F (PGF) measured by radioimmunoassay in amniotic fluid obtained by amniocentesis (●) and amniotomy (○) before the onset of labour. (Mitchell *et al.*, 1977c.)

A discontinuous rise in PGE level at 36 weeks of gestation has, however, been observed by Dray and Frydman (1976) in samples taken by amniocentesis. In labour, the concentration of PGF increases more than that of PGE (Keirse and Turnbull, 1973; Keirse *et al.*, 1974; Dray and Frydman, 1978).

The raised levels of PGF and PGFM in amniotic fluid obtained by amniotomy suggest a local control of prostaglandins consistent with our subsequent finding

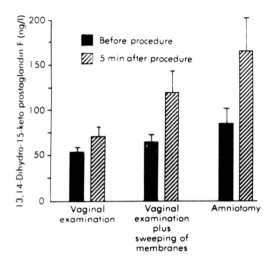

Fig. 5. Peripheral plasma concentrations of PGFM (mean ± S.E.M.) in women in late pregnancy before (solid bars) and 5 min after (hatched bars) vaginal examination, vaginal examination plus sweeping of membranes, and amniotomy. (Mitchell *et al.*, 1977a.)

that peripheral plasma levels of PGFM are elevated within 5 min of amniotomy, or even vaginal examination alone (Mitchell *et al.*, 1977d) (Fig. 5). That the greatest increase in PGFM levels should be found after amniotomy is not surprising since the fetal membranes are significant sources of prostaglandins (Macdonald *et al.*, 1974; Keirse and Turnbull, 1976; Mitchell *et al.*, 1978b).

Gustavii has also been convinced of the importance of a local mechanism controlling parturition involving the decidual membrane and the fetal membranes, and in a recent paper (Gustavii, 1978) has re-emphasized the hypothesis that labilization of decidual lysosomes releases phospholipase A_2, which catalyses hydrolytic cleavage of the 2-position of glycerophospholipids. Fatty acids at the 2-position, such as arachidonic acid, are precursors of prostaglandins, which he postulates will then be formed in increasing amounts, to bring about labour.

Gustavii had previously suggested that progesterone stabilizes lysosomes, thereby preventing release of phospholipase A_2. Schwarz *et al.* (1974) found that the cytosol of chorioamnion homogenates contained a progesterone binding protein, in low concentration before 38 weeks of pregnancy, but in much higher concentrations at term. It differs from cytosol progesterone receptors and transcortin. Schwarz *et al.* propose that this specific progesterone binding protein competes with lysosomes for progesterone, which causes a local withdrawal of progesterone, independent of maternal plasma levels and the lysosomes become unstable. The cause for the rapid accumulation of this progesterone binding protein at term is unknown.

The basic supposition in this concept is that the rate-limiting step in prostaglandin synthesis is the availability of free fatty acid substrates. It should be noted, however, that human amniotic fluid contains a vast excess of arachidonic acid over the levels of PGE and PGF (Keirse *et al.*, 1977) and that a similar pattern is found in uterine tissues (Keirse, 1975). It is, therefore, unlikely that precursor availability is the only rate-limiting step in prostaglandin biosynthesis within the human uterus, although the intracellular availability of arachidonic acid to prostaglandin synthesizing enzymes is unknown and may prove an important determining factor.

Recently, Maathius and Kelly (1978) have demonstrated that the concentrations of prostaglandins in human decidual tissue (conceptual age 3–10 weeks) are lower than those measured in the endometrium at any stage in the normal menstrual cycle. Apparently, the human conceptus is able to interfere with the endometrial synthesis or metabolism of PGE and PGF very soon after implantation. Extremely low levels of both PGF and PGE (0.025 μg/g) were found in endometrium obtained from a pregnancy with a conceptual age of about 17 days. Endometrial histology was indistinguishable from that in the late secretory phase, but in the absence of pregnancy, prostaglandin levels would be about 200 times greater in this phase than were actually found. In the non-pregnant state, high levels of oestradiol and progesterone relate to high levels of prostaglandin F.

These findings, coupled with the great excess of arachidonic acid over PGE and PGF in amniotic fluid and uterine tissues in late human pregnancy, described by Keirse *et al.*(1977), suggest that pregnancy maintenance in man may depend on the nearly complete inhibition of the prostaglandin synthetase enzyme system in certain critical intrauterine tissues, possibly fetal membranes and, in particular, decidua. An endogenous inhibitor of prostaglandin synthesis has been found in the α-globulin fraction of human plasma (Saeed *et al.*, 1977) and one might speculate that the inhibitor could prove to be a protein of placental or trophoblastic origin. Clarification of the mechanism which inhibits prostaglandin synthesis so effectively in human pregnancy deserves high priority.

CONCLUSIONS

To summarize, the many studies outlined in this review show that parturition in man, unlike that in the sheep or several other species, is not preceded by a sudden change in maternal levels of oestrogens or progesterone, and that the role of the fetus in initiating labour also seems much less dramatic and direct. Administration of corticosteroids suppresses maternal and fetal adrenal function and causes a fall in oestrogen levels in the mother; there is no activation of placental 17α-hydroxylation by corticosteroid administration as in the sheep, with progesterone falling and oestrogens rising over a short period of time.

Human pregnancy appears to be maintained by a mechanism which inhibits prostaglandin synthesis within the uterus. Compared with the sheep, human myometrium is relatively sensitive to prostaglandins throughout pregnancy. Initiation of labour may, therefore, depend on the release from inhibition of prostaglandin synthesis in tissues such as the fetal membranes, and decidua. In late pregnancy the mechanism is readily activated by local trauma.

The nature of the factor which inhibits prostaglandin synthesis remains uncertain. It may be a protein of placental or trophoblastic origin, or it may be progesterone, stabilizing the decidual lysosomes until its effect is overcome at term by rapidly increased production of a specific progesterone binding protein which, in effect, causes local progesterone withdrawal in the fetal membranes.

Once synthesis of PGE, PGF and prostacyclin begins to increase in the uterus, they can bring about all the aspects of progressive labour, inducing powerful co-ordinated uterine activity (possibly stimulating the formation of gap junctions) and causing the changes in the connective tissue of the cervix which, together with the muscular activity of the uterine fundus, produces softening and progressive dilatation of the cervix.

This concept accords quite closely with the proposal by Liggins *et al.* (1977b) that "the onset of labour in man is mainly the outcome of a genetically determined maturational event in the amnion and/or chorion. The fetus itself and the mother may modulate, but rarely control, the time of birth."

REFERENCES

Anderson, A. B. M. (1976). *In* "Prevention of Fetal Handicap through Ante-natal Care (A. C. Turnbull and F. P. Woodford, eds), Vol. 3, pp. 137–148, Associated Scientific Publishers, Amsterdam.

Anderson, A. B. M., Flint, A. P. F. and Turnbull, A. C. (1975). *Journal of Endocrinology* **66**, 61.

Ash, R. W., Challis, J. R. G., Harrison, F. A., Heap, R. B., Illingworth, D. V., Perry, J. S. and Poyser, N. L. (1973). *In* "Fetal and Neonatal Physiology" (Comline *et al.*, eds), pp. 551–561, Cambridge University Press, London.

Bassett, J. M. and Thorburn, G. D. (1969). *Journal of Endocrinology*, **44**, 285.

Beitins, I. Z., Kowarski, A., Shermeta, D. W., De Lemos, R. and Migeon, C. J. (1970). *Paediatric Research* **4**, 129.

Cawson, M. J., Anderson, A. B. M., Turnbull, A. C. and Lampe, L. (1974). *Journal of Obstetrics and Gynaecology of the British Commonwealth* **81**, 737.

Csapo, A. I., Knobil, E., Van der Molen, H. J. and Wiest, W. G. (1971). *American Journal of Obstetrics and Gynecology* **110**, 630.

Currie, W. B., Wong, M. S. F., Cox, R. I. and Thorburn, G. D. (1973). *Memoirs of the Society for Endocrinology* **20**, 95.

Dray, F. and Frydman, R. (1976). *American Journal of Obstetrics and Gynecology* **126**, 13.

Dray, F. and Frydman, R. (1978). *In* "Pre-natal Endocrinology and Parturition", INSERM Symposium, pp. 121–135, INSERM, Paris.

Fairclough, R. J. and Liggins, G. C. (1975). *Journal of Endocrinology* **67**, 333.

Fencl, M. and Tulchinsky, D. (1975). *New England Journal of Medicine* **292**, 133.

Fitzpatrick, R. J. (1977). *In* "The Fetus and Birth" (J. Knight and M. O'Connor, eds), pp. 31–39, Elsevier/Excerpta Medica/North Holland, Amsterdam.

Flint, A. P. F., Anderson, A. B. M., Steele, P. A. and Turnbull, A. C. (1975a). *Biochemical Society Transactions* **3**, 1189.

Flint, A. P. F., Forsling, M. L., Mitchell, M. D. and Turnbull, A. C. (1975b). *Journal of Reproduction and Fertility* **43**, 551.

Gant, N. F., Hutchinson, H. T., Siiteri, P. K. and Macdonald, P. C. (1971). *American Journal of Obstetrics and Gynecology* **111**, 555.

Garfield, R. E., Rabidean, S., Challis, J. R. G. and Daniel, E. E. (1979). *American Journal of Obstetrics and Gynecology* **133**, 308.

Gautray, J. P., Jolivet, A., Dhen, N., Vielk, J. P. and Tajchner, G. (1974). *In* "Avortement et Parturition Provoques" (M. J. Bosc, R. Palmer and Cl. Sureau, eds), pp. 227–238, Masson, Paris.

Gennser, G., Ohrlander, S. and Eneroth, P. (1977). *In* "The Fetus and Birth" (J. Knight and M. O'Connor, eds), pp. 401–420, Elsevier/Excerpta Medica/ North Holland.

Gréen, K., Bygdeman, M., Toppozada, M. and Wiqvist, N. (1974). *American Journal of Obstetrics and Gynecology* **120**, 35.

Gustavii, B. (1978). *In* "Prenatal Endocrinology and Parturition" INSERM Symposium, pp. 93–101, INSERM, Paris.

Hibbard, B. M., Sharma, S. C., Fitzpatrick, R. J. and Hamlett, J. D. (1974). *Journal of Obstetrics and Gynaecology of the British Commonwealth* **81**, 35.

Hillier, K., Calder, A. A. and Embrey. M. P. (1974). *Journal of Obstetrics and Gynaecology of the British Commonwealth* **81**, 257.

Honnebier, W. J. and Swaab, D. F. (1973). *Journal of Obstetrics and Gynaecology of the British Commonwealth* **80**, 577.

Jones, C. T., Boddy, K. and Robinson, J. S. (1977). *Journal of Endocrinology* **72**, 293.

Karim, S. M. M. and Devlin, J. (1967). *Journal of Obstetrics and Gynaecology of the British Commonwealth* **74**, 230.

Keirse, M. J. N. C. (1975). D. Phil. thesis, University of Oxford.

Keirse, M. J. N. C. and Turnbull, A. C. (1973). *Journal of Obstetrics and Gynaecology of the British Commonwealth* **80**, 970.

Keirse, M. J. N. C. and Turnbull, A. C. (1975). *British Journal of Obstetrics and Gynaecology* **82**, 887.

Keirse, M. J. N. C. and Turnbull, A. C. (1976). *British Journal of Obstetrics and Gynaecology* **83**, 146.

Keirse, M. J. N. C., Flint, A. P. F. and Turnbull, A. C. (1974). *Journal of Obstetrics and Gynaecology of the British Commonwealth* **81**, 131.

Keirse, M. J. N. C., Hicks, B. R., Mitchell, M. D. and Turnbull, A. C. (1977). *British Journal of Obstetrics and Gynaecology* **84**, 937.

Leong, M. K. H. and Murphy, B. E. P. (1976). *American Journal of Obstetrics and Gynecology* **124**, 471.

Liggins, G. C. (1969). *Journal of Endocrinology* **42**, 323.

Liggins, G. C., Kennedy, P. C. and Holm, L. W. (1967). *American Journal of Obstetrics and Gynecology* **98**, 1080.

Liggins, G. C., Forster, S., Grieves, S. A., and Schwarz, A. L. (1977b). *Biology of Reproduction* **16**, 39.

Liggins, G. C., Fairclough, R. J., Grieves, S. A., Kendall, J. Z. and Knox, B. S. (1973). *Recent Progress in Hormone Research* **29**, 111.

Liggins, G. C., Fairclough, R. J., Grieves, S. A., Forster, C. S. and Knox, B. S. (1977a). *In* "The Fetus and Birth" (J. Knight and M. O'Connor, eds), pp. 5–25, Elsevier/Excerpta Medica/North Holland, Amsterdam.

Louis, T. M., Challis, J. R. G., Robinson, J. S. and Thorburn, G. D. (1976). *Nature, London* **264**, 797.

Maathius, J. B. and Kelly, R. W. (1978). *Journal of Endocrinology* **77**, 361.

Macdonald, P. C., Schulz, F. M., Duenholter, J. H., Gant, N. F., Jimenez, J. M., Pritchard, J. A., Porter, J. C. and Johnston, J. M. (1974). *Obstetrics and Gynecology* **126**, 13.

Madill, D. and Bassett, J. M. (1973). *Journal of Endocrinology* **58**, 75.

Mahajan, D. K. and Samuels, L. T. (1975). *Steroids* **24**, 217.

Mati, J. K. G., Horrobin, D. F. and Bramley, P. S. (1973). *British Medical Journal* ii, 149.

Mitchell, M. D. and Flint, A.P. F. (1977). *Prostaglandins* **14**, 611.

Mitchell, M. D., Flint, A. P. F. and Turnbull, A. C. (1975). *Prostaglandins* **9**, 47.

Mitchell, M. D., Flint, A. P. F. and Turnbull, A. C. (1977a). *Journal of Reproduction and Fertility* **48**, 189.

Mitchell, M. D., Sors, H. and Flint, A. P. F. (1977b). *Lancet, ii,* 558.

Mitchell, M. D., Bibby, J., Hicks, B. R. and Turnbull, A. C. (1978b). *Prostaglandins* **15**, 377.

Mitchell, M. D., Keirse, M. J. N. C., Anderson, A. B. M. and Turnbull, A. C. (1977c). *British Journal of Obstetrics and Gynaecology* **84**, 35.

Mitchell, M. D., Flint, A. P. F., Bibby, J., Brunt, J., Arnold, J. M., Anderson, A. B. M. and Turnbull, A. C. (1977d). *British Medical Journal ii,* 1183.

Mitchell, M. D., Flint, A. P. F., Bibby, J., Brunt, J., Arnold, J. M., Anderson, A. B. M. and Turnbull, A. C. (1978a). *Journal of Clinical Endocrinology and Metabolism* **46**, 947.

Murphy, B. E. P. (1973). *American Journal of Obstetrics and Gynecology* **115**, 521.

Murphy, B. E. P., Patrick, J. and Denton, R. L. (1975). *Journal of Clinical Endocrinology and Metabolism* **40**, 164.

Nwosu, U. C., Wallach, E. E. and Bolognese, R. J. (1976). *Obstetrics and Gynecology* **47**, 137.

Rees, L. H., Jack, P. M. B., Thomas, A. L. and Nathanielsz, P. W. (1975). *Nature, London* **253**, 274.

Rush, R. W., Keirse, M. J. N. C., Howat, P., Baum, J. D., Anderson, A. B. M. and Turnbull, A. C. (1976). *British Medical Journal ii,* 965.

Saeed, S. A., McDonald-Gibson, W. J., Cuthbert, J., Copas, J. L., Schneider, C., Gardiner, P. J., Butt, N. M. and Collier, H. O. J. (1977). *Nature, London* **270**, 32.

Salmon, J. A. and Amy, J. J. (1973). *Prostaglandins* **4**, 523.

Samuelsson, B. (1974). *In* "Les Prostaglandines", INSERM Symposium, pp. 21–41, INSERM, Paris.

Schwarz, B. E., Vanatta, P., Siiteri, P. K. and Macdonald, P. C. (1974). *Gynecologic Investigation* **5**, 21.

Siiteri, P. K. and MacDonald, P. C. (1966). *Journal of Clinical Endocrinology* **26**, 751.

Silman, R. E., Chard, T., Lowry, P. J., Smith, I. and Young, I. M. (1976). *Nature, London* **260**, 716.

Silman, R. E., Holland, D., Chard, T., Lowry, P. J., Hope, J., Rees, L. H., Thomas, A. and Nathanielsz, P. (1979). *Journal of Endocrinology* **81**, 19.

Steele, P. A., Flint, A. P. F. and Turnbull, A. C. (1976). *Journal of Endocrinology* **69**, 239.

Thorburn, G. D., Challis, J. R. G. and Robinson, J. S. (1977). *In* "Biology of the Uterus" (R. M. Wynn, ed.), pp. 653–732, Plenum Press, New York.

Turnbull, A. C. (1978). *In* "Prenatal Endocrinology and Parturition", INSERM Symposium, pp. 77–92 INSERM, Paris.

Turnbull, A. C., Patten, P. T., Flint, A. P. F., Keirse, M. J. N. C., Jeremy, J. Y. and Anderson, A. B. M. (1974). *Lancet* **1**, 101.

Turnbull, A. C., Anderson, A. B. M., Flint, A. P. F., Jeremy, J. Y., Keirse, M. J. N. C. and Mitchell, M. D. (1977). *In* "The Fetus and Birth" (J. Knight and M. O'Connor, eds), pp. 427–452, Elsevier/Excerpta Medica/North Holland, Amsterdam.

OVARIAN FUNCTION IN PREGNANT WOMEN AT TERM

B. Acar, R. Fleming and J. R. T. Coutts

Department of Obstetrics and Gynaecology, The University of Glasgow, Royal Maternity Hospital, Rottenrow, Glasgow G4 ONA, Scotland

INTRODUCTION

Luteectomy in pregnant women 6 weeks after ovulation neither causes abortion nor a significant drop in peripheral plasma progesterone (P) levels (Csapo *et al.*, 1974). However, both *in vitro* (Le Maire *et al.*, 1968) and *in vivo* (Le Maire *et al.*, 1970) it has been demonstrated that corpora lutea of late gestation and term pregnancy secrete P. Weiss and Rifkin (1975) further established that during the early puerperium the human corpus luteum actively secreted P but neither oestradiol (E_2) nor oestrone (E_1). These authors also observed that non-luteal ovarian tissues secreted E_2 during the puerperium.

The present study was carried out to investigate further the relationships between steroid hormones from luteal and non-luteal ovaries in women at term pregnancy and to examine any possible role in this steroidogenesis for human chorionic gonadotrophin (hCG).

MATERIALS AND METHODS

Patients and Samples

Thirty-six patients with term pregnancies (35 singleton; 1 twin) being delivered by caesarean section (27 elective, nine following failure to progress after labour induction) were studied after informed consent had been obtained. The patients received either general (Pentothal) or epidural (Marcain) anaesthesia.

Serono Symposium No. 35, "The Human Placenta", edited by A. Klopper, A. Genazzani and P. G. Crosignani, 1980. Academic Press, London and New York.

Table I. Details of radioimmunoassays.

Hormone	Antigen [a]	Major cross-reactions (%)	Assay precision (%) Intra	Inter
Progesterone	Progesterone-11α-hemisuccinate	Deoxycorticosterone, 11 20α-Dihydroprogesterone, 1.2	±13	±13
Oestradiol	Oestradiol-6-(O-carboxy methyl)oxime	Oestriol, 11 Oestriol, 12	11	11
Oestrone	Oestrone-6-(O-carboxy methyl)oxime	All < 0.1	10	6
Androstenedione	Androstenedione-7α-succinate	5α-Androstenedione, 70 Testosterone, 0.5	6	12
Testosterone	Testosterone-11α-hemisuccinate	5α-Dihydrotestosterone, 3 5β-Dihydrotestosterone, 2 19-Nortestosterone,29	11	8
hCG	hCG	LH, 100	6	Single assay

[a]All steroid antigens are BSA-linked.

Gestational age was determined by ultrasonic examination, clinical examination and from the menstrual history. The mean gestation was 279.3 ± 7.1 (s.d.) days (range 261–292 days). Bilateral ovarian and peripheral venous blood samples were collected immediately after removal of the fetus and suturing of the uterine wall. Blood samples were collected from each patient in the following order: right ovarian vein simultaneously with peripheral vein (antecubital vein) followed immediately by the left ovarian vein. The ovary containing the corpus luteum was identified by observation. The delay between delivery of the placenta and collection of the last blood sample was 23.1 ± 4.4 (s.d.) min (range 16–32 min).

Assay Methods

Blood samples in lithium heparin tubes were centrifuged within 30 min of collection and the plasma samples were separated and stored at $-20\,^{\circ}$C until assay. Using sensitive, specific, precise radioimmunoassays each plasma sample was analysed for its content of P, E_2, E_1, androstenedione (A), and testosterone (T). In addition, the levels of hCG in the peripheral plasma samples were also determined. Table I lists details of the radioimmunoassays used: the antigens to which antisera were raised, the cross-reactivity of antisera, and the reliability criteria of the assays in which these samples were analysed. All samples were assayed in triplicate; in the case of steroid hormone assays the three different samples from one patient were assayed in the same assay.

Steroid assays incorporated dextran-coated charcoal to separate free and antibody-bound fractions, whilst the hCG assay employed a standard double-antibody technique.

RESULTS

Figure 1 shows the key used in the succeeding figures to represent peripheral, corpus luteum-containing ovary (CL) and the contralateral, non-corpus luteum-

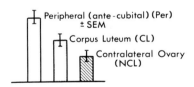

Fig. 1. Key showing symbols used in succeeding figures to depict peripheral samples, samples from the vein draining the ovary containing the corpus luteum and samples from the vein draining the contralateral ovary.

containing ovary (NCL). Figures 2, 3 and 4, show the mean concentrations ± s.e.m. for these three samples from all 36 patients for P, E_1 and E_2 and A and T, respectively.

Progesterone

When the Student's *t*-test was applied to the data (Fig. 2) on paired samples (*n* = 36), the P levels in the CL ovarian venous plasma were significantly higher than those in either the NCL ovarian venous or the peripheral plasmas (*p* < 0.001

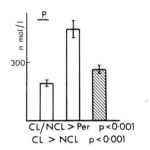

Fig. 2. Progesterone levels, mean ± S.E.M., from all 36 patients in peripheral and ovarian venous plasmas (for key see Fig. 1).

for both). In addition the P levels in the plasma from the NCL ovarian vein were significantly higher than those in peripheral plasma (*p* < 0.001).

The levels of P observed in the CL ovarian venous plasmas were similar to those found in our laboratory in CL ovarian venous plasma samples from normally cycling patients during the luteal phase (Macnaughton *et al.*, 1979).

Oestradiol, Oestrone, Androstenedione and Testosterone

The NCL and CL venous plasma levels for each of the hormones E_2, E_1, A and T were both significantly greater than the peripheral plasma levels of the same hormones (*p* < 0.001 for all four hormones; *n* = 36; paired data). However, there

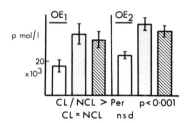

Fig. 3. Mean levels ± S.E.M. of oestrone (OE_1) and oestradiol (OE_2), from all 36 patients, in peripheral and ovarian venous samples (for key see Fig. 1).

were no significant differences (*n* = 36 for each; paired data) between the levels of any hormone in the two ovarian venous samples (see Figs 3 and 4).

The levels of E_2, E_1 and T found in the ovarian venous plasmas at term in this study were considerably higher than those found in our laboratory in ovarian venous plasma at any stage during the menstrual cycle (Coutts *et al.*, 1979). The

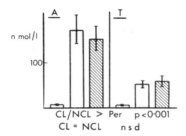

Fig. 4. Androstenedione (A) and testosterone (T) levels (mean ± S.E.M.) from all 36 patients in peripheral and ovarian venous samples (for key see Figure 1).

A levels found in ovarian venous plasmas here were similar to those found by us during the luteal phase in the CL ovarian vein (Macnaughton *et al.*, 1979) but were much higher in the NCL ovarian vein than those observed in it at any stage of the menstrual cycle.

In all of the paired data examinations there were a few exceptions (e.g. two patients P in CL less than peripheral; four patients P in NCL less than peripheral; three patients E_2 in CL less than peripheral; four patients E_2 in NCL less than peripheral). However, the exceptional cases differed for the different hormones, thus indicating that the ovarian venous levels were reflecting ovarian steroidogenesis and were not the results of contamination with residual placental blood.

hCG

The levels of hCG in the peripheral plasma samples were variable with mean concentrations of 8490 ± 1164 (S.E.M.) IU/l. These values are similar to values

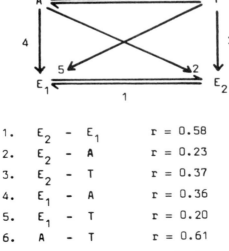

1.	E_2	– E_1	r = 0.58
2.	E_2	– A	r = 0.23
3.	E_2	– T	r = 0.37
4.	E_1	– A	r = 0.36
5.	E_1	– T	r = 0.20
6.	A	– T	r = 0.61

Fig. 5. Correlation coefficient (*r*) between oestrogen and androgen levels in paired data from ovarian venous plasmas (*n* = 72).

often observed in term human pregnancy. No significant correlations were obtained between hCG concentrations in peripheral plasmas and the concentrations of any of the steroid hormones either in peripheral plasmas or in ovarian venous plasmas.

Relationships between Different Steroid Hormones

The relationships between the different steroid hormones were investigated by examining their relative concentrations within each of the three compartments for each patient. P levels did not correlate significantly with the levels of any of the other hormones in any compartment. Since very similar patterns were noted with respect to production of E_2, E_1, A and T by both ovaries, the relationships between these hormones were investigated. Having established no difference between the CL and the NCL ovarian venous levels the data for these hormones were combined to give 72 values for correlation studies. The results of correlation data are shown in Fig. 5.

DISCUSSION

The results of this study show that at term the human corpus luteum of pregnancy secretes P in amounts which are roughly equivalent to the production by the active corpus luteum of the luteal phase of the reproductive cycle. This concurs with previous investigators' findings *in vitro* (Le Maire *et al.*, 1968) and *in vivo* (Le Maire *et al.*, 1970; Weiss and Rifkin, 1975).

Since the P levels in the CL ovary did not correlate significantly with the circulating levels of hCG the maintenance of progesterone secretion by the corpus luteum does not appear to be a direct trophic effect of hCG. Weiss and Rifkin (1975) also observed that ovarian tissues apart from the corpus luteum elaborated E_2 but not E_1. The present study demonstrates that non-luteal ovarian tissue from both ovaries is responsible for production of E_2, E_1, A and T and also that the NCL containing ovary produces some P although an insignificant amount by comparison to the CL ovary. The production of ovarian E_2 confirms the results of Weiss and Rifkin (1975) but that of E_1 is contrary to their conclusions. On close examination of these authors' limited data, however, it appears that had they examined paired data they would have obtained similar results with regard to E_1 to those reported in this study. The levels of oestrogens and androgens which were found in both ovarian veins, with the exception of the A level in the CL ovary, were much greater than those found in ovarian venous plasmas obtained at any stage of the menstrual cycle. Similarly the level of P in the NCL ovarian vein was also greater than that seen at any stage of the menstrual cycle in this vessel. It is impossible to decide from the type of study reported here which non-luteal ovarian tissues might have been responsible for elaboration of these steroids. Potential sources might be Graafian follicles, which have been frequently observed— up to 8 mm in diameter—in ovarian tissue at term (A.D.T. Govan, personal communication) and ovarian tissue luteinized by the high levels of hCG.

The lack of significant correlations between the peripheral levels of hCG and the levels of any of the other steroid hormones, either ovarian or peripheral, suggests that the latter explanation is not true and other factors may be involved.

The similar patterns observed in the three compartments with respect to E_2, E_1, A and T suggest that the same ovarian tissues might be responsible for secretion of both androgens and oestrogens.

The data correlating the C_{18} and C_{19} steroid concentrations in ovarian venous plasma show that both the 17a-hydroxysteroid dehydrogenase and the aromatase enzymes are equally active for both of their potential substrates (Fig. 5), indicating that ovarian E_2 during the early puerperium may be synthesized via either A or T.

REFERENCES

Coutts, J.R.T., Gaukroger, J. M., Samad Kader, A. and Macnaughton, M. C. (1979). *Journal of Reproduction and Fertility* Suppl. 28, in press.

Csapo, A. I., Pulkinnen, M. O. and Kaihola, H. L. (1974). *American Journal of Obstetrics and Gynecology* **118**, 985.

Le Maire, W. J., Rice, B. F. and Savard, K. (1968). *Journal of Clinical Endocrinology* **28**, 1249.

Le Maire, W. J., Conly, P. W., Moffett, A. and Cleveland, W. W. (1970). *American Journal of Obstetrics and Gynecology* **108**, 132.

Macnaughton, M. C., Samad Kader, A., Gaukroger, J. M. and Coutts, J.R.T. (1979). *Journal of Reproduction and Fertility* Suppl. 28, in press.

Weiss, G. and Rifkin, I. (1975). *Obstetrics and Gynecology* **46**, 557.

ENDOCRINE CHANGES IN TWIN PREGNANCY

R. L. TambyRaja and S. S. Ratnam

University of Singapore, Singapore

INTRODUCTION

Animal research over the past 10 years has provided substantial data to support the thesis that the steroid hormones of the fetoplacental unit play a role in the onset of labour. In view of the early onset of labour in twin pregnancy and its contribution to higher perinatal mortality, it seemed worthwhile to undertake serial measurements of the levels of plasma 17β-oestradiol, progesterone, and oestriol in uncomplicated twin pregnancy. The accounts of twin pregnancy in the English literature have changed but little in the past 25 years since Bender (1952) advocated that, "The object of antenatal care in twin pregnancy should be to prevent as far as possible the premature onset of labour. To this end, it is suggested that every woman with a twin pregnancy should be admitted to hospital for bed rest."

Advancing obstetrical knowledge related to the endocrinology of pregnancy and myometrial contractility have opened new avenues of therapy.

PATIENTS AND METHODS

The patients were selected from volunteers attending a research antenatal clinic. All were certain of their last menstrual period and were attended during pregnancy by the individual research worker. The diagnosis of twins was con-

Serono Symposium No. 35, "The Human Placenta", edited by A. Klopper,
A. Genazzani and P. G. Crosignani, 1980. Academic Press, London and New York.

firmed by ultrasound or abdominal radiography. The pregnancies were reviewed after delivery. Ten patients diagnosed before 30 weeks with normal pregnancies who delivered infants weighing more than 2500 g were selected for study.

Heparinized blood samples were taken weekly from each patient. The plasma was immediately separated from the cells by centrifugation and stored at $-15\,^{\circ}$C until assay. Plasma progesterone, 17β-oestradiol, and oestriol were assayed in duplicate by radioimmunoassay using specific antibodies. Unconjugated 17β-oestradiol was measured by the radioimmunoassay method of Hotchkiss et al. (1971) using an antiserum raised in rabbits against 17β-oestradiol-6-(carboxymethyl)oxime–bovine serum albumin. Plasma total oestriol was measured by a modification of the radioimmunoassay of Wilson (1973) using an antiserum against oestriol-6-(O-carboxymethyl)oxime-bovine serum albumin. The method has been previously described (Chew et al., 1976). Progesterone was assayed in duplicate by means of the radioimmunoassay method of Devilla et al. (1972) using an antiserum generated in sheep by the injection of 11-hydroxy-progesterone hemisuccinate conjugated to bovine serum albumin. Control samples taken during the steroid assays showed that the intra- and interassay coefficients of variation were less than 15%.

Fifty patients in whom the diagnosis of twin pregnancy was confirmed by ultrasound or abdominal X-ray examination were treated with salbutamol from the time of diagnosis. Tablets of 4 mg were given three times per day; the dose was increased to 8 mg three times a day at the next weekly antenatal attendance if the pulse rate remained at 100 beats/min or less. Of the 50 patients, six were excluded in view of pregnancy complications (antepartum haemorrhage and severe pre-eclampsia) and two were lost to follow up. A control group matched for age and parity consisted of 42 women with twin pregnancies in whom the diagnosis was made before 30 weeks and who were treated with traditional bed rest. They spent at least 2 weeks in the antenatal ward, were allowed toilet facilities and given only haematinic supplements. Effectiveness of therapy was judged in terms of length of gestation, birthweight and perinatal mortality.

RESULTS

Plasma oestradiol and oestriol (Figs 1 and 2) showed an increase from the 30th week. The increase was steeper between the 34th and 36th weeks. The increase in both oestrogens showed the same pattern and reached a peak around 36 weeks. The mean plamsa level ($\pm$ s.e.m.) of oestradiol at 30 weeks was 19.3 $\pm$ 0.52 ng/ml reaching a peak of 39.21 $\pm$ 3.35 ng/ml at 36 weeks. Similarly, plasma oestriol rose from 155 $\pm$ 15.4 ng/ml to a peak value of 336 $\pm$ 31.6 ng/ml at 38 weeks. The individual variations were more marked for plasma oestriol. Plasma progesterone levels (Table II, Figure 3) showed little variation in the last 10 weeks of pregnancy, ranging from 203 $\pm$ 9.5 ng/ml to 387 $\pm$ 36.2 ng/ml. There was no decline in level before the onset of labour. The ratio of plasma progesterone to 17β-oestradiol remained under 12.1 in the last 4 weeks of pregnancy.

On salbutamol treatment there was a lower level of plasma oestradiol for each week of gestation from 21.9 ng/ml at 30 weeks, to a peak level of 34.2 ng/ml at 36 weeks (Table I). The difference from the untreated control was, however, not

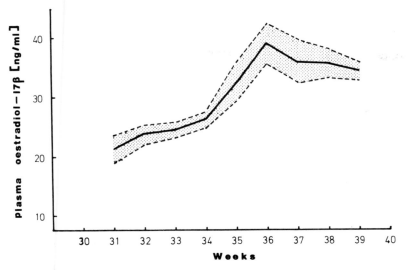

Fig. 1. Serial plasma levels of unconjugated 17β-oestradiol in twin pregnancy. Mean values ± S.E.M. are shown.

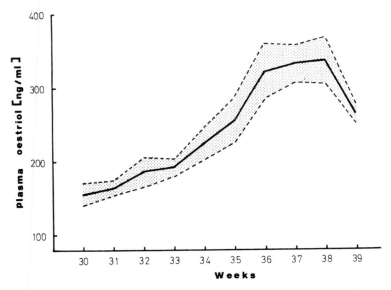

Fig. 2. Serial plasma levels of total oestriol in twin pregnancy. Mean values ± S.E.M. are shown (in nanograms per millilitre).

statistically significant. Similarly, there was no significant depression of plasma oestriol. Plasma progesterone levels in the salbutamol group were not higher than the controls (Table II).

The mean period of gestation at delivery was 258 days for the control group

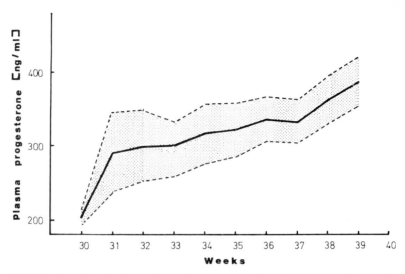

Fig. 3. Serial plasma levels of unconjugated progesterone in twin pregnancy. Mean values ±
S.E.M. are shown (in nanograms per millilitre).

receiving bed rest and 271 days for the salbutamol group ($p < 0.001$). Moreover,
the mean birthweight of the group having bed rest at 2326 g was significantly
lower than the mean birthweight of 2729 g in the salbutamol-treated patients
($p < 0.001$). What is more remarkable is that there was not a single neonatal
death due to prematurity and hyaline membrane disease in the babies born to the
salbutamol-treated mothers, although 36 of the 84 babies weighed less than
2500 g. It is also significant that only four of the salbutamol-treated babies
weighed less than 2000 g and no infant weighed less than 1500 g. In contrast, all
six babies who did not survive in the bed rest group weighed less than 2000 g
although they had no congenital malformations. The perinatal mortality of 11.9%
in the salbutamol group was considerably lower than the rate of 71.4% in the
group having bed rest.

DISCUSSION

It is interesting that the mean plasma oestradiol levels in twin pregnancies are
higher than those reported from this laboratory (Chew and Ratnam, 1976) and
levels in a similar study by Turnbull *et al*. (1974). The two oestrogens reached
their peak 2 weeks before the highest level reported in singleton pregnancies. It
is of significance (TambyRaja *et al*., 1974, 1975; Iwasaki and Sugato, 1976)
that an early rise in oestrogen levels predisposes to preterm parturition in that the
mean duration of gestation in twins is shorter by 2 weeks (Guttmacher, 1939).

Plasma progesterone levels were almost double those reported for single
pregnancies. There was no significant fall in the maternal plasma progesterone
before the onset of labour. The high levels of this hormone until the end of
pregnancy indicates continuing placental function. The high progesterone levels
may have been related to the continuance of pregnancy (Csapo *et al*., 1974) in

Table I. Mean serial oestradiol ± S.E.M. (in nanograms per millilitre).

Group	Gestation (weeks)				
	30	31	32	33	34
Control	19.3 ± 0.5	21.2 ± 2.3	23.9 ± 1.7	24.3 ± 1.4	26.4 ± 1.4
Salbutamol	21.9 ± 2.5	19.2 ± 3.6	17.5 ± 3.9	25.6 ± 4.2	22.2 ± 2.2
Group	Gestation (weeks)				
	35	36	37	38	39
Control	32.6 ± 3.3	39.2 ± 3.4	36.0 ± 3.5	36.0 ± 2.4	34.6 ± 1.6
Salbutamol	29.8 ± 4.7	34.2 ± 5.2	23.8 ± 4.6	30.8 ± 2.4	26.8 ± 0.9

Table II. Mean serial progesterone ± S.E.M. (in nanograms per millilitre).

Group	Gestation (weeks)				
	30	31	32	33	34
Control	203 ± 9.4	291 ± 54.0	297 ± 48.7	297 ± 36.4	318 ± 41.5
Salbutamol	247.1 ± 62.3	224.3 ± 20.3	266.3 ± 18.9	292.3 ± 34.9	260.3 ± 29.6
Group	Gestation (weeks)				
	35	36	37	38	39
Control	321 ± 39.1	335 ± 32.7	331 ± 30.7	363 ± 36.5	387 ± 36.2
Salbutamol	273.8 ± 25.2	315.0 ± 27.5	322.8 ± 20.8	330.7 ± 38.1	289.4 ± 70.8

the face of factors such as stretch (Poyser *et al.*, 1971) and oestrogens (Liggins and Grieves, 1971; TambyRaja, 1979) which increase prostaglandins and uterine activity. The reason for the fall in plasma oestrogens during salbutamol therapy is uncertain. It may in part be associated with the mechanism of the onset of preterm labour. The observation may represent yet another action of betasympathomimetic agents, as salbutamol reduces potassium levels in women in preterm labour (Smith and Thompson, 1977).

The heavier babies born to salbutamol-treated mothers could have resulted from increased uteroplacental blood flow, and induced diabetic state, or an altered fat metabolism. Morris *et al.* (1955) has demonstrated decreased uterine blood flow in twins, which may account for the high incidence of fetal growth retardation. The increase in uterine blood flow during beta-adrenergic therapy (Brettes *et al.*, 1976) may play a major role in improving fetal weight. In preliminary studies, we have not detected significant alteration of carbohydrate metabolism in mothers receiving salbutamol. It seems likely that, in this instance, Pederson's (1974) hypothesis of maternal hyperglycaemia, inducing fetal hyperinsulinism and macrosomia, is not tenable. The elevated triglyceride and cholesterol levels suggests that in man lipolysis is mediated by β_2-receptors (Goldberg *et al.*, 1975).

Szabo and Szabo's (1974) suggestion of fatty acids being a metabolic fuel to the fetus has recently been confirmed (Wynn and Oakley, 1978). Goldberg *et al.* (1975) have shown increases in fatty acid levels following administration of salbutamol. In pregnant diabetics, higher plasma levels of free fatty acids lead to gradient-dependent diffusion with transfer of free fatty acid across the placenta. Whether a subtle diabetic state leads to fetal hyperinsulinism by a direct action of the fetal pancreas or lipolysis that causes fetal macrosomia is only speculative.

REFERENCES

Bender, S. (1952). *Journal of Obstetrics and Gynaecology of the British Empire* **59**, 510.

Brettes, J. P., Renaud, R. and Gantar, R. (1976). *American Journal of Obstetrics and Gynecology* **124**, 164.

Chew, P. C. T., Ratnam, S. S. and Salmon, J. A. (1976). *Journal of Endocrinology* **71**, 267.

Chew, P. C. T. and Ratnam, S. S. (1976). *Journal of Endocrinology* **69**, 163.

Csapo, A. I., Pohanka, O. and Kaihola, H. L. (1974). *British Medical Journal i*, 137.

Devilla, G. O., Roberts, K. D., Wiest, W. G., Mikail, G. and Flickinger, G. (1972). *Journal of Clinical Endocrinology* **35**, 458.

Goldberg, R., Joffe, B. I., Bersohn, I., Van Os, M., Krut, L. and Seftel, H. C. (1975). *South African Postgraduate Journal* **51**, 53.

Guttmacher, A. F. (1939). *American Journal of Obstetrics and Gynecology* **38**, 277.

Hotchkiss, J., Atkinson, L. E. and Knobil, E. (1971). *Endocrinology* **89**, 117.

Iwasaki, H. and Sugato, Y. (1976). *In* "Proceedings of the VIIIth World Congress of Gynaecology and Obstetrics", p. 104, Excerpta Medica, Amsterdam.

Liggins, C. L. and Grieves, S. A. (1971). *Nature, London* **232**, 629.

Morris, N., Osborn, S. B. and Wright, H. P. (1955). *Lancet i*, 323.

Pederson, M. I. (1974). *In* "Studies on Carbohydrate Metabolism in Newborn Infants of Diabetic Mothers", p. 48, Copenhagen.

Poyser, N. L., Horton, E. W., Thomson, C. J. and Lo, S. M. (1971). *Nature, London* **230**, 526.

Smith, S. R. and Thompson, D. (1977). *British Journal of Obstetrics and Gynecology* **84**, 344.

Szabo, A. J. and Szabo, O. (1974). *Lancet* **2**, 498.

TambyRaja, R. L., Anderson, A. B. M. and Turnbull, A. C. (1974). *British Medical Journal* **4**, 67

TambyRaja, R. L., Turnbull, A. C. and Ratnam, S. S. (1975). *Australian and New Zealand Journal of Obstetrics and Gynaecology* **15**, 191.

TambyRaja, R. L. (1979). (in press).

Turnbull, A. C., Patten, P., Anderson, A. B. M., Kierse, M. J. N. C. and Jeremy, J. Y. (1974). *Lancet i*, 101.

Wilson, G. R. (1973). *Clinica chimica acta* **46**, 297.

Wynn, V. and Oakley, N. W. (1978). *In* "Proceedings of 6th Asia Oceania Congress of Endocrinology".

LIPID AND FATTY ACID COMPOSITION OF AMNIOTIC FLUID AND FETAL BLOOD DURING LABOUR

G. C. Di Renzo, G. Salvioli, A. Bartolamasi and A. Mambrini

Istituto di Clinica Ostetrica e Ginecologica and
Istituto di Clinica Medica Generale e Terapia Medica, Università di Modena,
Via Del Pozzo 71, 41100 Modena, Italy

INTRODUCTION

The amount of lipid in amniotic fluid of normal subjects increases progressively with gestational age and is maximal in labour at term (Das *et al.*, 1975). The fatty acid composition differs between individual lipid classes and palmitic acid is the major fatty acid at labour (Singh and Zuspan, 1973). The ratio of the quantity of lecithin to the quantity of sphingomyelin (L/S ratio) in the phospholipids extracted from the amniotic fluid was greater than 2 after 34 weeks and reaches a maximum at term; serving as an index of the fetal lung maturity (Gluck *et al.*, 1971). Moreover, during labour a selective increase of free fatty acid has been demonstrated (MacDonald *et al.*, 1974; Filshie and Anstey, 1978), and also of F prostaglandins (Kierse *et al.*, 1974) as well as L/S ratio (Whittle *et al.*, 1977). Except for the last investigation, all these studies evaluate the differences between samples taken from patients who were delivered spontaneously and those who underwent caesarean section before the onset of labour. Moreover, the increase of L/S ratio during labour is controversial (Craven *et al.*, 1976; Cabero *et al.*, 1976; Whittle *et al.*, 1977).

Therefore we have carried out an investigation to establish the amount of lipid (cholesterol, triglycerides, phospholipids), the lecithin/sphingomyelin (L/S) ratio

Serono Symposium No. 35, "The Human Placenta", edited by A. Klopper,
A. Genazzani and P. G. Crosignani, 1980. Academic Press, London and New York.

and the fatty acid composition (in per cent) of total lipids, of lecithin and of sphingomyelin in amniotic fluid during labour, examining serial samples from the same subjects. The same parameters have been estimated in umbilical cord plasma at delivery.

PATIENTS AND METHODS

Sixteen patients, who gave full and informed consent, were admitted to the study, the ages ranged from 18 to 35 years (mean 26.4); parity ranged from 0 to 2 (mean 0.3) and 75% were primigravida. The gestational ages were between 38 and 41 weeks (mean 39.3); birthweights ranged from 2800 to 4100 g with a mean of 3483; Apgar score at first minute ranged from 6 to 10 with a mean of 8.9; in all cases spontaneous labour followed 1-3 h from spontaneous rupture of membranes; all were delivered vaginally of liveborn infants.

Amniotic fluid specimens were collected as follows: by amnioscope at the time of the first vaginal examination and following rupture of membranes: during labour about every 3 h by intrauterine polyethylene catheter inserted per vaginum (10 cases); and at delivery. All samples were free from contamination with blood or meconium. In all newborns, samples of blood were taken immediately after delivery from the cord vein.

Amniotic fluid (4 ml) or plasma (2 ml) was extracted with 30 ml chloroform-methanol (2:1 v/v) containing 0.05% butylhydroxytoluene to prevent lipid oxidation. Cholesterol, phospholipids and triglycerides were determined in the chloroform phase, using conventional methods. An aliquot of lipid extract was employed for separation of lecithin and sphingomyelin using thin layer chromatography with precoated silica gel G plates. The solvent system was chloroform–methanol–water (65:25:4, v/v). Fractions of interest (L and S), were identified using iodine vapour and scraped off. An aliquot was digested for phosphorus determination by the method of Bartlett (1959). Another aliquot was used for the transesterification reaction in a Teflon-capped glass tube by adding 2.5 ml of methanol and 0.1 ml of concentrated sulphuric acid. The samples were heated at 60 °C for 3 h and at the end the methyl esters of fatty acids were extracted by adding 2 ml of water and 8 ml of isooctane. The isooctane phase was evaporated and an aliquot injected into a Packard gas chromatograph model 420 equipped with a U-shaped glass column filled with 10% SP-2330 on 100/120 Supelcoport and operating at 191 °C The individual fatty acid methyl esters were identified by comparison with the relative retention time of a standard fatty acid. The peak areas were determined with a Hewlett-Packard model 3380A integrator. Individual free fatty acids (FFA) were determined in duplicate amniotic fluid specimens by the gas chromatographic method of Hagenfeldt (1966), employing heptadecanoic acid as internal standard. The values for arachidonic acid are expressed in microequivalents per litre. The results were analysed using a Student's paired *t*-test.

RESULTS

In amniotic fluid total cholesterol, phospholipids and triglycerides show high levels at term with a slight but non-significant decrease during labour (Table I). On the other hand, L/S ratio and free arachidonic acid increase markedly during

Table I. Lipid and free fatty acid content and L/S ratio of amniotic fluid during labour.

		Cholesterol (mg/dl)	Phospholipids (mg/dl)	Triglycerides (mg/dl)	Free arachidonic acid (μequiv/l)[a]	L/S ratio[b]
Before labour	Mean	58.6	39.6	43.8	1.69	2.79
	± S.D.	13.4	5.9	7.9	0.84	1.46
At delivery	Mean	52.4	35.6	41.6	2.92	6.10
	± S.D.	10.9	4.8	9.1	0.81	2.60

[a] $p < 0.02$ [b] $p < 0.01$.

Table II. Fatty acid composition of lecithin of amniotic fluid during labour.

Fatty acid[a]	Before labour[b]	At delivery[b]
16:0	61.2 ± 8.6	60.8 ± 7.9
16:1	6.2 ± 1.2	5.7 ± 1.0
18:0	3.9 ± 0.9	4.1 ± 1.6
18:1	11.9 ± 1.8	12.4 ± 1.2
18:2	5.0 ± 0.5	4.8 ± 0.6
20:3	1.2 ± 0.1	1.3 ± 0.1
20:4	6.1 ± 0.9	7.0 ± 0.8

[a] Number of carbon atoms: number of double bonds.
[b] Percentages of total fatty acids ± S.D.

Table III. Lipid content of newborn plasma (at delivery).

	Mean ± S.D. (mg/dl)
Cholesterol	57.1 ± 15.6
Phospholipids	63.2 ± 9.7
Triglycerides	34.1 ± 10.7

labour. The rise is statistically significant (Table I). No variation is detected in fatty acid composition of total lipid of lecithin (Table II) and sphingomyelin.

The amount of cholesterol, triglyceride and phospholipid in fetal plasma is shown in Table III. The fatty acid compositions of both plasma cholesterol esters and phospholipids show a high percentage of arachidonic (20:4) and eicosatrienoic (20:3) acids (Table IV).

Table IV. Fatty acid composition of cholesterol esters and of phospholipids in newborn plasma (at delivery).

Fatty acid[a]	Cholesterol esters[b]	Phospholipids[b]
16:0	19.4 ± 2.1	31.5 ± 2.1
16:1	4.9 ± 1.0	1.0 ± 0.1
18:0	2.8 ± 0.2	12.2 ± 1.9
18:1	29.8 ± 3.8	13.1 ± 2.2
18:2	28.0 ± 4.6	12.6 ± 2.8
20:3	1.8 ± 0.2	6.6 ± 0.8
20:4	11.3 ± 2.8	21.1 ± 2.7

[a] Number of carbon atoms: number of double bonds.
[b] Percentage of total fatty acids ± S.D.

DISCUSSION

Our findings are in agreement with those found in the literature for the lipid content of either amniotic fluid or newborn plasma (Wille and Phillips, 1971; Girault *et al.*, 1974; Das *et al.*, 1975; Whittle *et al.*, 1977; Schindler *et al.*, 1978). Small differences may be accounted for by the different methods used for extraction of lipids. It is necessary to point out the difference in the amount of free arachidonic acid of amniotic fluid between our samples and those of Filshie and Anstey (1978). They found mean levels of 2.56 μequiv/l in eight specimens of amniotic fluid taken at elective caesarean section and of 3.86 μequiv/l in five samples taken from caesarean section in labour. The difference was not statistically significant. The authors write that, although the number of samples were small, they have observed similar findings with serial samples of amniotic fluid collected from a larger series of patient before and during labour, but the figures are not given. Moreover, the method of Filshie and Anstey (extraction with chloroform and methylation with BF_3-methanol) may be incorrect because by using chloroform some triglycerides are extracted and BF_3-methanol is a trans-methylating mixture. In our method diazomethane is used as methylating agent, so avoiding possible mistakes. This fact may explain the difference observed in free arachidonic acid content of amniotic fluid between the two studies. L/S ratio increased in all our cases during labour, confirming the data of Cabero *et al.* (1976). We were unable to demonstrate (possibly because of the small number of patients) the three patterns of change in the L/S ratio during labour described by Whittle *et al.* (1977). In accord with these authors we found that the increase in L/S ratio in labour generally reflects change in the lecithin concentrations, the sphingomyelin level remaining nearly constant. In the newborn, the fatty acid compositions of plasma cholesterol esters and phospholipids show a high concentration compared to normal adults or the mothers (Sprecher and Robertson, 1967; Lin and Horning, 1975; Filshie and Anstey, 1978). The percentage of linoleic acid in both lipid fractions is higher in the adult plasma, whereas arachidonic acid is higher in the newborn. In both maternal and fetal circulation palmitic acid is a constant proportion of all the fatty acid (Sprecher and Robertson, 1967; Filshie and Anstey, 1978). High arachidonic acid concentration may thus depend on synthetic activity in the placenta or might be preferentially transported across the placenta from the maternal to the fetal circulation (Elphick and Hull, 1976; Filshie and Anstey, 1978).

From these findings, the hypothesis of a selective increase of arachidonic acid in amniotic fluid for its utilization in the mechanism of initiation and maintenance of labour (MacDonald *et al.*, 1974) gains some support. Moreover, parturition may be considered a stimulus either for surfactant release or production, possibly through the rise in fetal cortisol (Whittle *et al.*, 1977).

REFERENCES

Bartlett, G. R. (1959). *Journal of Biological Chemistry* **234**, 466.

Cabero, L., Roses, A., Viscasillas, P., Quilez, M., Giralt, E. and Duran Sanchez, P. (1976). *British Journal of Obstetrics and Gynaecology* **83**, 452.

Craven, D. J., Khattab, T. Y. and Simons, E. M. (1976). *British Journal of Obstetrics and Gynaecology* **83**, 39.

Das, S. K., Foster, H. W., Adhikary, P. K., Mody, B. B. and Bhattacharyya, D. K. (1975). *Obstetrics and Gynecology* **45**, 425.

Elphick, M. C. and Hull, D. D. (1976). *Journal of Physiology, London* **264**, 751.

Filshie, G. M. and Anstey, M. D. (1978). *British Journal of Obstetrics and Gynaecology* **85**, 119.

Girault, A., Girault, M., Grosieux, P., Le Lirzin, R. and Rouchy, R. (1974). *Revue francais de la gynécologie* **69**, 187.

Gluck, L., Kulovich, M. V. and Borer, R. C. (1971). *American Journal of Obstetrics and Gynecology* **109**, 440.

Hagenfeldt, L. (1966). *Clinica chimica acta* **13**, 266.

Kierse, M. J. N. C., Flint, A. P. F. and Turnbull, A. C. (1974). *Journal of Obstetrics and Gynaecology of the British Commonwealth* **81**, 131.

Lin, S. N. and Horning, E. C. (1975). *Journal of Chromatography* **112**, 483.

MacDonald, P. C., Schultz, F. M., Duenhoelter, J. H., Gant, N. F., Jimenez, J. M., Pritchard, J. A., Porter, J. C. and Johnston, J. M. (1974). *Obstetrics and Gynecology* **44**, 629.

Schindler, A. E., Anderer, M. and Liebich, H. M. (1978). *Archiv für Gynäkologie* **226**, 289.

Singh, E. J. and Zuspan, F. P. (1973). *American Journal of Obstetrics and Gynecology* **117**, 919.

Sprecher, H. and Robertson, A. (1967). *Journal of Laboratory and Clinical Medicine* **70**, 489.

Whittle, M. J., Hill, C. M. and Harkes, A. (1977). *British Journal of Obstetrics and Gynaecology* **84**, 500.

Wille, L. E. and Phillips, G. B. (1971). *Clinica chimica acta* **54**, 457.

PARTIAL PURIFICATION OF β-LIPOPROTEIN AND β-ENDORPHIN FROM HUMAN PLACENTAL EXTRACTS AND PLASMA LEVELS DURING PREGNANCY*

A. R. Genazzani, P. Tarli[1], F. Fraioli[2], F. Facchinetti, R. Pallini and C. Massafra

*Cattedra di Patologia Ostetrica e Ginecologica, University of Siena,
Via P. Mascagni 46, 53100 Siena,
[1] ISVT Sclavo, Research Centre, Via Fiorentina 1, 53100 Siena,
[2] V Clinica Medica, Policlinico and Umberto I, University of Rome, Italy*

INTRODUCTION

It has been suggested that during pregnancy the placenta shares (O'Sullivan, 1971) or mimics (Josimovich, 1974) some of the functions of the pituitary. The discovery and isolation from human placental tissue of several hormones such as chorionic gonadotrophin (hCG) (Bahl, 1969), thyrotrophin (hCT) (Hennen *et al.*, 1969) and somatomammotrophin (hCS) (Josimovich and MacLaren, 1962) strongly support this point of view. It has also been reported that the human placenta contains and synthesizes (Genazzani *et al.*, 1974, 1975) an ACTH-like peptide, human chorionic corticotrophin (hCC). This finding, together with the fact that adrenocorticotrophic hormone (ACTH) and β-lipotrophin (β-LPH) have been found in the same human pituitary cells (Pelletier *et al.*, 1977), and the recent observation that both ACTH and β-LPH are derived from the same glyco-protein precursor of molecular weight 31 000 daltons (Mains *et al.*, 1977) led us (Fraioli and Genazzani, 1979; Genazzani *et al.*, 1979) and other authors (Nakai *et al.*, 1978; Odagiri *et al.*, 1979) to investigate the presence of β-LPH and its 61–91 C-terminal fragment, β-endorphin (β-EP), in extracts of human placentae.

*Supported by the CNR project "Biology of reproduction".

Serono Symposium No. 35, "The Human Placenta", edited by A. Klopper,
A. Genazzani and P. G. Crosignani, 1980. Academic Press, London and New York.

Consistent amounts of immunoreactive material similar to both B-EP and β-LPH have been detected in human placental extracts (Genazzani *et al.*, 1979; Nakai *et al.*, 1978; Odagiri *et al.*, 1979); furthermore, when tested for parallelism of their dilution curves in an opioid radio-receptor assay (Fraioli and Genazzani, 1979), these extracts showed a close similarity to synthetic β-EP.

The present paper describes the extraction and partial purification of these hormones from human placentae, and their plasma levels in normal and pregnant women at different periods of gestation, in comparison with those found in plasma samples from cord blood.

MATERIALS AND METHODS

Placental Tissue. Extraction and Fractionation

Human placentae were subjected to the extraction and purification procedure previously described for pituitary glands (Li *et al.*, 1975, 1977). The process can be summarized as follows. Freshly delivered placentae were minced and carefully washed in cold isotonic saline solution to remove the blood. They were then homogenized in three volumes of acetone–hydrochloric acid (97.5: 2.5) in a Waring blender and a placental powder (PP) was prepared by adding another three volumes of cold acetone and settling overnight at 4 °C. The PP (5.8 mg/g placental tissue; protein content 48.3% on a weight basis) was characterized by gel chromatography of a Sephadex G-75 column (1.5 cm × 50 cm) equilibrated and eluted with 0.1% acetic acid and 0.01% bovine serum albumin (BSA). The chromatographic fractions were tested for their β-LPH and β-EP immunoreactive content.

Furthermore, the PP was dissolved in water at pH 3.0 and the solution brought to 6% saturation of NaCl. After centrifuging, the supernatant was brought to complete saturation with solid NaCl. The precipitate was suspended in water and desalted by ultrafiltration using an Amicon model 2000 apparatus equipped with an Amicon UM-05 membrane. The retained solution was lyophilized. The protein yield was 83.2% in comparison to the content of the parent PP. The powder was then dissolved in 0.01 M ammonium acetate solution (pH 4.6) and applied to a carboxymethyl cellulose (CMC) column (1.5 cm × 50 cm) previously equilibrated with the same solution.

After initial elution performed with the equilibrating solution, a pH and salt concentration gradient was started by adding 0.1 M ammonium acetate (pH 6.7) to a 500 ml mixing bottle containing the initial solution. The gradient was then increased by introducing 0.2 M ammonium acetate solution into the mixing bottle.

Fractions of 5 ml collected at a flow rate of 50 ml/h were monitored by optical density at 280 nm, pooled and lyophilized. Small aliquots of each fraction were tested by radioimmunoassay (RIA) for their β-EP and β-LPH content. The fractions containing β-LPH and β-EP immunoreactive materials were pooled and dissolved in 0.01 M ammonium acetate solution at pH 4.6 and applied to a second CMC column (1.5 cm × 20 cm). Ion-exchange chromatography was performed as previously described but fractions of 1.5 ml were collected. Pools of the fractions were lyophilized and tested for their content of β-LPH and β-EP by RIAs.

Plasma Samples: Collection, extraction and Chromatography

Twenty-six blood samples were taken from healthy pregnant women between the 9th and the 39th week of pregnancy, and 14 were obtained from healthy volunteers during the early follicular phase. Five cord blood samples were collected promptly after delivery. All samples were taken with heparin, immediately centrifuged at 4 °C and the plasma was stored in plastic tubes at −20 °C until assay.

Plasma (2.5 ml) was extracted with 150 mg glass powder as previously described (Facchinetti and Genazzani, 1979). The extracts, dissolved in 0.4 ml 0.1 M acetic acid, 0.01% BSA, were applied to a Sephadex G-75 column (1.5 cm × 45 cm) equilibrated and eluted with the same solution. The column was previously calibrated with ^{125}I-labelled β-LPH and β-EP. As reported elsewhere (Facchinetti and Genazzani 1979), the recovery after glass powder extraction and chromatography of 30 plasma samples was 54.0 ± 8.6% (mean ± standard deviation) for β-LPH and 54.9 ± 7.8% for β-EP, respectively.

Radioimmunoassay

A rabbit anti-β-EP serum, kindly supplied by Dr C. Pert (NIH, Bethesda, Md, U.S.A.), was used for both β-LPH and β-EP double antibody RIAs (Facchinetti and Genazzani, 1979) at different dilutions (1:3300 and 1:6800 respectively). Labelling of the peptides was performed by the chloramine T method (Greenwood *et al.*, 1963) and purification of the tracers was achieved using a 1 cm × 25 cm Sephadex G-75 column, eluted with 0.1 M acetic acid containing 0.01% BSA. Synthetic β-EP (Bachem Inc., Torrance, Calif., U.S.A.) and purified human β-LPH (generously supplied by Dr C. H. Li, San Francisco, Calif., U.S.A.) were used as standards and for labelling. The sensitivity of the assays was 6 pg and 15 pg for β-EP and β-LPH, respectively.

RESULTS

Partial Purification from Placental Extracts

The PP was submitted to Sephadex G-75 gel chromatography and the fractions were measured for their β-LPH and β-EP immunoreactive contents. The elution patterns reported in Fig. 1 indicate the existence of two separate peaks of immunoreactive materials with the same elution volumes of β-LPH and β-EP tracers. Moreover, the dilution curves of pooled, freeze-dried fractions corresponding to the elution volumes of β-LPH and β-EP show a close parallelism with those obtained from the reference materials (Fig. 2).

The PP contents of β-LPH and β-EP were 58.5 and 109.8 pg/mg protein, respectively. In order to purify both the peptides, the PP was submitted to NaCl precipitation, ultrafiltration and CMC column chromatography. The β-LPH and β-EP contents of the material before the CMC fractionation were 96.6 and 53.4 pg/mg of protein, respectively. The CMC elution pattern showed a series of peaks when the 280 nm optical density was monitored (Fig. 3). The fractions corresponding to the various peaks were pooled and freeze-dried, and, when tested in β-LPH and β-EP

A. R. Genazzani et al.

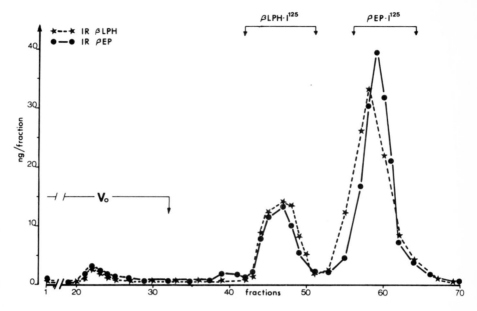

Fig. 1. Elution pattern of Sephadex G-75 gel filtration of PP. All fractions were tested for β-LPH (★– –★) and β-EP (●—●) immunoreactivity.

RIAs, showed the presence of immunoreactive material in fractions O, P and N, O, respectively (Table I). Other fractions presented minor amounts of β-LPH- and β-EP-like immunoreactive materials. A second CMC column chromatography was performed on the pooled I, N, O and P fractions, and the optical density at 280 nm and immunoreactive β-EP and β-LPH contents were also monitored (Fig. 4). Immunoreactive β-EP was found in pooled fractions 1, 2 and 8, the largest concentration being in fraction 2. Immunoreactive β-LPH was present in fractions 1, 2 and 3 (Table I).

Dilution curves of fractions 1 and 2 in the respective β-LPH and β-EP RIAs were performed, and a close parallelism was found between reference β-LPH and materials present in fraction 1 (Fig. 2(a)), and between reference β-EP and materials present in fraction 2 (Fig. 2(b)).

Furthermore, the dilution curves of fractions 1 and 2 were parallel to those performed on pooled fractions from PP Sephadex G-75 gel chromatography containing respectively β-LPH and β-EP immunoreactive materials (Fig. 2).

Plasma Levels in Normal Women and During Pregnancy

The β-LPH and β-EP plasma levels determined in healthy volunteers in the early follicular phase were 121 ± 15 and 31 ± 5 pg/ml (mean ± standard error), respectively (Table II). The range of β-LPH was 58–263 pg/ml, and that of β-EP was

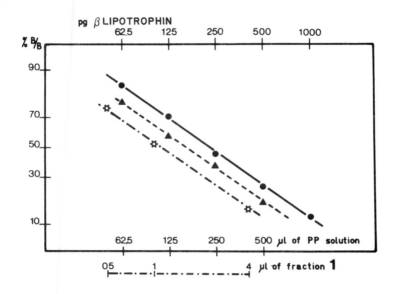

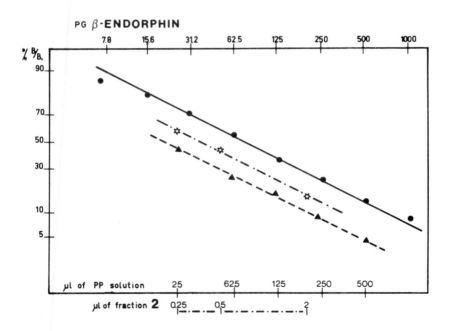

Fig. 2. β-EP and β-LPH RIAs: dilution curves of reference hormone (●——●) and pooled Sephadex G-75 gel chromatography (▲– – –▲) and CMC (✿–·–·✿) fractions.

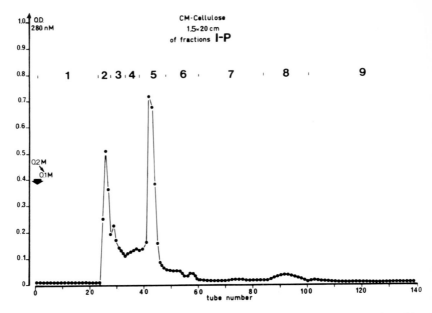

Fig. 3. CMC chromatography pattern of NaCl fractionated placental powder monitored by optical density at 280 nm.

Table I. β-LPH and β-EP immunoreactive material in fractions from CMC column chromatography of PP (part A) and in pooled I, N, O, P, fractions (part B) of the CMC fractionation.

Fractions		β-LPH (ng)	β-EP (ng)
A	I	N.D.	19.5
	N	7.6	92.5
	O	96.0	240.4
	P	35.0	4.8
B	1	56.0	22.0
	2	87.5	129.1
	3	40.0	N.D.
	8	N.D.	38.0

N.D., not detectable.

3–64 pg/ml. The ratio between β-LPH and β-EP on a molar basis was 1.37 ± 1.2 (range 0.84–2.42).

Table II also shows the results obtained in 26 pregnant women at different periods of gestation. The β-LPH ranged between 52 and 235 pg/ml, and β-EP

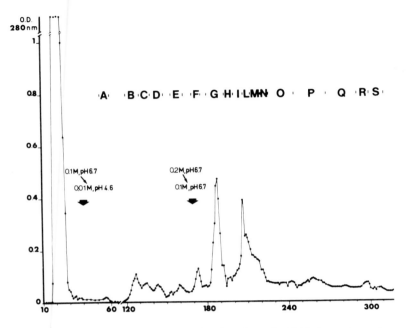

Fig. 4. CMC chromatographic pattern of I–P fractions from the CMC chromatography reported in Fig. 2.

ranged between 7 and 65 pg/ml, respectively. The molar ratio varied between 0.56 and 6.02.

In the plasma samples from cord blood, β-LPH ranged from 86 to 240 pg/ml, and β-EP from 16 to 85 pg/ml, the molar ratio varying from 0.94 to 2.14.

DISCUSSION

These findings confirm the presence in placental extracts of consistent amounts of both immunoreactive β-LPH and β-EP materials. As evaluated from the data obtained through Sephadex G-75 gel chromatography of PP, the placental contents of β-LPH and β-EP were 164 and 307 pg/g fresh, minced and washed tissue. Furthermore, additional information has been obtained: the elution volumes of the main peaks from the Sephadex column (coinciding with those of the corresponding reference peptides) and the parallelism shown in the RIA dilution curves, both indicate a close molecular similarity with the above-mentioned peptides, one of which (β-LPH), is of human pituitary origin. Moreover, parallelism was also exhibited by the materials eluted from the CMC column in the same conditions as those reported for β-LPH and β—EP of pituitary origin. This fact indicated that the application to placental extracts of the fractionation procedure reported for the isolation of pituitary peptides (Li *et al.*, 1975) seems suitable for the purifica-

Table II. Plasma levels of βLPH and βEP immunoreactive material in women at different periods of pregnancy, in cord blood and in healthy volunteers in early follicular phase.

Weeks	βLPH (pg/ml)	βEP (pg/ml)	M.R.[a]	N	βLPH (pg/ml)	βEP (pg/ml)	M.R.[a]
Pregnant women				*Cord Blood*			
9	132	18	2.44	1	157	39	1.33
10	90	11	2.72	2	240	85	0.94
15	115	25	1.53	3	202	40	1.68
16	204	48	1.42	4	106	16	2.14
17	89	16	1.85	5	86	18	1.02
18	55	16	1.15				
	214	36	1.98	*Non-pregnant women*			
	118	20	1.97	1	100	24	1.37
24	89	11	2.70	2	263	51	1.59
	170	20	2.83	3	58	13	1.49
28	116	20	1.93	4	140	41	1.14
	124	65	0.63	5	82	3	2.10
29	126	34	1.23	6	72	13	1.91
32	197	17	3.86	7	101	28	1.21
33	100	59	0.56	8	140	47	0.99
34	77	15	1.71	9	101	36	0.93
	155	53	0.97	10	96	38	0.84
35	52	9	1.93	11	200	64	1.04
36	141	25	1.88	12	86	21	0.93
	90	7	4.29	13	166	45	1.23
	221	26	2.83	14	87	12	2.42
37	116	25	1.55				
	229	44	1.73				
	139	34	1.36				
39	233	17	4.57				
	235	13	6.02				

[a]Ratio between the molar concentrations of β-LPH and β-EP.

tion of placental β-LPH and β-EP without affecting their immunological characteristics, when these are compared to the reference peptides and to the corresponding hormones present in the placental powder and in the plasma of pregnant women (A. R. Genazzani *et al.*, unpublished results).

This fact is of particular interest, because the above-mentioned technique is generally used to obtain the pituitary hormones, and is therefore also potentially useful in obtaining all analogous placental hormones.

The plasma β-LPH levels in normal women (Tables II and III) are slightly higher than those reported by Wiedemann *et al.* (1977), Bachelot *et al.* (1977), Tanaka *et al.* (1978) and Krieger *et al.* (1977, 1979), while they correspond to those reported by Wardlaw and Frantz (1979) and by Höllt *et al.* (1979).

β-EP, which was not detected by Suda *et al.* (1978) in plasma of normal subjects, is consistently found in all the samples (Tables II and III), and its range corresponded

Table III. Normal plasma levels of β-LPH and β-EP reported in literature.

Authors	β-LPH			β-EP		
	Mean ± S.E.	Range	N	Mean ± S.E.	Range	N
Bachelot et al. (1979)[a]	19.9 ± 2.9	7–37	12			
Wiedemann et al. (1977)	72	29–145	9			
Nakao et al. (1978)	111.2 ± 17.4	52–150	5	5.8 ± 1.1	2.7–7.8	5
Jeffcoate et al. (1978)		25–200	8			
Suda et al. (1978)				Not detectable		3
Tanaka et al. (1978)[a]	58.0 ± 5.8		3			
Wardlaw and Frantz (1979)	114.0 ± 50.0[b]	54–161	5	21.0 ± 7.3	14–32	5
Krieger et al. (1979)	66.0 ± 5.8	28–115	24			
Höllt et al. (1979)		21–101	5		12–23	5
Wiedemann et al. (1979)					5–45	14
Present data	120.8 ± 56.3	58–263	14	31.1 ± 17.7	3–64	14

[a]Expressed as 1.22 MSH. [b]Mean ± S.D.

to that recently reported by Wardlwa and Frantz (1979) and by Wiedemann *et al.* (1979). Lower values have been reported by Nakao *et al.* (1978) and Csontos *et al.* (1979). These differences in absolute levels of the two peptides may be attributable to the use of different antisera and/or reference preparations. More homogeneous values are reported for the β-LPH/β-EP molar ratio in the plasma of normal subjects; in our experiments, this ratio was 1.37 ± 0.48 (mean ± S.D.).

During pregnancy, no pattern was observed in the plasma levels of β-LPH and β-EP. Values were in the same range as in non-pregnant subjects, the mean values being 139 ± 56 (mean ± S.D.) and 26 ± 15 pg/ml for β-LPH and β-EP, respectively; the molar ratio was 2.22 ± 1.27. The presence of significant amounts of both peptides, as well as the presence of ACTH in placental tissue (Genazzani *et al.*, 1975; Rees *et al.*, 1975; Odagiri *et al.*, 1979) and the capacity of trophoblastic cells to synthesize ACTH (Genazzani *et al.*, 1974; Liotta *et al.*, 1977), β-LPH and β-EP *in vitro* (Liotta and Krieger, 1980), suggest that placental tissue probably also synthesizes β-LPH and β-EP through a common precursor containing ACTH, as occurs in the pituitary gland (Mains *et al.*, 1977).

The data reported by Odagiri *et al.* (1979) showing the presence in placental extracts of high molecular weight components with the antigenic determinants of ACTH, β-LPH and β-EP, support the hypothesis of the existence of a common precursor.

The observation that plasma ACTH levels rise, beginning from the early stages of gestation (Genazzani *et al.*, 1975, 1976) to reach levels two to three times the normal (Genazzani *et al.*, 1972), while both β-LPH and β-EP plasma concentrations remain within the normal range, is open to several interpretations.

The presence of β-LPH and β-EP in the placental tissue does not *per se* imply that these peptides are secreted directly into the maternal or fetal circulation: they may be metabolized within the placenta itself, or bound by the opiate receptors present in the myometrium or other uterine tissues.

The existence in pregnancy of higher molar concentrations of ACTH than of β-LPH and β-EP is in agreement with the previously reported data concerning normal subjects of both sexes and patients with pituitary–adrenal diseases (Gilkes *et al.*, 1977, Liotta *et al.*, 1978; Krieger *et al.*, 1979). In this respect, Tanka *et al.* (1978) showed an equimolar ACTH and β-LPH secretion *in vivo* from the pituitary, although they and Liotta *et al.* (1978) demonstrated that the half-life of both endogenous and exogenous β-LPH is nearly twice that of ACTH. Furthermore, it is possible that, in pregnancy, the volumes of distribution and the metabolic clearance rates of the various hormones are not the same as in normal females, and that particular endocrine environments, i.e. the changes in adrenal steroid levels occurring during pregnancy (Genazzani *et al.*, 1976), can interefere in the metabolizing system of β-EP and other opioid peptides, as shown in experimental animals (Holaday *et al.*, 1979, Holaday and Loh, 1979).

As far as the β-LPH and β-EP values in cord blood are concerned, these were found to be high in three out of five subjects, in agreement with the data reported by Csontos *et al.* (1979). This fact may be indicative of phenomena causing fetal stress during labour and delivery, and our previous data on ACTH levels in cord blood vessels support this hypothesis (Genazzani *et al.*, 1976).

REFERENCES

Bachelot, I., Wolfsen, A. R. and Odell, W. D. (1977). *Journal of Clinical Endocrinology and Metabolism* **44**, 939–946.

Bahl, O. P. (1969). *Journal of Biological Chemistry* **244**, 575–583.

Csontos, K., Rust, M., Höllt, V., Mahr, W., Kromer, W. and Teschemacher, H. J. (1979). *Life Sciences* **25**, 835–844.

Facchinetti, F. and Genazzani, A. R. (1979). *In* "Radioimmunoassay of Drugs and Hormones in Cardiovascular Medicine" (A. Albertini, M. Da Prada and B. A. Peskara, eds), pp. 347–354, Elsevier North Holland, Amsterdam.

Fraioli, F. and Genazzani, A. R. (1979). *Obstetric and Gynecological Investigations* in press.

Genazzani, A. R., Ruedi, B., Aubert, M. L. and Felber, J. P. (1972). *Hormone Metabolism Research* **4**, 470–477.

Genazzani, A. R., Hurlimann, J., Fioretti, P. and Felber, J. P. (1974). *Experientia* **30**, 430–432.

Genazzani, A. R., Fraioli, F., Hurlimann, J., Fioretti, P. and Felber, J. P. (1975). *Clinical Endocrinology* **4**, 1–14.

Genazzani, A. R., Felber, J. P. and Fioretti, P. (1976). *Acta endocrinologia, Copenhagen* **83**, 800–810.

Genazzani, A. R., Facchinetti, F., Fraioli, F., Pallini, R. and Tarli, P. (1979). *In* "Psychoneuroendocrinology in Reproduction" (L. Zichella and P. Pancheri, eds), pp. 469–474, Elsevier North Holland, Amsterdam.

Gilkes, J. J. H., Rees, L. H. and Besser, G. M. (1977). *British Medical Journal* i, 996–998.

Greenwood, F. C., Hunter, W. M. and Glover, J. S. (1963). *Biochemical Journal* **89**, 114–123.

Hennen, G., Pierce, J. G. and Freychet, P. (1969). *Journal of Clinical Endocrinology and Metabolism* **29**, 581–594.

Holaday, J. W., Law, P. Y., Loh, H. H. and Li, C. H. (1979). *Journal of Pharmacology and Experimental Therapeutics* **208**, 176–183.

Holaday, J. W. and Loh, H. H. (1979). *Advances in Biochemical Psychopharmacology* **20**, 227–258.

Höllt, V., Müller, O. A. and Fahlbusch, R. (1979). *Life Sciences* **25**, 37–44.

Jeffcoate *et al.* (1978). *Journal of Clinical Endocrinology and Metabolism* **47**, 160.

Josimovich, J. B. and MacLaren, J. A. (1962). *Endocrinology* **71**, 209–220.

Josimovich, J. B. (1974). *American Journal of Obstetrics and Gynecology* **120**, 550–552.

Krieger, D. T., Liotta, A. and Li, C. H. (1977). *Life Sciences* **21**, 1771–1778.

Krieger, D. T., Liotta, A. S., Suda, T., Goodgold, A. and Condon, E. (1979). *Journal of Clinical Endocrinology and Metabolism* **48**, 566–571.

Li, C. H., Danho, W. O., Chung, D. and Rao, A. J. (1975). *Biochemistry* **14**, 947–952.

Li, C. H., Yamashiro, D., Chung, D., Doneen, B. A., Loh, H. H. and Tseng, L. (1977). *Annals of the New York Academy of Sciences* **297**, 158–166.

Liotta, A., Osathanondh, R. Ryan, K. J. and Krieger, D. T. (1977). *Endocrinology* **101**, 1552–1558.

Liotta, A. S., Li, C. H., Schussler, G. C. and Krieger, D. T. (1978). *Life Sciences* **23**, 2323–2330.

Liotta, A. S. and Krieger, D. T. (1980). This volume.

478   *A. R. Genazzani et al.*

Mains, R. E. Eipper, B. A. and Ling, N. (1977). *Proceedings of the National Academy of Sciences of the U.S.A.* **74**, 3014–3018.

Nakai, Y., Nakao, K., Oki, S. and Immura, M. (1978). *Life Sciences* **23**, 2013–2018.

Nakao, K., Nakai, Y., Oki, S., Horii, K. and Imura, H. (1978). *Journal of Clinical Investigation* **62**, 1395–1398.

Odagiri, E., Sherrell, B. J., Mount, C. D., Nicholson, W. E. and Orth, D. N. (1979). *Proceedings of the National Academy of Sciences of the U.S.A.* **76**, 2027–2031.

O'Sullivan, D. (1971). *Chemical Engineering News* **49**, (28) 35.

Pelletier, G., Leclerc, R., Labrie, F., Cote, J., Chretien, M. and Lis, M. (1977). *Endocrinology* **100**, 770–776.

Rees, L. H., Burke, C. W., Chard, T., Evans, S. W. and Letchworth, A. T. (1975). *Nature, London* **254**, 620–622.

Suda, T., Liotta, A. S. and Krieger, D. T. (1978). *Science, New York* **202**, 221–223.

Tanaka, K., Nicholson, W. E. and Orth, D. N. (1978). *Journal of Clinical Endocrinology and Metabolism* **46**, 883–890.

Wardlaw, S. L. and Frantz, A. G. (1979). *Journal of Clinical Endocrinology and Metabolism* **48**, 176–180.

Wiedemann, E., Saito, T., Linfoot, J. A. and Li, C. H. (1977). *Journal of Clinical Endocrinology and Metabolism* **45**, 1180–1111.

Wiedemann, E., Saito, T., Linfoot, J. A. and Li, C. H. (1979). *Journal of Clinical Endocrinology and Metabolism* **49**, 478–480.